Stefano Fanti – Mohsen Farsad – Luigi Mansi

Atlas of SPECT-CT

Stefano Fanti – Mohsen Farsad – Luigi Mansi

Atlas of SPECT-CT

Springer

Stefano Fanti, Prof. Dr.
University of Bologna
Policlinico S.Orsola-Malpighi
Dipto. Medicina Nucleare
Via Massarenti
40100 Bologna
Italy
fanti@orsola-malpighi.med.unibo.it

Luigi Mansi, Prof. Dr.
University of Naples
Ist. Scienze Radiologiche
Piazza Miraglia 2
80138 Napoli
Italy
luigi.mansi@unina2.it

Mohsen Farsad, MD.
Central Hospital Bozen
Nuclear Medicine
Via Pöhler
39100 Bolzano
Italy
mohsen.farsad@asbz.it

ISBN: 978-3-642-15725-7 e-ISBN: 978-3-642-15726-4

DOI: 10.1007/978-3-642-15726-4

Library of Congress Control Number: 2011928411

Cover design: eStudioCalamar, Spain

Printed on acid-free paper

Springer is part & Springer Science + Business Media (www.springer.com)

Acknowledgement

We would like to dedicate this book to all people who are tired of being told that nuclear medicine is the future: Nuclear Medicine is the present.

Contents

Contributors

Monica Agostini U. O. Medicina Nucleare, Azienda Sanitaria di Cesena, Cesena, Italy

Carina Mari Aparici Department of Radiology and Biomedical Imaging, University of California, San Francisco, CA, USA

Anca M. Avram Division of Nuclear Medicine/Radiology, University of Michigan Medical Center, Ann Arbor, MI, USA

Mirco Bartolomei U. O. Medicina Nucleare, Azienda Sanitaria di Cesena, Cesena, Italy

Chiara Basile Medical Physics, Servizio di Fisica Sanitaria, Azienda Ospedaliera S. Camillo Forlanini, Roma, Italy

Ambros J. Beer Department of Nuclear Medicine, Klinikum rechts der Isar der Technischen Universität München, Munich, Germany

Francesca Botta Unità di Fisica Sanitaria, Istituto Europeo di Oncologia, Milano, Italy
Medical Physics and Nuclear Medicine, European Institute of Oncology, Milano, Italy

Andreas K. Buck Department of Nuclear Medicine, Klinikum rechts der Isar der Technischen Universität München, Munich, Germany

Michela Casi U. O. Medicina Nucleare, Azienda Sanitaria di Cesena, Cesena, Italy

Angel Soriano Castrejón Department of Nuclear Medicine, Universitary General Hospital of Ciudad Real, Ciudad Real, Spain

Marta Cremonesi Unità di Fisica Sanitaria, Istituto Europeo di Oncologia, Milano, Italy
Medical Physics and Nuclear Medicine, European Institute of Oncology, Milano, Italy
Medical Physics Department, Istituto Europeo di Oncologia, Milano, Italy

Vincenzo Cuccurullo U.O. Medicina Nucleare, Seconda Università di Napoli, Napoli, Italy

Concetta De Cicco Divisione di Medicina Nucleare, Istituto Europeo di Oncologia, Milano, Italy
Medical Physics and Nuclear Medicine, European Institute of Oncology, Milano, Italy

Francesco De Lauro U. O. Medicina Nucleare, Azienda Sanitaria di Cesena, Cesena, Italy

Amalia Di Dia Unità di Fisica Sanitaria, Istituto Europeo di Oncologia, Milano, Italy
Medical Physics and Nuclear Medicine, European Institute of Oncology, Milano, Italy

Fernando Di Gregorio U.O. Medicina Nucleare, Azienda Ospedaliera Santa Maria della Misericordia di Udine, Udine, Italy
Nuclear Medicine, University Hospital, Udine, Italy

Ryan A. Dvorak Division of Nuclear Medicine/Radiology, University of Michigan Medical Center, Ann Arbor, MI, USA

Paola Erba U.O. Medicina Nucleare, Azienda Ospedialiero-Universitaria Pisana, Pisa, Italy

Jure Fettich Department of Nuclear Medicine, University Medical Centre of Ljubljana, Ljubljana, Slovenia

Albert Flotats Department of Nuclear Medicine, Universitat Autònoma de Barcelona, Hospital de la Santa Creu i Sant Pau, Barcelona, Spain

José Manuel Cordero Garcia Department of Nuclear Medicine, Universitary General Hospital of Ciudad Real, Ciudad Real, Spain

Victor Manuel Poblete García Department of Nuclear Medicine, Universitary General Hospital of Ciudad Real, Ciudad Real, Spain

Onelio Geatti U.O. Medicina Nucleare, Azienda Ospedaliera Santa Maria della Misericordia di Udine, Udine, Italy
Nuclear Medicine, University Hospital, Udine, Italy

Andor W. J. M. Glaudemans Department of Nuclear Medicine and Molecular Imaging, University Medical Center Groningen, Groningen, The Netherlands

Henrik Gutte Department of Clinical Physiology, Nuclear Medicine and PET, Copenhagen University Hospital, Copenhagen, Denmark

Randall Hawkins Department of Radiology and Biomedical Imaging, University of California, San Francisco, CA, USA

Ken Herrmann Department of Nuclear Medicine, Klinikum rechts der Isar der Technischen Universität München, Munich, Germany

Marina Hodolic Department of Nuclear Medicine, University Medical Centre of Ljubljana, Ljubljana, Slovenia

Cornelis A. Hoefnagel Department of Nuclear Medicine, The Netherlands Cancer Institute and Academical Medical Center, Amsterdam, The Netherlands

Eugenio Inglese U. O. Medicina Nucleare, Ospedale Maggiore della Carità di Novara, Novara, Italy

Andreas Kjær Department of Clinical Physiology, Nuclear Medicine and PET, Copenhagen University Hospital, Copenhagen, Denmark

Marco Krengli U. O. Medicina Nucleare, Ospedale Maggiore della Carità di Novara, Novara, Italy

Torsten Kuwert Clinic of Nuclear Medicine, University of Erlangen-Nuremberg, Erlangen, Germany

Elena Lazzeri U.O. Medicina Nucleare, Azienda Ospedialiero-Universitaria Pisana, Pisa, Italy

Gianfranco Loi U. O. Medicina Nucleare, Ospedale Maggiore della Carità di Novara, Novara, Italy

Lucio Mango Servizio di Fisica Sanitaria, Azienda Ospedaliera S. Camillo Forlanini, Roma, Italy Medical Physics, Azienda Ospedaliera S. Camillo Forlanini, Roma, Italy

Luigi Mansi University of Naples, Ist. Scienze Radiologiche, Piazza Miraglia 2, Napoli, Italy

Agustín Ruiz Martínez Department of Nuclear Medicine, Universitat Autònoma de Barcelona, Hospital de la Santa Creu i Sant Pau, Barcelona, Spain

Vincenzo Mattone U. O. Medicina Nucleare, Azienda Sanitaria di Cesena, Cesena, Italy

Jann Mortensen Department of Clinical Physiology, Nuclear Medicine and PET, Copenhagen University Hospital, Copenhagen, Denmark

Massimiliano Pacilio Servizio di Fisica Sanitaria, Azienda Ospedaliera S. Camillo Forlanini, Roma, Italy
Medical Physics Department, Azienda Ospedaliera S. Camillo Forlanini, Rome, Italy

Giovanni Paganelli Divisione di Medicina Nucleare, Istituto Europeo di Oncologia, Milano, Italy
Medical Physics and Nuclear Medicine, European Institute of Oncology, Milano, Italy

Pier Francesco Rambaldi U.O. Medicina Nucleare, Seconda Università di Napoli, Napoli, Italy

Prado Talavera Rubio Department of Nuclear Medicine, Universitary General Hospital of Ciudad Real, Ciudad Real, Spain

Ivan Santi U. O. Medicina Nucleare, Policlinico S. Orsola-Malpighi, Bologna, Italy

Youngho Seo Department of Radiology and Biomedical Imaging, University of California, San Francisco, CA, USA

Alberto Signore Nuclear Medicine, 2nd Faculty of Medicine, Università Sapienza di Roma, Roma, Italy
Department of Nuclear Medicine and Molecular Imaging, University Medical Center Groningen, University of Groningen, Groningen, The Netherlands

Ana María García Vicente Department of Nuclear Medicine, Universitary General Hospital of Ciudad Real, Ciudad Real, Spain

John Patrick Pilkington Woll Department of Nuclear Medicine, Universitary General Hospital of Ciudad Real, Ciudad Real, Spain

Ka Kit Wong Division of Nuclear Medicine/Radiology, University of Michigan Medical Center, Ann Arbor, MI, USA
Department of Nuclear Medicine, VA Ann Arbor Healthcare System, Ann Arbor, MI, USA

Chapter 1 SPECT-CT: Importance for Clinical Practice

Luigi Mansi, Vincenzo Cuccurullo, and Pier Francesco Rambaldi

Contents

S. Fanti et al., *Atlas of SPECT-CT*,
DOI: 10.1007/978-3-642-15726-4_1, © Springer-Verlag Berlin Heidelberg 2011

1.1 The Diagnostic World Before Hybrid Machines

Diagnostic imaging in the twentieth century was mainly based on two separate universes: (1) the morpho-structural, where information on anatomy and structures is acquired, having pathology as the gold standard, and (2) the functional, where normal and altered functions are analyzed, with pathophysiology as the reference.

In the "old medicine," these universes existed and were observed separately, like with mono-ocular vision, only capable of seeing half of the whole view; therefore, using a single eye, incomplete information was gathered. To overcome this handicap, traditional diagnostic imaging can use information acquired separately by visual comparison, but this approach is affected by many limitations, mainly because of the subjective nature of the analysis.

In the last decades, the incredibly fast development of technology and computers led to a revolution that almost killed analogical imaging, creating a new world only occupied by digital data. In this scenario, a major improvement has been obtained with so-called *fusion imaging*, allowing the overlap of digital scans acquired using different techniques and/or performed on different days. The main consequence, with the possibility of overlapping PET (or SPECT) and CT images, has been achieving a fused image combining morpho-structural and functional data together. In other words, it has become possible to obtain information containing the advantages but not the disadvantages of the single procedures taken alone, allowing higher diagnostic accuracy.

However, despite the advanced level reached by computerized techniques, major problems in the post-processing of fusion imaging, i.e., because of the retrospective rigid registration, still exist. In particular, limited anatomical accuracy in the fused image (up to 1 cm and more), mainly due to the unsatisfactory reproducibility of positioning in different sessions and to technical issues, is achievable. Moreover, when CT is acquired separately with respect to radionuclide procedures, no measured attenuation correction can be reliably obtained for PET and SPECT in a short time, also creating errors in accurate quantitative analysis. Furthermore, acquiring two studies at different times causes a delay in the duration of the whole diagnostic process, having effects on the timeliness of the diagnosis. This condition can have both medical consequences, because of the possibility of hindering diagnostic and therapeutic strategies, and economic ones, because of time spent in the hospital, waiting lists, and the cost for the full medical treatment.

1.2 The Advent of Hybrid Systems

With respect to the post-processing problems present in fusion imaging, the availability of hybrid machines, i.e., a CT (or, in the near future, a MR) and a PET (or SPECT) scanner working together, led to a major revolution. The main advantage is the highly precise anatomical accuracy of the fused image (averaging 1° mm), with the two studies being acquired simultaneously with the patient immobile on the same bed. Moreover, a reliable attenuation correction, and therefore an accurate quantitative analysis, is achievable. All these advantages are obtained with a shorter duration of the whole procedure, allowing an earlier diagnosis. It has to be pointed out that some minor technical problems still exist in the hybrid machines, mainly because of the technical differences between CT and nuclear medicine (NM) procedures. However, many solutions, such as respiratory gating, are already being used in clinical practice, and every day new methods are being developed to further improve the whole system in order to optimize the final result.

1.3 SPECT-CT, Parallels and Divergences with Respect to PET-CT

The initial commercial development of SPECT-CT was based on joining a state-of-the-art SPECT and a low-resolution standard axial CT. Major applications were focused on CT-based attenuation correction in cardiology and oncology, with further emphasis, mainly in oncology, on a better localization of hot spots. Therefore, the first steps in the history of SPECT-CT were parallel to those for PET-CT. Also for PET, the earliest rationale for the use of hybrid systems was the possibility to obtain a faster measured attenuation correction with CT. A major improvement was the reduction in the whole body imaging time by replacing the slowly rotating rod source (which took several minutes per bed position) with the much faster CT scan, taking typically less than 1–2° min for the entire body.

However, while today PET-CT, even including a diagnostic multislice CT (MSCT), has virtually replaced stand-alone PET, the situation is completely different for SPECT-CT. Despite evidence that combined modalities, such as for PET, can improve the reader's confidence and therefore diagnostic accuracy, there are currently relatively few SPECT-CT machines. This discrepancy is based on many factors. First, a hybrid machine costs more than a SPECT alone, and therefore its cost-effectiveness needs to be demonstrated. Furthermore, the need for a more space and, considering the X-rays produced by CT, radioprotection can eventually create unfavorable conditions and/or additional costs. Having recently overcome the fear of a Tc-99m supply shortage, the major competitors concerning more widespread use of SPECT-CT scanners are PET and/or other alternative procedures (ultrasound, MSCT, magnetic resonance) because of their clinical capabilities. In fact, although PET is unquestionably increasing its presence in diagnostics daily, also the other radiological alternative procedures with respect to SPECT are reinforcing and/or enlarging their operative field. This means that there are many reasons to support the development of a diagnostic imaging department based on radiological techniques and PET-CT, without the need for "traditional" nuclear medicine based on gamma emitters.

1.4 Clinical Role for Gamma Emitters in the Third Millennium

To determine the clinical role of SPECT-CT, we have to include this goal in a more general discourse on the value of gamma emitters for diagnostic purposes. This is a mandatory premise because of the certain improvement achievable by SPECT-CT, with anatomical localization added to functional data to transform unclear medical treatment with reliable nuclear medicine. It has to be emphasized that the potential added contribution of CT to SPECT can be even higher than the value of combining CT with PET because of the poorer resolution and higher noise of images acquired with gamma emitters.

Therefore, the main question to be answered in this chapter is: can we assume that there will be a future for SPECT-CT like for PET-CT, defining the hybrid system as a new standard, starting from a clinical value already verifiable in the present that will continue into the near future?

Considering the chapters that will follow, presenting some of the most important clinical applications showing the role of the hybrid system, we want discuss and report here the general situation, justifying the continued use of gamma emitters in the PET era.

1.5 Gamma Emitters With or Without SPECT

To demonstrate the effectiveness of SPECT-CT, first an analysis of whether gamma emitters will continue to play a clinical role will be analyzed, despite the increased use of more effective and/or appealing PET procedures, which is growing every day.

The situation will certainly develop in institutions that do not have PET scanners that developing optimal conditions in facilities with a PET scanner but without a cyclotron, where at least part of the clinical indications will continue to be assessed using gamma tracers.

In this context, the best situation will involve using procedures that allow better cost-effectiveness for gamma emitters, in the presence of strong and consolidated clinical indications. This condition affects many radionuclide studies, such as those in cardiology, inflammation and infection, neuropsychiatry, orthopedics, nephrology, and endocrinology; many of these are supported by a high diagnostic accuracy or prognostic value, in the presence of wider diffusion and lower costs with respect to PET. In some cases, as in dynamic studies (renal scintigraphy, cystoscintigraphy, gastrointestinal transits, hepatobiliary scintigraphy, etc.) or as a premise for radioguided surgery, gamma emitters will probably continue to be a first choice also in the near future. Further indications could develop or find a wider diffusion, such as the use of gamma emitters in pre-therapeutic dosimetry, where their longer decay time with respect to the corresponding positron tracers may allow more reliable tumor and whole body dose calculations. Pre-therapeutic studies could become an important field of interest, as already took place for I-131, giving value to an individual dosimetry calculated for I-131 MIBG (using I-123 MIBG), Y-90 octreotide (In-111 octreotide), Y-90 zevelin (In-111 zevelin), I-131 bexxar (I-123 bexxar), etc.

Further technological improvements could also better define a possible clinical role of studies with gamma emitters as a guide to biopsy or interventional therapies; new indications could be derived from the definition of the biological target in radiotherapy; applications could clearly emerge as a consequence of the development of new tracers, including antibodies, antibiotics, neurotransmitters, radiomolecules involved in apoptosis or in neoangiogenesis, and all radiocompounds existing in new territories designed by genomics, proteomics, and the emerging molecular biology. In this direction, we have to remember not only the great practical advantages of Tc-99m, but also the radiochemical value of I-123 to label innovative biomolecules, or of In-111, when a slow biokinetic has to be studied. New and original indications could be derived from the diffusion of novel techniques, such as using multiple energies and dual imaging, allowing, for example, to study metabolism (and/or receptors) and perfusion in cardiology simultaneously.

To all these indications, implemented applications for old radiotracers can be added. We need only remember the role of Tc-99m sestamibi in defining drug resistance and apoptosis, or the possibility to acquire original pathophysiological information in heart and brain diseases using cardiac scintigraphy with I-123 MIBG. And certainly old techniques such as the thyroid scan, Meckel's diverticulum detection, testing of bleeding and angiomas using red blood cells, etc., will remain part of the diagnostic armamentarium.

The continuation of a clinical role for gamma emitters will be strongly supported by technological developments, introducing new cameras, detectors, software, and procedures allowing faster and more effective scans with a sensitivity and resolution increased by five- to ten-fold and more. This is already happening in nuclear cardiology, but will also evolve in other fields because of the introduction of dedicated cameras.

A relevant impulse to the expansion of radionuclide studies with gamma emitters could also be its introduction as a "major procedure" in emergency departments. In the following, we will present a general discussion (since this issue is not specifically treated in the other chapters of this book) about how demonstrating the cost-effectiveness of gamma emitters in emergency departments can provide a primary motivation to acquire a SPECT-CT.

1.6 Nuclear Medicine in the Emergency Department (A Useful Location for a SPECT-CT)

The clinical role of nuclear medicine is based on its own capabilities compared to those of alternative procedures. Its value can be unique and/or complementary, answering not only diagnostic queries, but also questions related to the prognosis and therapy; in this way an individual course and more effective therapeutic strategy can be better defined. But no role is possible when a procedure is not available.

Therefore, the value of nuclear medicine in emergency departments is negatively conditioned by its absence in first aid stations. With the necessity for speed in emergency situations, a role for a procedure not available 24 h a day, 365 days a year, and not located where the emergency has to be diagnosed and treated, cannot be supported.

If we analyze the main criteria for the organization of a diagnostic imaging department for emergencies, we indentify the main constitutive elements as the location of resources, work load, type of required services, and costs, including instruments and personnel. The facility has to be organized as rationally and efficiently as possible. Therefore, a standard department is traditionally based on the presence of a few machines, able to provide results as quickly and cost-effectively as possible for the large majority of events. This means that traditional radiology, such as ultrasounds and a MSCT, needs to be present. A significant improvement can be added by the availability of angiographic techniques, which can also be interventional procedures; conversely, they are considered not cost-effective, too complicated, and too slow in answering the demands of both nuclear medicine and MRI. As a vicious circle, being only rarely present in the diagnostic imaging services of emergency department, radionuclide procedures do not demonstrate evidence-based effectiveness, being too far from the initial clinical request. The problem increases when a 24 h nuclear medicine service is not available, causing further delays by adding "unnecessary dangerous minutes" because of the time for the patient, technician, and physician to arrive at the facility, the time to prepare the radiocompound, etc., all of which make reaching the clinical assessment too slow. A partial solution could be given by telenuclear medicine, allowing a remote interpretation of emergency studies by an on-call expert, but this does not solve all the problems.

Therefore, nuclear medicine is not considered useful in emergency situations, although it has major advantages, being feasible in all patients without absolute contraindications in the presence of clinical justification. Moreover, radionuclide techniques do not require preparation or pre-diagnostic examinations, are not operator-dependent, and permit the best functional imaging, whole body, and quantitative analysis, providing unique capabilities with respect to all the alternative techniques.

The question at this point is: if we solve all the "practical" problems described above, is there a clinical role for nuclear medicine in emergency departments? The answer is probably yes, if there is evidence of many strong and well-defined indications (Table 1.1).

Referring to the literature, and a wider and deeper analysis of reasons justifying these applications, we want to emphasize here that radionuclide techniques using gamma emitters can contribute both when the fastest diagnosis and choice of a therapeutic approach are requested and when a best diagnosis and therapy are achievable because there is no critical urgency. In fact, nuclear medicine can play a relevant role, adding a prognostic evaluation, better monitoring, and a more precise determination of the time of discharge. Considering

Table 1.1 Main indications for nuclear medicine in emergency departments

• Chest pain: Pulmonary embolism, myocardial infarction
• Cerebral emergencies: Cerebrovascular accidents, brain death, head traumas, ictal epilepsy
• Acute inflammation/infection
• Abdominal bleeding
• Trauma
• Transplants
• Skeletal, hepatobiliary, renal, endocrine emergencies
• Acute scrotal pain
• Pulmonary aspiration

human resources and facilities, nuclear medicine can therefore be cost-effective, playing a major role, for example, avoiding admission for false emergencies and reducing the number of quick discharges with related increased risks, causing deaths and/or future costs because of damages and the consequent need for rehabilitation.

In the following, some of the most important information for emergency nuclear medicine is reported. At present, this information is only "practically" feasible using gamma emitters, as PET tracers are not immediately available on demand.

1.6.1 Chest Pain

1.6.1.1 Myocardial Infarct

It has been clearly demonstrated in facilities with a nuclear medicine division in the emergency department that myocardial scintigraphy (MS), because of a higher accuracy with respect to ECG and ultrasound, can help to better define the diagnostic and therapeutic strategies. In particular, it reduces the number of erroneous admissions for false emergencies, i.e., for patients without a myocardial infarct (MI); conversely, it increases the number of correct admissions, including up to 50–65% of subjects with a non-diagnostic ECG misdiagnosed as having MI. As a further advantage, MS distinguishes 2–8% of patients at risk for a too early discharge, causing a three times higher probability of death and significantly higher costs for rehabilitation and/or new major events. With respect to savings, it has also been calculated that the presence of a nuclear medicine division in the emergency department reduces costs for false emergencies by 5%. In this way a gain in the order of tens of millions of Euros per year can be obtained.

As a further indication, it has to be remembered that gated-SPECT using perfusion tracers is an accurate, reliable, and easy method to evaluate cardiac perfusion and function in all circumstances required in emergency.

1.6.1.2 Pulmonary Embolism

Although today in many institutions the first-line examination in patients with suspicious pulmonary embolism is MSCT with contrast media, up to 25% of patients cannot be recruited using this procedure, which shows toxicity and/or collateral effects, including death. Perfusion lung scintigraphy (PLS), with or without a complementary ventilatory scan, is feasible in all patients without absolute contraindications in the presence of a clinical advantage and does not requires pre-test examinations; the scan is affected by a very high negative predictive value, also showing good accuracy, mainly in younger patients. Moreover, it can add complementary information to MSCT, better defining the severity and extension of the alveolar-capillary function of each lung; finally PLS reliably defines the efficacy of therapeutic procedures, both medical and interventional.

1.6.2 Cerebral Emergencies

1.6.2.1 Cerebrovascular Accidents (CVA)

MSCT is the first-line procedure in these patients, but a cerebral blood flow study with gamma tracers (CBF-SPECT) can be an alternative or complementary study for an early and accurate diagnosis (also in reversible ischemia), for defining the vasodilatory reserve (diamox test), contributing to the prognostic information based on location, extension, and severity, and for differentiating between nutritional reperfusion versus luxury perfusion; similarly, a better selection and monitoring of patients undergoing interventional approaches can be obtained.

1.6.2.2 Head Trauma

CT is also the first-line procedure for head trauma. CBF-SPECT can be an alternative or complementary procedure for early and accurate diagnosis (also for patients with negative CT results); moreover, it can add prognostic information based on location, extension, and severity, also providing an explanation for the behavioral and psychological sequelae present in the large majority of patients with brain injuries.

1.6.2.3 Brain Death

The role of techniques, also planar, using gamma emitters to define brain death can be very relevant. CBF radiotracers are concentrated only by the living brain, permitting a reliable confirmatory test of brain death (as a complement or alternative to transcranial Doppler US, somatosensory-evocated potentials, EEG, and angiography) to shorten the clinical observation time. Together with being accurate, reproducible, and technically easy, a further advantage compared to angiographic techniques using contrast media is the absence of toxic effects that can be present using radiological iodinated compounds, affect kidney function, which can lead to the need for transplants.

1.6.2.4 Ictal Epilepsy

CBF-SPECT is a very reliable method to diagnose and localize the epileptic focus before surgery. If injected during or immediately after an acute event, a higher uptake of the CBF radiotracer is observed at the level of the critical area, allowing a detection sometimes not possible with other procedures.

1.6.3 Bone Scan in Emergencies

A mistake in detecting a bone fracture is one of the most frequent causes of legal malpractice trials. Bone scintigraphy can perform a primary role because of its very high sensitivity, mainly in the presence of a mismatch between symptoms and treatment, taken as the first-line examination; similarly, incremental information can be acquired in unconscious poly-traumatized patients. Bone scintigraphy can also help exclude bone involvement or define disease activity in patients affected with conditions such as tendinitis, rheumatoid arthritis, and sacroileitis, while significant clinical improvement can be achieved in the identification of child abuse. Useful information can be acquired about territory borderlines with respect to the emergency, such as the differential diagnosis of the age of fractures in traumatized patients, to reliably recognize the "actual damage" as opposed to that caused by old injuries. An interesting application can also be found in military medicine to exclude bone pain simulation.

1.6.4 Hepatobiliary Emergencies

Hepatobiliary scintigraphy permits reliable functional evaluation of the hepatobiliary system, today also contributing to the detection of duodenogastric reflux, biliary leakage, and fistula. It can play a role in monitoring patients undergoing bowel surgery, and can also help diagnose biliary atresia in pediatric patients and biliary colic when negative at ultrasounds. The most important indication in emergency medicine is the reliable diagnosis of acute cholecystitis. There is strong evidence that cholescintigraphy is significantly more accurate than US in the diagnosis of acute acalculous cholecystitis.

1.6.5 Acute Inflammation Infection

Useful information can be obtained using traditional studies, such as bone, renal, and biliary scintigraphy.

The use of radiolabeled white blood cells (WBC) is too complex for routine use in emergencies, but can be proposed in the presence of clinical suspicion, mainly for post-surgical patients. WBC can detect acute appendicitis in subjects with equivocal clinical findings also in the presence of non-typical and/or difficult locations, such as retrocoecal; moreover, it can show perforation reliably and early.

1.6.6 Abdominal Bleeding

The Tc-99m pertechnetate scan is the first-line procedure for abdominal bleeding in pediatric patients because of its high accuracy in detecting Meckel's diverticulum. In adults, application of radiolabeled red blood cell (RBCs) can precede angiography because of the high negative predictive value; this also has a diagnostic potential in patients with absence of active rapid bleeding, negative or inconclusive endoscopy for whom invasive procedures are contraindicated (as in an immediate post-surgical phase).

1.6.7 Transplants

Nuclear medicine can play a primary role in transplant units to define brain death, to recruit donors, and to evaluate early and complications reliably, and is available for patients undergoing renal, cardiac, hepatic, and pulmonary transplants using standard examinations. The possible role of WBCs to detect infections should also be remembered.

1.6.8 Trauma

Being ancillary and/or an alternative to more effective procedures, radionuclide techniques in abdominal and pelvic traumas can provide useful data for skeletal pathologies and, as previously reported, head traumas. A complementary role can be demonstrated in all cases when dynamic information can better define the clinical pattern, such as using renal or hepatobiliary scintigraphy to define altered function, leakage, and fistula.

1.6.9 Post-surgical Emergencies

Nuclear medicine, as previously described, can play an alternative, original, and/or complementary role in many post-surgical complications. Using radionuclide procedures, it is possible to detect and/or evaluate the clinical relevance of trauma, fistula, leakage, bleeding, and sepsis. Moreover, they can reliably define cardiovascular and renal complications and diagnose pulmonary embolism. Finally, as previously reported, CBF radiotracers can be an important tool contributing to the definition of brain death.

1.6.10 Miscellaneous

Radionuclide procedures can play a role in many renal emergencies, such as transplants, acute renal failure, non-diagnosed obstructive uropathy, and acute infection. Important information can be obtained in patients with acute scrotal pain, correctly determining the need for surgical therapy.

In pediatrics, unique information can be achieved to detect pulmonary aspiration in newborns, evaluating reflux after the administration of milk labeled with Tc-99m.

Also, in strict emergency situations, nuclear medicine can contribute to diagnosing diseases such as acute thyroiditis and pheocromocytoma.

1.7 Why a SPECT-CT in Emergency Departments?

In the above, the clinical effectiveness of radionuclide procedures using gamma radiotracers in urgent situations has been demonstrated. Therefore, the absence of nuclear medicine in emergency departments is not because it is not useful, but can rather mainly be explained by structural, organizational, and economic issues. If we solve these problems without changing the rationale of emergency departments, we could improve the entire clinical result.

Our proposal is that the best way to include nuclear medicine in the diagnostic imaging section of emergency departments is to transform MSCTs into SPECT-CTs. A gamma camera/SPECT, as part of the hybrid machine, can significantly increase the diagnostic accuracy, also providing further original and/or complementary information that can reduce the number of mistakes and/or better define therapeutic strategies.

1.8 Can SPECT-CT Be Cost-Effective?

To answer to this question, we first need to have evidence of the clinical effectiveness, defining a role in comparison with alternative procedures, both radiological and PET-CT. Similarly, we need to specify when the hybrid machine should be implemented clinically instead of a SPECT alone. Together with this evaluation, we have to calculate whether the cost is justifiable and sustainable.

Evaluation of the clinical usefulness in different fields will be the subject of the next chapters, describing the most important applications of SPECT-CT. Also the contribution of the implementation in emergency medicine has to be taken into account. At the end of this book, we hope the readers will have sufficient information to evaluate the improvements achievable with a SPECT-CT in order to make decisions about its acquisition.

To make a more rational and pragmatic evaluation, a cost analysis also has to be performed. Concerning the necessary costs, that a relevant percentage of the value of hybrid machines is determined by the radiological component needs to be remembered. Only considering diagnostic CT, it has to be pointed out that a more expensive MSCT, with at least 16 slices (preferably 64) or more, is only mandatory for research or when angiographic data, such as for coronary CT, are requested. This means that satisfactory and less expensive results (also in terms of radioprotection) can also be obtained routinely in the large majority of institutions with systems with a MSCT with less than 16 slices.

Therefore, to correctly evaluate the cost-effectiveness and to determine the best and most productive technological acquisition for SPECT-CT, we have to take into account the dimension and mission of the institution (general hospital, cardiology, oncology, emergency, research, private practice, pediatrics, etc.). We hope that reading this book will show that SPECT-CT can significantly enhance the field of nuclear medicine.

Suggested Reading

Blackmore CC. Evidence-based imaging in trauma radiology: where we are and how to move forward. Acta Radiol. 2009; 50(5):482–9.

Bülow H, Schwaiger M. Nuclear cardiology in acute coronary syndromes. Q J Nucl Med Mol Imaging. 2005;49(1):59–71.

Freeman LM, Stein EG, Sprayregen S, Chamarthy M, Haramati LB. The current and continuing important role of ventilation-perfusion scintigraphy in evaluating patients with suspected pulmonary embolism. Semin Nucl Med. 2008;38(6):432–40.

Gallagher MJ, Ross MA, Raff GL, Goldstein JA, O'Neill WW, O'Neil B. The diagnostic accuracy of 64-slice computed tomography coronary angiography compared with stress nuclear imaging in emergency department low-risk chest pain patients. Ann Emerg Med. 2007;49(2):125–36.

Joffe AR, Lequier L, Cave D. Specificity of radionuclide brain blood flow testing in brain death: case report and review. J Intensive Care Med. 2010;25(1):53–64.

Mansi L, Rambaldi PF, Cuccurullo V, Varetto T. Nuclear medicine in emergency. Q J Nucl Med Mol Imaging. 2005; 49(2):171–91.

Sivit CJ. Contemporary imaging in abdominal emergencies. Pediatr Radiol. 2008;38 Suppl 4:S675–8.

Wackers FJ. Chest pain in the emergency department: role of cardiac imaging. Heart. 2009;95(12):1023–30.

Chapter 2 SPECT-CT: Technology and Physics

Agustín Ruiz Martínez

Contents

S. Fanti et al., *Atlas of SPECT-CT*,
DOI: 10.1007/978-3-642-15726-4_2, © Springer-Verlag Berlin Heidelberg 2011

Single photon emission computed tomography (SPECT) is an imaging technique that uses a gamma camera to produce a functional 3D distribution of a photon emitter radionuclide within the body, whereas computed tomography (CT) uses an external source of x-rays to produce anatomical 3D images. From a clinical point of view, therefore, a combined SPECT/CT system could provide both functional and anatomical images. At the same time, it can also accurately generate an attenuation correction of the SPECT images. From a technological point of view, although each technique is based on a different physical process to acquire the data (emission of radiation by the patient in SPECT and transmission of radiation through the patient in CT), the two have similarities in image formation and image reconstruction processes.

2.1 SPECT

A SPECT study is divided into two phases: acquisition and processing. In the acquisition phase, the gamma camera rotates around the patient in a series of steps, and a planar image, called a projection, is obtained for each angular position. In the processing phase, these planar images are reconstructed into 3D images by means of mathematical algorithms.

The gamma camera requires a set of parameters to perform the acquisition phase of the study. Some of these parameters are significant because they are related to the image quality: counts per projection (or time per projection, depending on the study), total rotation around the patient, pixel matrix size and detector-patient distance. The greater the number of counts per projection is, the better the quality of the image. However, this may involve excessively long acquisition times, and artifacts may appear because of patient motion. As acquisition time can be optimized by using multi-head gamma cameras, currently commercially available SPECT systems are dual-head.

The total rotation around the patient is usually 90°, 180° or 360°, and the total number of projections may vary from 60 to 128. The acquisition pixel matrix should be of the same order as the number of projections to avoid the appearance of star artifacts, so that SPECT data are typically acquired in 64×64 pixel matrices, although in some specific applications 128×128 pixel matrices can be used. To obtain an acceptable image quality, the patient-detector distance should be as small as possible. The use of automatic patient contour detection systems, if these are available, or the choice of elliptical orbits can optimize the patient-detector distance.

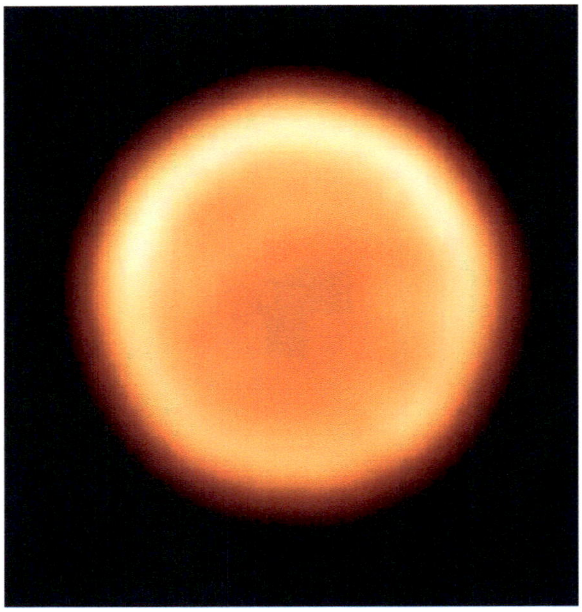

Fig. 2.1 Uniform cylinder without AC correction

In the processing phase, there are several methods to reconstruct three-dimensional sections from planar images. The most common method is the filtered back-projection (FBP), but in certain studies iterative methods such as maximum likelihood expectation maximization/ordered subset expectation maximization (MLEM/OSEM) can lead to better results. It is also necessary to use mathematical image filters to obtain an image of adequate quality. However, filters alter raw images, so the choice of a particular filter and its parameters depends on the physical characteristics of the organ under study and the purpose of the study.

An important issue to consider in SPECT is the attenuation of photons within the organ under study, or within the patient. Attenuation may lead to images being reconstructed with apparently less activity at the center of the image, when distribution of activity in the organ is actually uniform (Fig. 2.1). The attenuation can be corrected by using mathematical algorithms, such as the Chang filter, but improper use of this algorithm may cause undesirable effects, such as activity overestimation at the center of the image (Fig. 2.2). Attenuation correction using transmission is the optimal method, and it can be performed with an external encapsulated source or with an x-ray source, usually a CT (Fig. 2.3).

Several types of artifacts may appear using the SPECT technique. They may be related to instrumentation, patient, study acquisition or data processing.

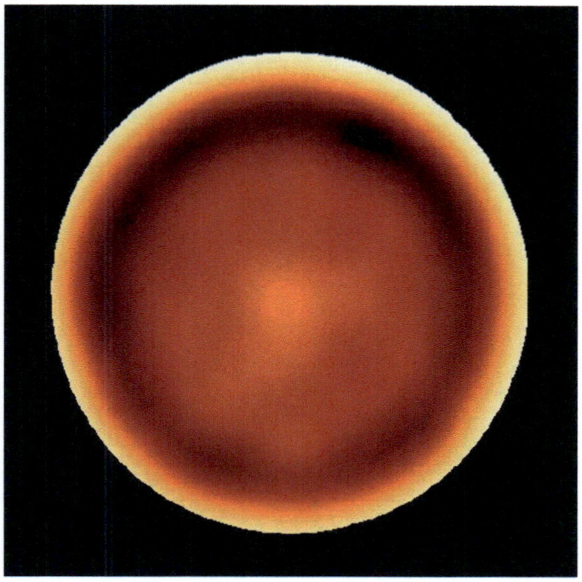

Fig. 2.2 Improper Chang AC correction

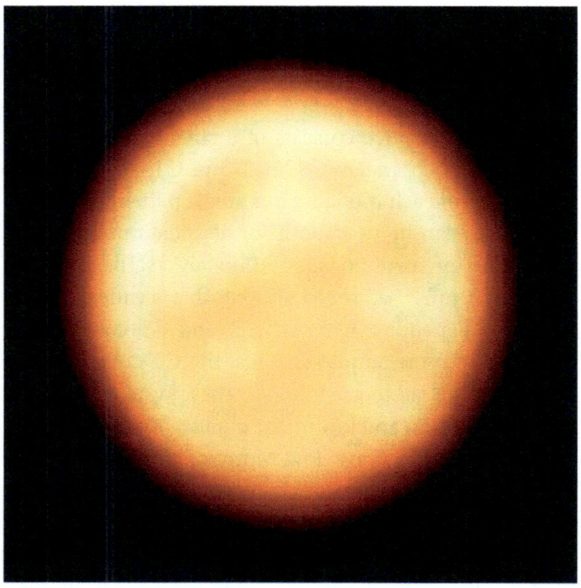

Fig. 2.3 Uniform cylinder with CT AC correction

Flood field non-uniformity can lead to the appearance of whole or partial rings. In dual-head systems, differences in flood uniformity between the two detectors can also cause artifacts, even when individual head flood uniformities are correct. Image blurring is another common artifact and can be caused by patient motion, but also by instrumentation errors such as an erroneous center of rotation (COR) or a gamma-camera head tilt. Partial volume artifacts are typical of tomographic techniques and are due to insufficient data to reconstruct the image, such as too short a scan range or too small a field of view (FOV) in the case of SPECT. Other artifacts can be associated with inadequate reconstruction data, such as the choice of an improper filter or an incorrect application of filter parameters, which can lead to excessive smoothing or introduce noise in the image. There is no perfect filter, but an optimal one would provide maximum resolution while avoiding the introduction of artifacts.

2.2 CT

The process of obtaining an image of organs, tissues or structures inside the human body using x-rays is based on the different attenuations experienced by the radiation beam as it passes through materials with a different attenuation coefficient. This image is a transmission map of x-ray photons.

In the case of CT, an x-ray source performs a continuous rotation around the patient and, using a detection system located behind the patient, a profile of the beam attenuation (transmission) within the patient is obtained for each angular position. These attenuation measurements are used to generate a transversal array of attenuation coefficients by means of a filtered back-projection algorithm or some other tomographic reconstruction technique. After assigning a gray scale to the attenuation coefficient array, images representing the anatomy of the body are obtained.

As with SPECT, several parameters are needed to perform a CT study. In this case, the basic parameters are the kV, mA and pitch (ratio between the field size in the z-axis and the distance covered by the imaging table). For image reconstruction, the matrices are typically 256×256 or 512×512 with pixel sizes representing 0.5–2.0 mm of tissue. Mathematical filters are also needed, and their choice depends on the characteristics of the body region under exploration: brain studies need filters that enhance sharp variations, whereas abdominal studies need filters specially adapted to soft tissues.

The use of multidetector computed tomography (MDCT) devices is now increasing. These devices allow acquisition of 256–320 simultaneous slices in just 0.35–0.25 s rotation time. The maximum number of slices in hybrid systems (SPECT/CT or PET/CT), however, is 64. As well as faster acquisition times, these MDCT devices can provide very high quality images, though they may also increase the radiation doses to patient.

CT image quality can also be degraded by the presence of artifacts. The causes of these may be similar to those in the SPECT technique, but they may also be due to the physics involved in CT image formation. An x-ray beam spectrum is polyenergetic, that is, it is composed of photons with a range of energies. As the beam passes through an object, its average energy increases because the lower energy photons are absorbed, and only higher energy photons reach the detector. The beam is "hardened" and can then produce two types of artifacts: cupping artifacts (more intense beams on the outside of a homogeneous area) and, between dense objects, streaks and dark bands. Partial volume artifacts can arise as a consequence of an incomplete covering of an organ, tissue or structure, like in SPECT, and also because the different materials inside a voxel are represented by a single attenuation coefficient, which is the average of all the attenuation coefficients. Another physics effect that can lead to streaks in the image is photon starvation: when the beam passes through high attenuation areas, such as the shoulder, the number of photons reaching the detector is insufficient, and the corresponding projections for these angles are very noisy. Artifacts may also be caused by the device itself, such as the appearance of rings if a detector is uncalibrated. The appearance of shadows or streaks in the image may be the consequence of patient motion, but in CT studies the streaking artifacts may also result from the presence of metals inside the patient in the scan area (Fig. 2.4).

Helical scanning can also lead to artifacts when the anatomical structures show sharp variations along the z direction, causing the image to appear distorted in the transversal plane. This is because helical reconstruction needs an interpolation process at points located in the z direction (cranio-caudal) that have not been reached by the x-ray beam; in other words, the missing information at these points is obtained from the nearest irradiated points. Since the interpolation process is more complex in the case of MDCT helical scanning, the associated distortion is also more complex and may have the appearance of a windmill. In MDCT devices, as the number of slices that can be acquired simultaneously increases, the collimation along the z axis is greater, and therefore the x-ray beam is cone-shaped rather than fan-shaped, producing an effect similar to partial volume artifacts. CT systems are now equipped with hardware devices and software corrections to minimize the vast majority of the artifacts that may arise.

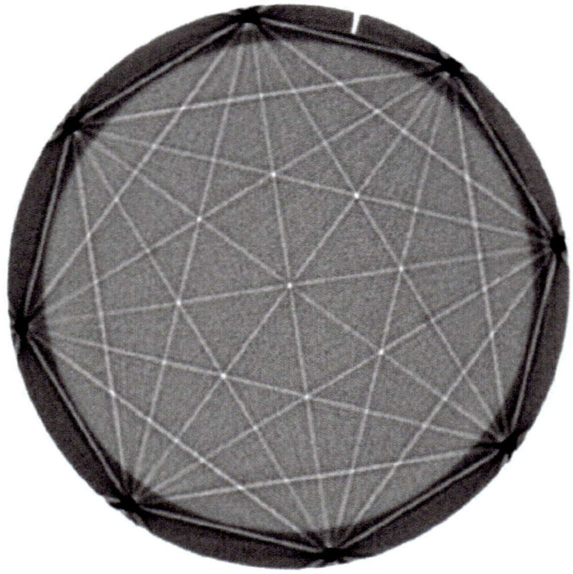

Fig. 2.4 Streak artifacts, due to metal screws, on a PMMMA phantom

2.3 SPECT/CT

A SPECT/CT device consists of a single unit that integrates these two systems, SPECT and CT, allowing data acquisition of each modality in a single patient study. The CT images can be used both for attenuation correction (AC) and for anatomical location (AL). The range of SPECT/CT units commercially available is wide, and performance depends on the SPECT and CT components installed. In more simple systems, the CT component is basically included to provide AC. These systems have low spatial resolution and low image quality, but the radiation dose to the patient is also low. More sophisticated systems incorporate MDCT, and they can perform high-resolution CT studies together with complex SPECT studies, such as CT coronary angiography with myocardial perfusion SPECT. The system generally used in most hospitals, nevertheless, is a dual-head gamma camera that incorporates a CT that has been optimized for AC and AL.

In the case of using CT for SPECT attenuation correction, it is necessary to reduce the resolution of CT data to match those of SPECT. Furthermore, since the effective energy of the x-ray beam is about 70 keV and the attenuation varies with energy, the CT attenuation map must be converted to the radionuclide photon energy used in SPECT (in most cases 140 keV photons emitted by ^{99m}Tc).

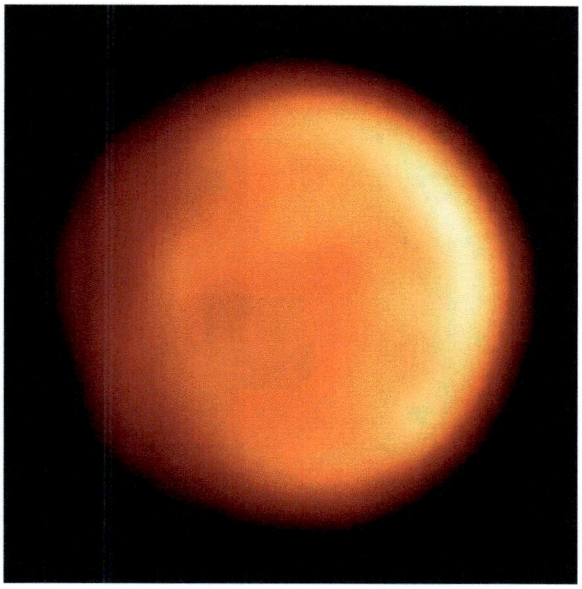

Fig. 2.5 Incorrect AC due to a misalignment between TC and SPECT

The use of CT data for the AC provides several advantages. The statistical noise associated with the AC is lower with CT than with other techniques, such as transmission with encapsulated sources, because the photon flux provided by the CT is higher. The total time to perform the study is significantly reduced because of the fast acquisition speed of CT. The anatomical images acquired with CT can be merged with the emission images to provide functional anatomical maps for precise localization of radiotracer uptake. The process of aligning the SPECT and CT images, in order to fuse them and analyze them, is called spatial registration.

SPECT/CT not only has the artifacts generated by each of the two imaging systems, but also has those that arise from the fusion of the two devices. The main issue to consider in SPECT/CT is the misalignment between the CT and SPECT images, which may be due to a technical problem with equipment (either hardware or software). Co-registration should therefore be checked regularly. Patient motion in the time interval between CT and SPECT acquisitions can also cause an incorrect spatial registration between the two images sets, and may involve inaccurate attenuation correction (Fig. 2.5) and incorrect correlation between anatomical and functional imaging. To avoid this potential problem, manufacturers tend to provide software for the correction and adjustment of the alignment of the two data sets.

Suggested Reading

Barrett JF, Keat N. Artifacts in CT: recognition and avoidance. RadioGraphics. 2004;24:1679–91.

de Cabrejas ML, Pérez AM, Giannone CA, Vázquez S, Marrero G. SPECT. Una guía práctica. Comité de Garantía de Calidad del Alasbimn. Mayo 1992.

Delbeke D, Coleman RE, Guiberteau MJ, et al. Procedure guideline for SPECT/CT imaging 1.0. J Nucl Med. 2009;47: 1227–34.

McQuaid SJ, Hutton BF. Source of attenuation-correction artefacts in cardiac PET/CT and SPECT/CT. Eur J Nucl Med Mol Imaging. 2008;35:1117–23.

Nuñez M. Cardiac SPECT. Alasbimn J. 2002;5(18): Article No. AJ18-13.

Patton JA, Turkington TG. SPECT/CT physical principles and attenuations correction. J Nucl Med Technol. 2008; 36:1–10.

Puchal Añé R. Filtros de imagen en Medicina Nuclear. Nycomed Amersham: Ediciones Eurobook; 1997.

Sociedad Española de Física Médica, Sociedad Española de Medicina Nuclear y Sociedad Española de Protección Radiológica. Protocolo Nacional del Control de Calidad en la Instrumentación en Medicina Nuclear. 1999.

Chapter 3 SPECT-CT for Tumor Imaging

Carina Mari Aparici,
Anca M. Avram, Angel Soriano Castrejón,
Ryan A. Dvorak, Paola Erba, Jure Fettich,
José Manuel Cordero Garcia,
Victor Manuel Poblete García,
Randall Hawkins, Marina Hodolic,
Prado Talavera Rubio, Youngho Seo,
Ana María García Vicente,
John Patrick Pilkington Woll,
and Ka Kit Wong

Contents

S. Fanti et al., *Atlas of SPECT-CT*,
DOI: 10.1007/978-3-642-15726-4_3,

3.1 Octreotide SPECT-CT

Angel Soriano Castrejón (✉), José Manuel Cordero Garcia, Victor Manuel Poblete García, John Patrick Pilkington Woll, and Ana María García Vicente

Somatostatine receptor scintigraphy (SRS) with somatostatine analogs is nowadays established as a first-line tool in the detection, staging and evaluation of the response of neuroendocrine tumors (NETs) and some neural crest tumors, yielding much better results than conventional imaging techniques [1] as many subtypes of these tumors overexpress a high density of somatostatine receptors at the cell surface [2, 3]. This overexpression of the somatostatin receptors, however, may also be present in some other tumors, such as differentiated thyroid carcinoma, lung cancer, breast cancer, meningiomas, well-differentiated astrocytomas, pituitary tumors, lymphoma and several others [4–7]. Some benign conditions, mainly related to the presence of inflammatory cells, i.e., in thyroidal oftalmopathy [8], may also show an increased expression of these surface receptors.

Six types of somatostatin receptors have been cloned, namely sst_1–sst_5, with sst_2 spliced to yield sst_{2A} y sst-$_{2B}$, with all somatostatine analogs having high affinity for the receptors sst_2 and sst_5, and varying affinity for types sst_3 and sst_4. They are G-protein-coupled receptors on the cell membrane that recognize the ligand and generate a transmembrane signal. The hormone-receptor complexes have the ability to be internalized. The vesicles formed fuse to lysosomes, degradating the hormone and recycling the receptor [9].

The short plasmatic half-life of somatostatine (about 3 min) has promoted the development of analogs with longer half-lives, suited to the clinical use. The most widely used somatostatine analog for SRS is [^{111}In]-diethylene triamine pentacetate acid [DTPA]-octreotide, a somatostatine-derivated octapeptide coupled to a chelant (DTPA) that shows a high affinity for receptor subtype 2 and 5, probably internalized after its binding to the receptor with residualization of the ^{111}In label, which would account for the good 24 h tumor-to-background ratio.

Thus, the biomarker analyzed by these somatostatine analogs is the overexpression of these receptors, offering functional information about this particular molecular characteristic, and evaluating the amount of viable tumoral tissue before and after treatment, or allowing the selection of those patients that could be candidates for the therapeutic use of somatostatine analogs.

Normal scintigraphic features include visualization of thyroid, spleen, liver, kidneys and, in some patients, pituitary gland. The pituitary, spleen and kidney visualization is due to receptor binding, while a tubular reabsorption mechanism mainly accounts for the renal uptake. The radiopharmaceutical is physiologically eliminated by renal clearance, although hepatobiliary clearance is also present, which causes the presence of the tracer in the bowel. The physiological urinary and intestinal elimination is responsible for the majority of doubtful or misinterpreted studies. Ongoing treatment with somatostatine-receptor blockers may cause a diminished spleen or liver uptake, but, in the presence of tumor with expression of these receptors, even high doses of unlabeled octreotide may not result in complete receptor occupancy [10, 11].

Although both conventional scintigraphy and SPECT imaging offer functional information of the greatest importance, not achievable by other means, the physical properties inherent to radionuclide imaging, such as photon attenuation, scattered radiation or partial volume effect, are responsible for its poor spatial resolution. Also, the lack of an adequate anatomical landmark can be a potential source of misinterpretation of the images, with the specificity of the technique being reduced at sites of physiological uptake [12]. All these shortfalls are significantly reduced by the use of hybrid SPECT-CT cameras, disposable versions of which have been available in clinical daily practice since 1999. Their widespread use has increased slowly but steadily. The hybrid equipment improves the quality of the images using the CT as a source of attenuation correction and at the same time provides useful anatomical information [13, 14]. The improvement achieved in the diagnostic accuracy of SRS by the use of SPECT-CT, when compared with the planar and SPECT images, has been reported by several groups [15–18], mainly reducing the false-positives results especially in areas of physiological uptake or elimination.

3.1.1 Neuroendocrine tumors

Neuroendocrine tumors are rare neoplasms that account for 2% of all tumors. They originate from neuroendocrine cells that are thought to arise from common precursor cells of the embryological neural crest and that can be found throughout the human body. Each type of cell produces a characteristic hormone and expresses its own protein markers, and the endocrine effect is mainly

	^{111}In-octreotide	^{123}I-MIBG	^{18}F-DOPA	^{18}FDG
Abdominal carcinoid	78% (76–82%, 720)	63% (54–72%, 125)	87% (80–93%, 116)	–
Pancreatic islet cell carcinoma	67% (56–77%, 99)	–	41% (36–47%, 22)	–
Pheochromocytoma	63% (51–73%, 14)	79% (68–82%, 161)	100% (75–100%, 14)	–
Merkel cell tumors	78% (51–92%, 20)	–	–	–
Medulary thyroid carcinoma	48% (42–57%, 168)	–	66% (52–80%, 48)	75% (67–82%, 128)
Neuroblastoma	63% (53–72%, 105)	84% (79–89%, 204)	–	–
Paraganglioma	94% (85–98%, 77)	69% (58–78%, 87)	100% (76–100%, 10)	–
Bronchial carcinoids	71% (52–86%, 31)	–	–	–
Small cell lung cancer	56% (38–71%, 40)	–	–	95% (88–98%, 96)

paracrine, being involved in the regulation of a large variety of body functions mainly because of the secretion of the so-called *biogenic amines* (serotonine, catecholamines, adrenocorticotropic hormone, growth hormone, substance P, prostaglandins, etc.). Thus, neuroendocrine tumors can arise almost anywhere, although they are more often found in the gastrointestinal (56%) and bronchopulmonary (12%) tracts [19].

Although classically classified according to the embryological organ from which they arise, the most recent World Health Organization (WHO) classification is based on histological characteristics, such as cellular grade, size and location of the primary tumor, local invasiveness and production of biological active substances [20], with the term *carcinoid* being replaced by *neuroendocrine tumor*. Globally, they are divided into well differentiated with a low grade of malignancy, well differentiated more aggressive tumors, poorly differentiated with a high grade of malignancy and mixed exocrine-endocrine tumors.

The most frequent behavior of these tumors is a slow growth, with a long survival time in spite of finding metastasis at the time of the diagnosis, but some of the tumors may be more aggressive, leading to a shorter survival. Some clinical symptoms, such as flushing or diarrhea, may be the initial presentation of the disease, although the diagnosis is only confirmed by histopathological examination, often followed by inmunohistochemical staining.

Although the so-called gastroenteropancreatic tumors are more frequently found, neuroendocrine neoplasms include neural crest tumors such as pheochromocytoma, derived from the cathecolamine-secreting chromafin cells of the adrenal medulla, which may be associated with inherited syndromes (MEN type II, von Hippel-Lindau syndrome, neurofibromatosis) and is metastasic in 10% of the cases, paraganglioma or neuroblastoma, a mainly pediatric tumor that accounts for 10% of the tumors in children and for which an accurate initial diagnosis is key for the final result.

A broad variety of therapeutic options are possible now for patients with neuroendocrine tumors, including surgery as the only curative alternative when it can be performed, palliative surgical procedures, chemoembolization or systemic treatment using Interferon or chemotherapy. Non-radioactively labeled somatostatine analogs or inclusive, radionuclide therapies with somatostatine analogs bound to ^{177}Lu, ^{90}Y, ^{131}I or ^{111}In can also be used, obtaining stabilization of the disease in around the 40% of the patients and partial regression in approximately 30% [4, 21]. Knowledge of the receptor expression status is of great interest not only for the staging and restaging after treatment, but also for the possible planning and follow-up of these recent therapies, as the expression of SRS makes these tumors suitable for treatment with somatostatine analogs. However, some tumors may suffer a dedifferentiation, with lost of expression of somatostatine receptors, with a low sensitivity in the SRS that would make them not appropriate for treatment [22].

Different tracers other than somatostatine analogs have been used in the investigation of this type of tumor, having shown very good results in specific subtypes [13]. Thus, ^{123}I-MIBG, an analog of guanetidine that accumulates in the presinaptic vesicles of the sympathomedullary system, represents a first-choice modality in functioning phaeochromocytomas, paragangliomas and neuroblastomas [23]. Moreover, the recent development of PET tracers, including ^{18}F-FDG [24, 25], ^{18}F-FDOPA [26, 27]or ^{68}Ga-[1,4,7,10-tetraazacyclododecane-1,4,7,10-tetraacetic acid]-1-Nal3-octreotide (^{68}Ga-DOTA-NOC) [28, 29] have broadened the possibilities of studying NETs. The table summarizes the sensitivities obtained from the literature for different types of tumors with the more widely used SPECT and PET tracers, modified from a recent review by

Koopmans et al. [30] (in brackets, the calculated confidence interval and the number of patients included).

3.1.2 Conclusion

SRS is the best tool for the detection, initial staging, evaluation of treatment response and even therapy planning of NETs.

SPECT/CT improves the accuracy significantly, offering invaluable anatomical information for a correct interpretation of scintigraphic findings, and facilitates performing a better attenuation correction.

References

1. Chiti A, Fanti S, Savelli G, Romeo A, Bellanova B, Rodari M, et al. Comparison of somatostatin receptor imaging, computed tomography and ultrasound in the clinical management of neuroendocrine gastro-entero-pancreatic tumors. Eur J Nucl Med. 1998;25:1396–403.
2. Oberg K. Molecular imaging in diagnosis of neuroendocrine tumors. Lancet Oncol. 2006;7:790–2.
3. Kwekkeboom DJ, Krenning EP, Scheidhauer K, Lewington V, Lebtahi R, Grossman A, et al. ENETS Consensus Guidelines for the Standards of Care in Neuroendocrine Tumors: somatostatin receptor imaging with 111In-pentetreotide. Neuroendocrinology 2009;90:184–9.
4. Gotthardt M, Dijkgraaf I, Boerman OC, Oyen WJ. Nuclear medicine imaging and therapy of neuroendocrine tumors. Cancer Imaging. 2006;31:S178–84.
5. Virgolini IJ, Gabriel M, von Guggenberg E, Putzer D, Kendler D, Decristoforo C. Role of radiopharmaceuticals in the diagnosis and treatment of neuroendocrine tumors. Eur J Cancer. 2009;45 Suppl 1:274–91.
6. García Vicente A, García Del Castillo E, Soriano Castrejón A, Alonso Farto J. Olfactory esthesioneuroblastoma: scintigraphic expression of somatostatin receptors. Rev Esp Med Nucl. 1999;18:367–70.
7. García Vicente A, Soriano Castrejón A, Alonso Farto J, Soler E, García del Castillo E. Merkel cell carcinoma. Utility of scintigraphy with 111In-DTPA-pentetreotide. Rev Esp Med Nucl. 1999;18:287–91.
8. Moncayo R, Baldissera I, Decristoforo C, Kendler D, Donnemiller E. Evaluation of immunological mechanisms mediating thyroid-associated ophthalmopathy by radionuclide imaging using the somatostatin analog 11 1In-octreotide. Thyroid 1997;7:21–9.
9. Hofland LJ, Lamberts SW. The pathophysiological consequences of somatostatin receptor internalization and resistance. Endocr Rev. 2003;24:28–47.
10. Kwekkeboom DJ, Reubi JC and Krenning EP. Peptide receptor scintigraphy in oncology. In: Ell PJ, Gambhir SS, editors. Nuclear medicine in clinical diagnoses and treatment. 3rd ed. London: Churchill-Livingstone; 2004. p. 97–106.
11. Banzo Marraco J, Prats Rivera E, Pazola Alba P, Tardín Cardoso L, Andres Gracia A, Santapau Traveria A. Diagnóstico y seguimiento de los tumores neuroendocrnos del tracto gastrointestinal mediante gammagrafía de receptores de somatostatina. In: Soriano Castrejón A, Martín Comín J, García Vicente AM, editors. Medicina Nuclear en la práctica clínica. Madrid: Aula Médica; 2009. p. 667–74.
12. Chowdhury FU, Scarsbrook AF. The role of hybrid SPECT-CT in oncology: current and emerging clinical applications. Clin Radiol. 2008;63:241–51.
13. Schilacci O, Danieli R, Manni C, Simonetti G. Is SPECT/CT with hybrid cameras useful to improve scintigraphy imaging interpretation? Nucl Med Comm. 2004;25:705–10.
14. Lucignani G, Bombardieri E. Progress and challenges in neuroendocrine and neural crest tumors: molecular imaging and therapy. Eur J Nucl Med Mol Imaging. 2009;36:2081–8.
15. Castaldi P, Rufini V, Treglia G, Bruno I, Perotti G, Stifano G, et al. Impact of 111In-DTPA-octreotide SPECT/CT fusion images in the management of neuroendocrine tumors. Radiol Med. 2008;113:1056–67.
16. Even-Sapir E, Keidar Z, Sachs J, Engel A, Bettman L, Gaitini D, et al. The new technology of combined transmission and emission tomography in evaluation of endocrine neoplasms. J Nucl Med. 2001;42:998–1004.
17. Krausz Y, Keidar Z, Kogan I, Even-Sapir E, Bar-Shalom R, Engel A, et al. SPECT/CT hybrid imaging with 111In-pentetreotide in assessment of neuroendocrine tumors. Clin Endocrinol. 2003;59:565–73.
18. Pfannenberg AC, Eschmann SM, Horger M, Lamberts R, Vonthein R, Claussen CD, et al. Benefit of anatomical-functional image fusion in the diagnostic work-up of neuroendocrine neoplasms. Eur J Nucl Med Mol Imaging. 2003;30:835–43.
19. Modlin IM, Lye KD, Kidd M. A 5-decade analysis of 13,715 carcinoid tumors. Cancer 2003;97:934–59.
20. Solcia E, Kloppel G, Sobin LH, et al. Histologic typing of endocrine tumors. WHO International Histological Classification of Tumors. 2nd ed. Heidelberg: Springer; 2000.
21. van Essen M, Krenning EP, Kam BL, de Jong M, Valkema R, Kwekkeboom DJ. Peptide-receptor radionuclide therapy for endocrine tumors. Nat Rev Endocrinol. 2009;5:382–93.
22. Zhang X, Cai W, Cao F, Schreibmann E, Wu Y, Wu JC, et al. 18F-Labeled bombesin analogs for targeting GRP receptor-expressing prostate cancer. J Nucl Med. 2006;47:492–501.
23. Vik TA, Pfluger T, Kadota R, Castel V, Tulchinsky M, Farto JC, et al. (123)I-mIBG scintigraphy in patients with known or suspected neuroblastoma: results from a prospective multicenter trial. Pediatr Blood Cancer. 2009;52:784–90.
24. Beuthien-Baumann B, Strumpf A, Zessin J, Bredow J, Kotzerke J. Diagnostic impact of PET with 18F-FDG, 18F-DOPA and 3-O-methyl-6-[18F]fluoro-DOPA in recurrent or metastatic medullarythyroid carcinoma. Eur J Nucl Med. 2007;34:1604–9.
25. Timmers H, Kozupa A, Chen C, Carrasquillo JA, Ling A, Eisenhofer G, et al. Superiority of fluorodeoxyglucose positron emission tomography to other functional imaging techniques in the evaluation of metastatic SDHB-associated pheochromocytoma and paraganglioma. J Clin Oncol. 2007;25:2262–9.

26. Koopmans KP, de Vries EG, Kema IP, Elsinga PH, Neels OC, Sluiter WJ, et al. Staging of carcinoid tumors using 18F-DOPA positron emission tomography: a diagnostic accuracy study. Lancet Oncol. 2006;7:728–34.
27. Koopmans KP, Neels OC, Kema IP, Elsinga PH, Sluiter WJ, Vanghillewe K, et al. Improved staging of patients with carcinoid and islet cell tumors with 18F-dihydroxyphenyl-alanine and 11C-5-hydroxy-tryptophan positron emission-tomography. J Clin Oncol. 2008;26:1489–95.
28. Ambrosini V, Campana D, Bodei L, Nanni C, Castellucci P, Allegri V. 68Ga-DOTANOC PET/CT clinical impact in patients with neuroendocrine tumors. J Nucl Med. 2010;51:669–73.
29. Lopci E, Nanni C, Rampin L, Rubello D, Fanti S. Clinical applications of 68Ga-DOTANOC in neuroendocrine tumors. Minerva Endocrinol. 2008;33:277–81.
30. Koopmans KP, Neels ON, Kema IP, Elsinga PH, Links TP, de Vries EG, et al. Molecular imaging in neuroendocrine tumors: molecular uptake mechanisms and clinical results. Crit Rev Oncol Hematol. 2009;71:199–213.

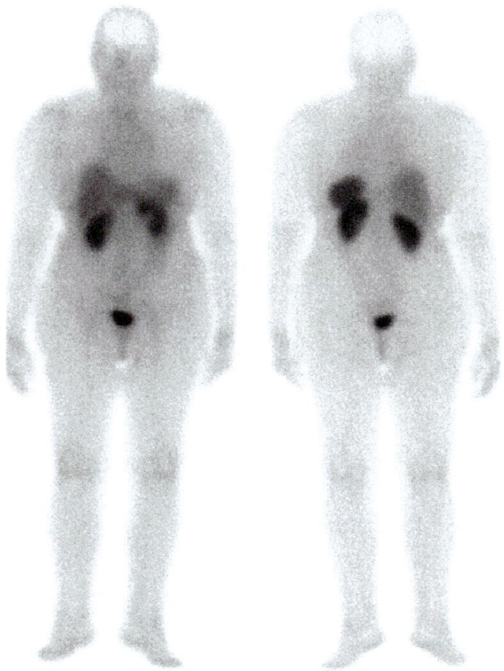

^{111}In octreotide findings

Total body planar images and abdominal SPECT-CT obtained 24 h after the intravenous administration of 222 MBq of ^{111}In octreotide show a normal distribution of the radiotracer without pathological uptake in the pelvic region. The final diagnosis was lymphocele.

Teaching point

^{111}In octreotide is an effective tool for depicting adenopatic masses. SPECT-CT allows to correlate morphologic alterations with functional data.

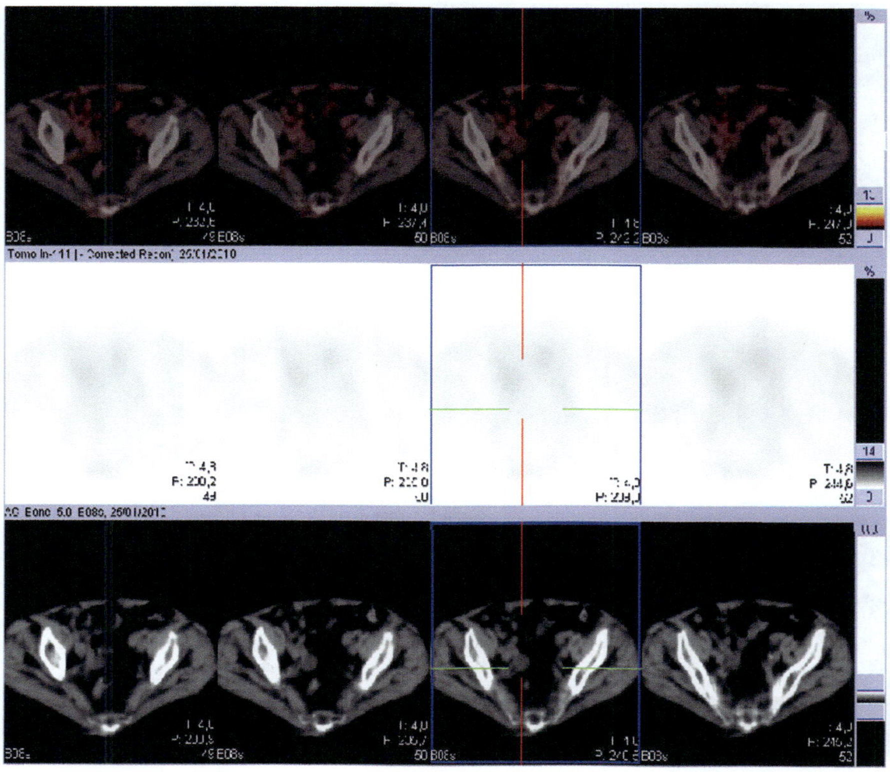

A patient diagnosed of a poorly differentiated carcinoid intestinal tumor (pT3 N0M0).

After surgery the ultrasound showed a solid mass in the right iliac territory suspicious of being a metastasis versus lymphocele.

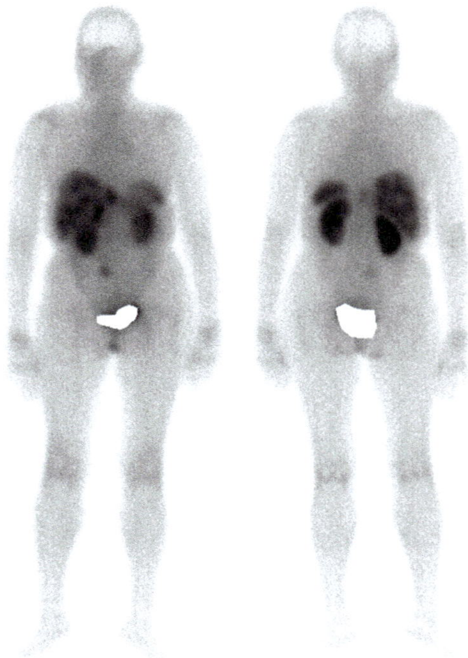

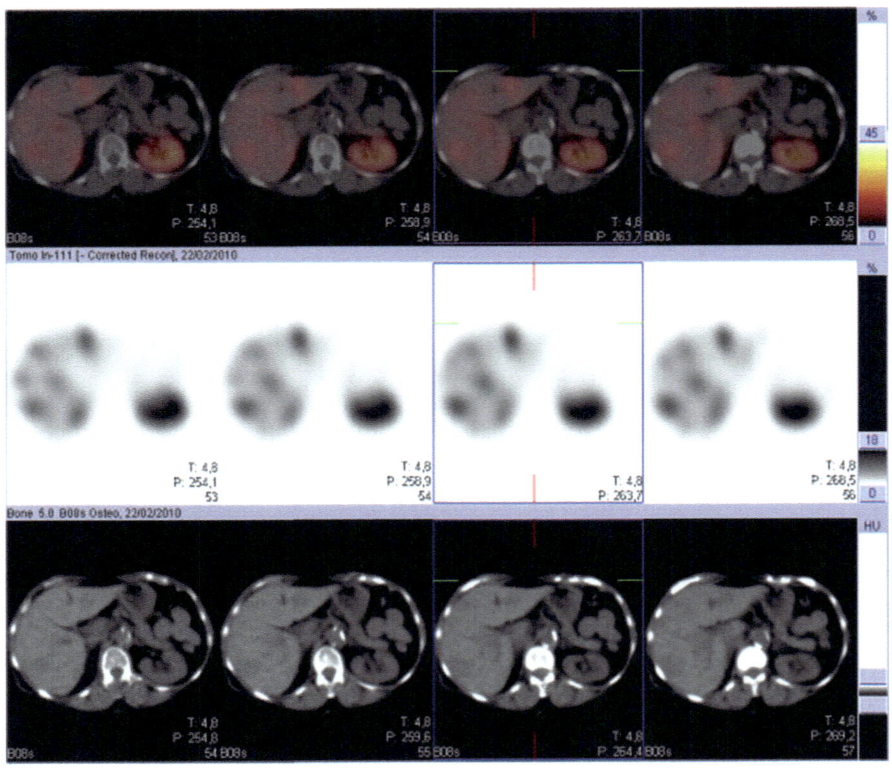

A patient diagnosed of an advanced carcinoid tumor with liver metastases of unknown origin determined by conventional diagnostic techniques.

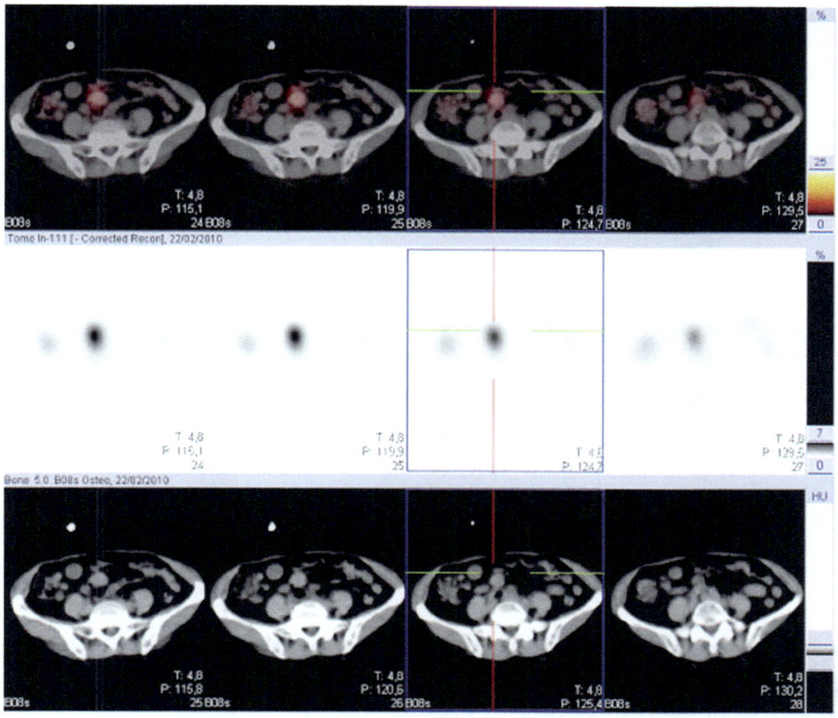

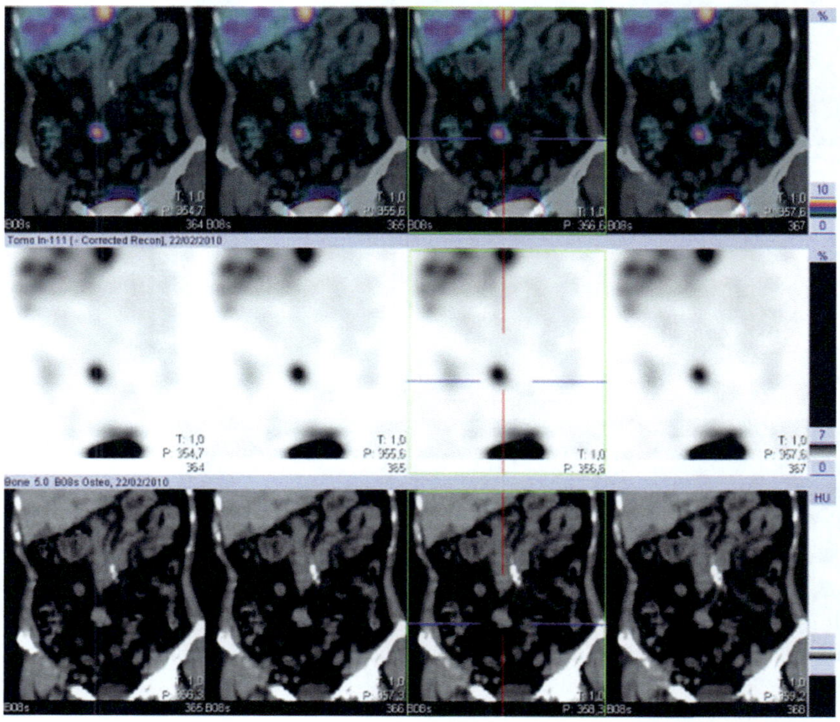

^{111}In octreotide findings

Total body planar images and abdominal SPECT-CT obtained 24 h after the intravenous administration of 222 MBq of ^{111}In octreotide show multiple hepatic lesions and a central abdominal lesion corresponding to adenopathy or implant (25 × 19 mm) close to the right common iliac territory.

Teaching point

The detection and staging of a carcinoid tumor and hepatic metastases are indications for using ^{111}In octreotide scintigraphy. This technique allows the correct classification of abdominal lesions and is useful to differentiate between primary and secondary lesions.

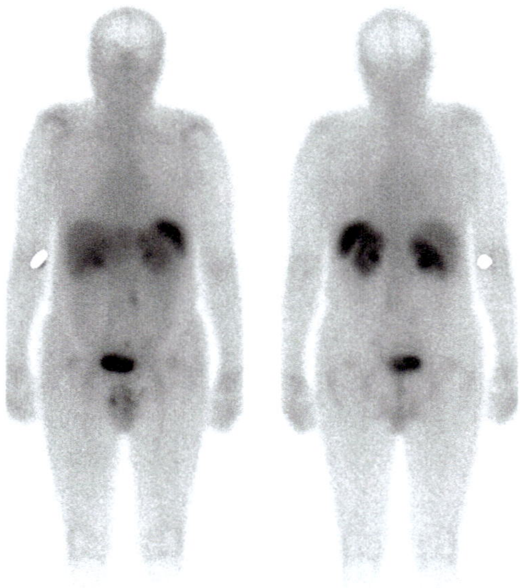

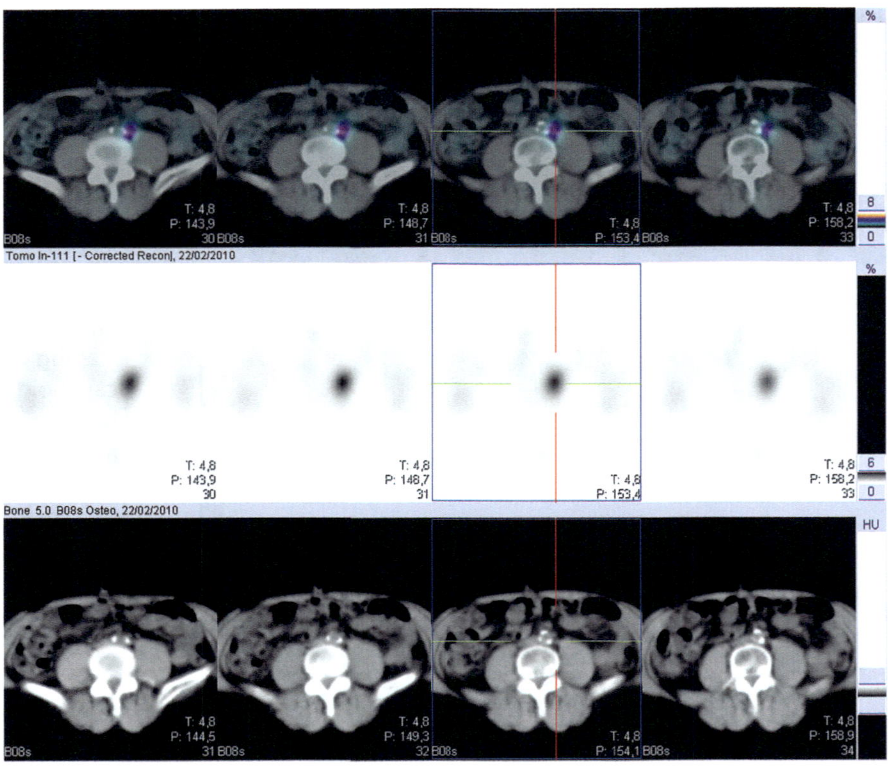

A patient who underwent gastric neuroendocrine tumor resection.

^{111}In octreotide findings

Total body planar images and abdominal SPECT-CT obtained 24 h after the intravenous administration of 222 MBq of ^{111}In octreotide show abdominal uptake. Fusion images show uretheral correspondence, eliminating the diagnosis of lymphadenopathy.

Teaching point

SPECT-CT fusion images are useful in the correct evaluation of small structures close to areas of physiological uptake or elimination.

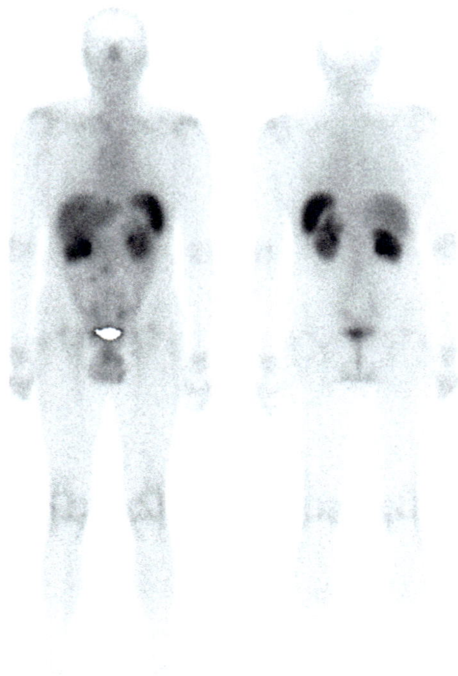

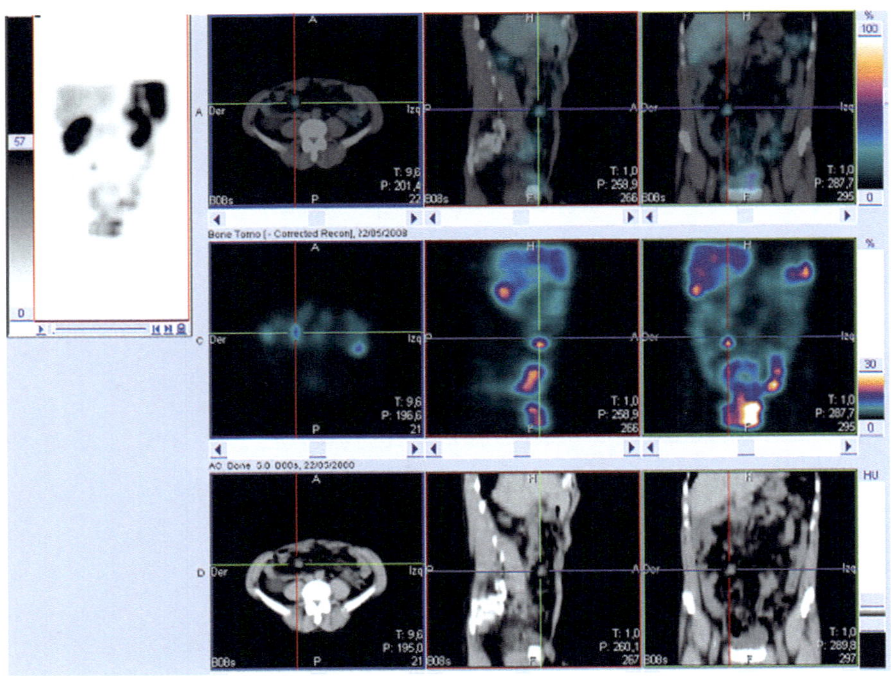

A patient diagnosed and surgically treated (right hemicolectomy) because of a low grade carcinoid tumor with lymph node affection (T3N2M1). The patient was treated with Somatuline® and followed up with octreotide scintigraphy.

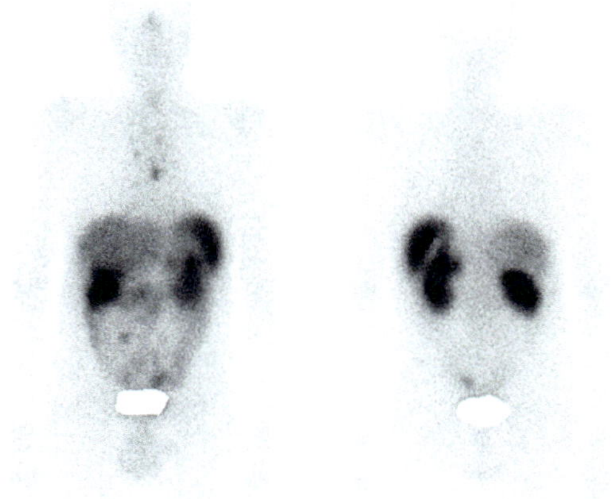

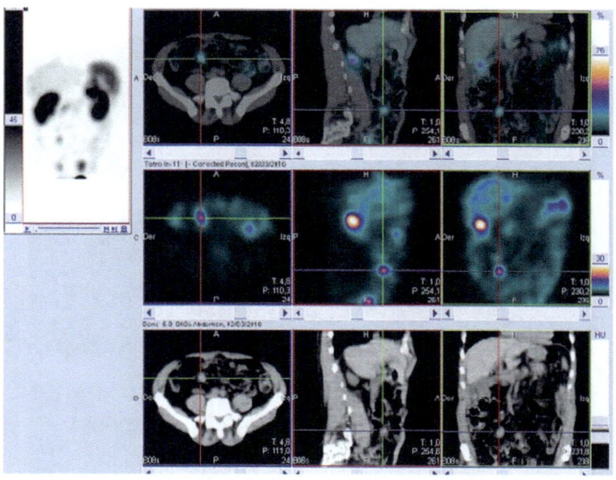

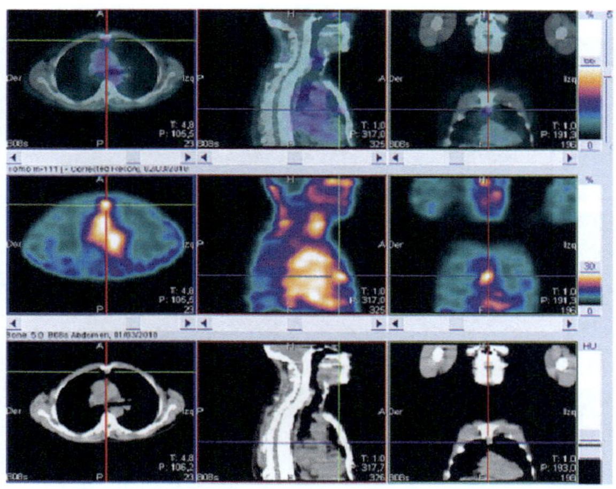

^{111}In octreotide findings

Total body planar images (the ones on page 12 were performed in 2008 and the ones on this page in 2010). Abdominal and thoracic SPECT-CT image corresponding to the last study, obtained 24 h after the intravenous administration of 222 MBq of ^{111}In octreotide, shows multiple lesions in mediastinum and abdomen with mesenteric implants and lymhadenopathies in the right iliac area corresponding to progression of the disease with respect to the previous study.

Blood analysis shows an increase in the levels of chromogranin (from 188 to 215 ng/ml).

Teaching point

The use of SPECT-CT images allows a better evaluation of new lesions in the control of patients with pathological octreotide scans.

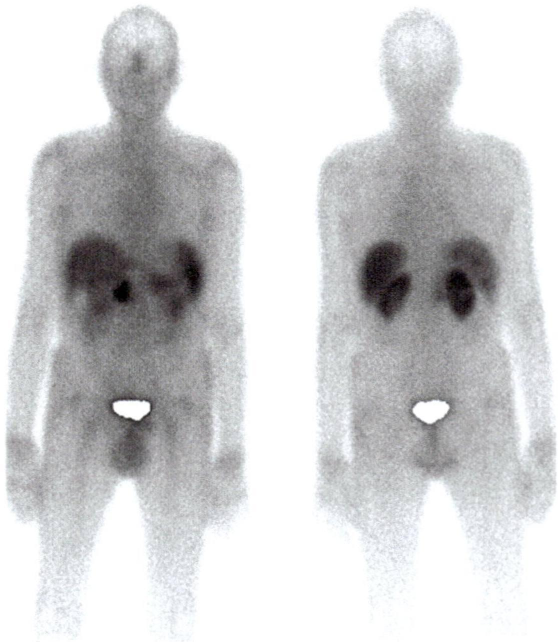

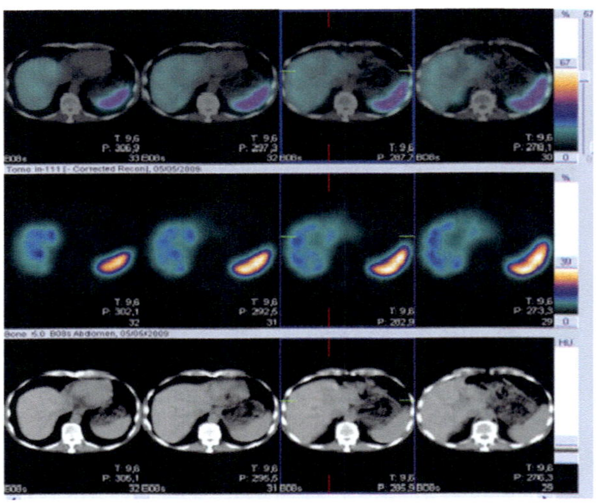

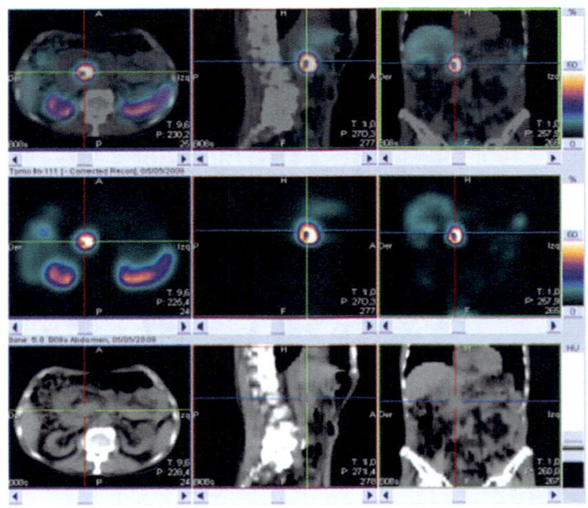

A patient diagnosed with locally advanced neuroendocrine pancreatic tumor with mesenteric vein infiltration and being treated with somatostatine analogs. During the follow-up, the CT image showed hepatic metastasis and persistent increased levels of chromogranin that rose from 230 ng/ml in beginning of 2009 to approximately 900 ng/ml in 2010.

Images show a comparison of the studies performed in 2009 (*page 14*) and 2010 (*page 15*).

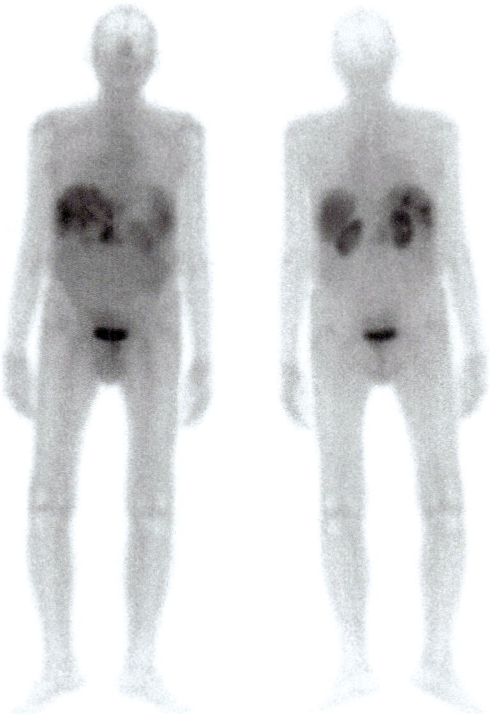

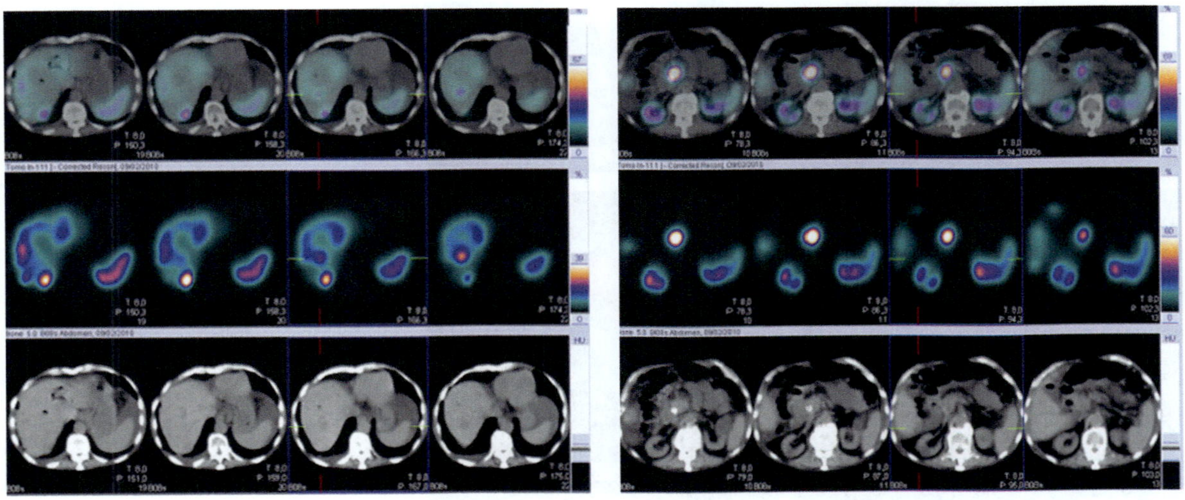

^{111}In octreotide findings

Bottom images: Total body planar images and abdominal SPECT-CT images obtained 24 h after the intravenous administration of 222 MBq of ^{111}In octreotide show new hepatic lesions and persistence of pancreatic disease with respect to the previous study corresponding to progression.

Teaching point

^{111}In octreotide scintigraphy is a useful tool in the follow-up of advanced neuroendocrine tumors and in the evaluation of treatment response.

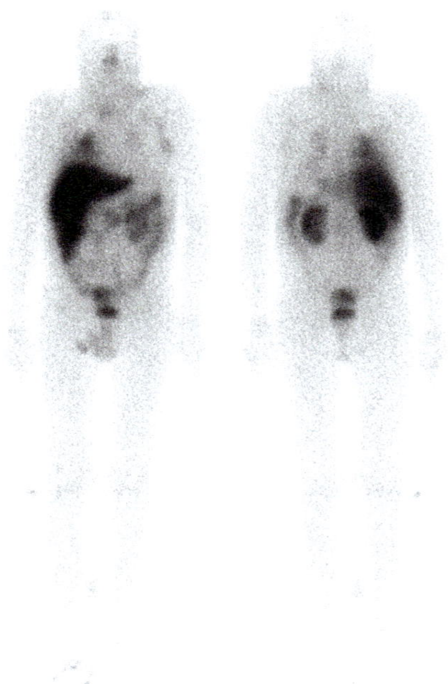

A patient diagnosed with a giant cell neuroendocrine tumor of the lung and with a clinical history of splenectomy because of a traffic accident. He was subject to an extension imaging study to determine the appropriate treatment.

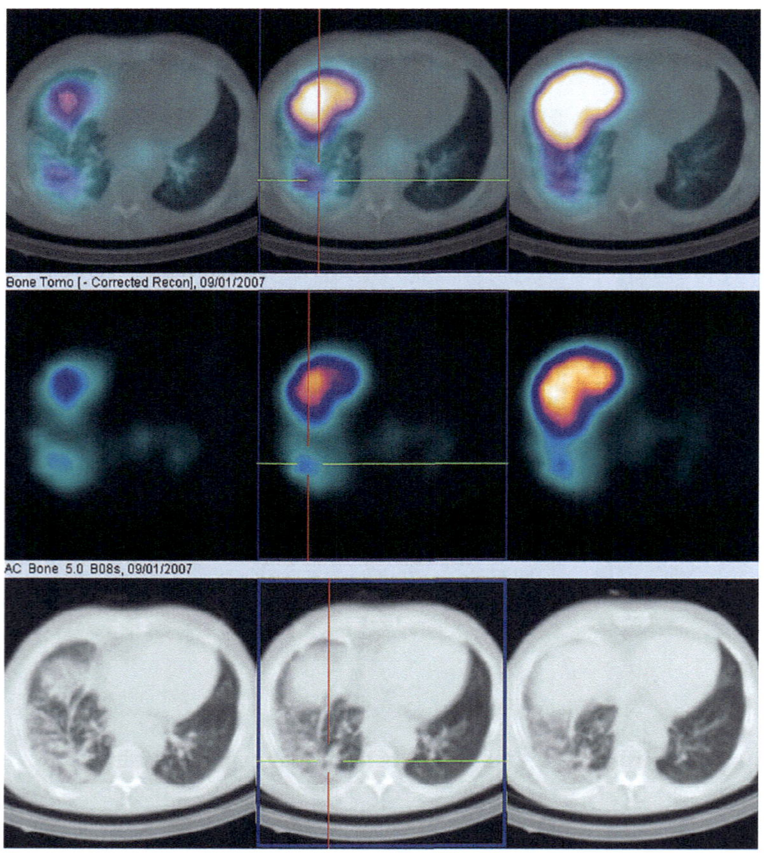

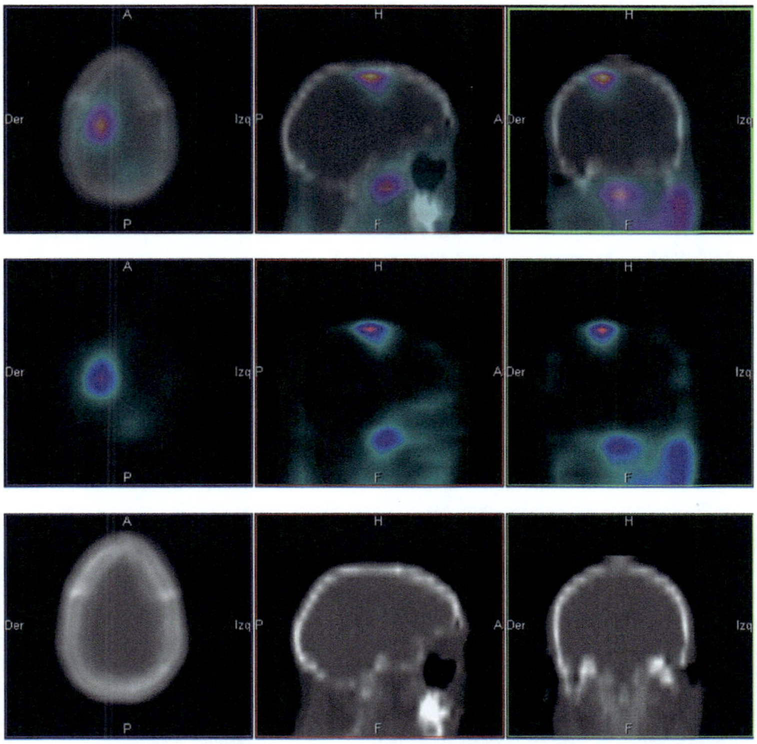

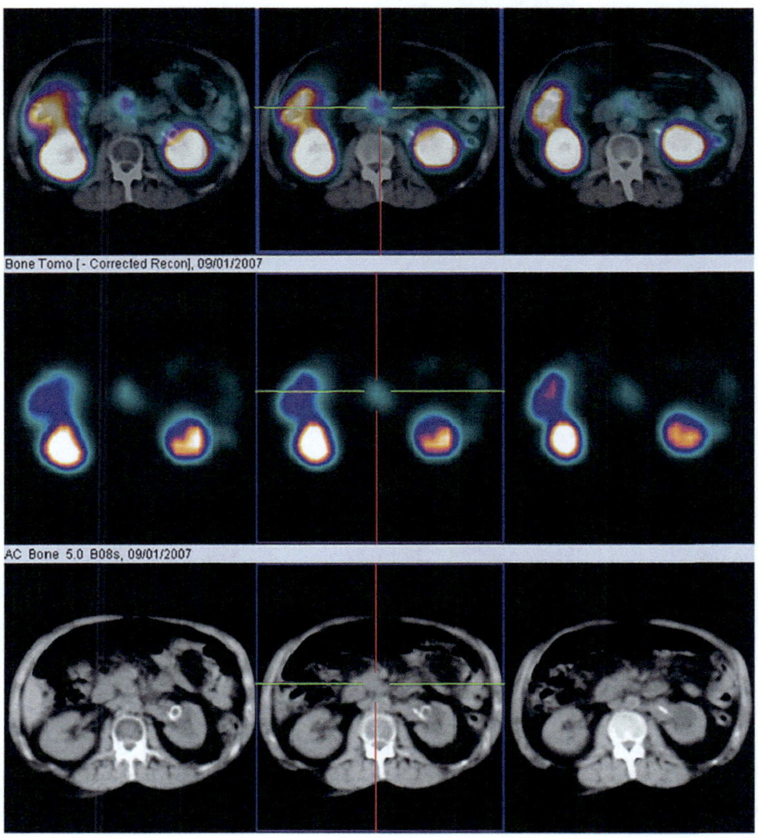

^{111}In octreotide findings

Total body planar images and thoracic, abdominal and head SPECT-CT obtained 24 h after the intravenous administration of 370 MBq of ^{111}In octreotide show increased expression of somatostatin analogs on the base of the right lung according to the primary tumor, in the mesenteric region and also on the right parietal bone, compatible with metastasic dissemination of the tumor.

Teaching point

^{111}In octreotide total body planar exploration determines the correct extension of the disease due to the unsuspected diagnosis of the skull metastases. SPECT/CT establishes the location of the bone involvement and a more accurate evaluation of abdominal lesions.

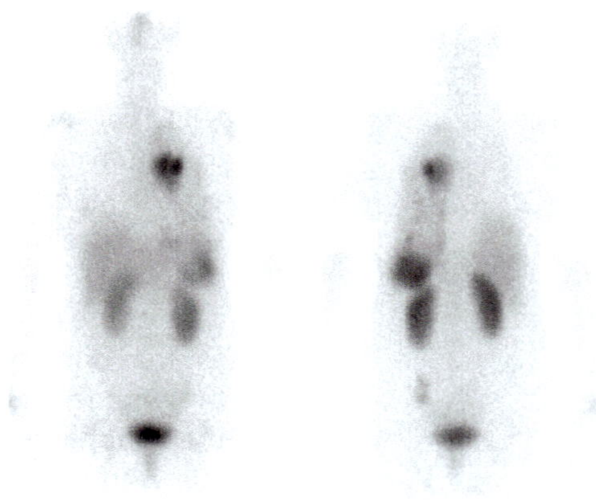

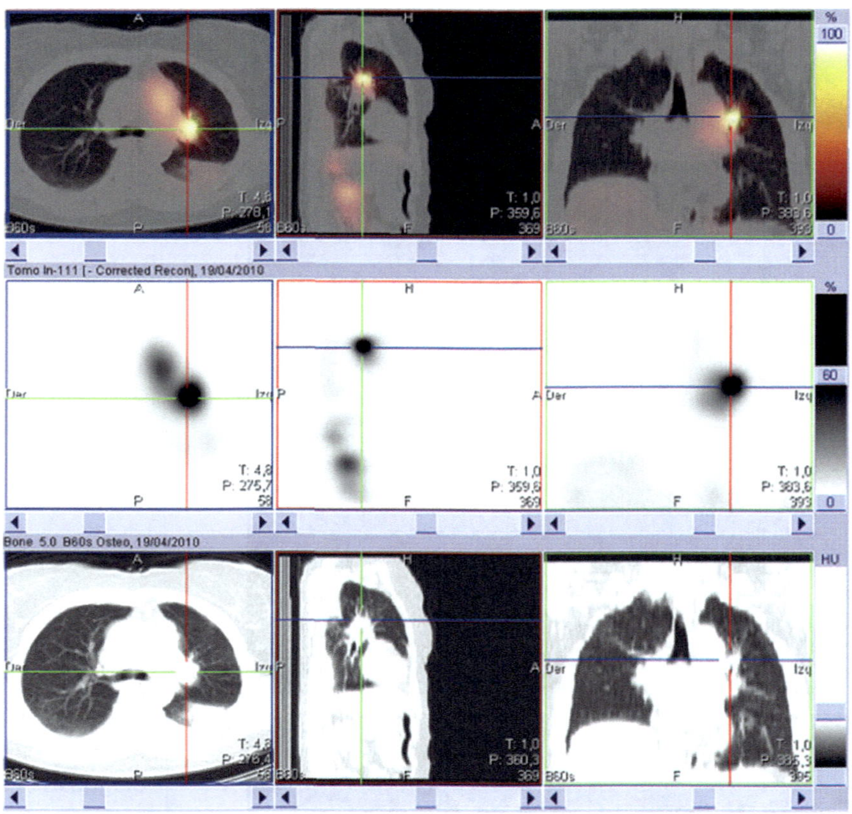

A patient with an 85-mm necrotic tumoral mass in the upper left lobe in contact with the ascending aorta and completely covering the left pulmonary artery. Furthermore, left pleural involvement and a 24-mm left suprarenal nodule are found.

Fine-needle aspiration (FNA) results of the pulmonary lesion are compatible with giant cell neuroendocrine carcinoma.

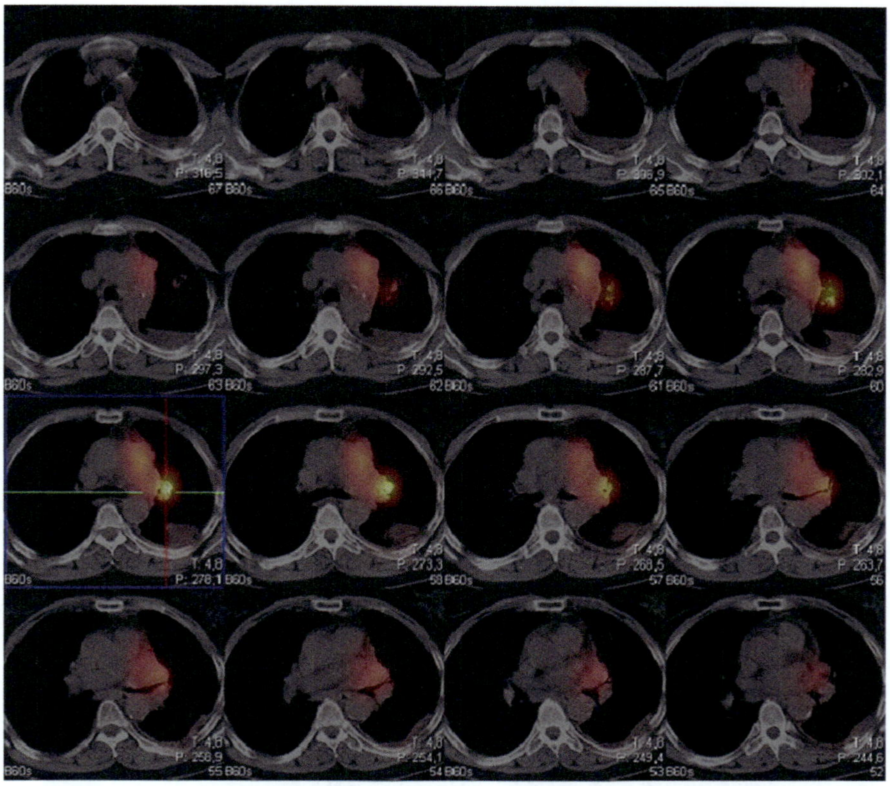

^{111}In octreotide findings

Total body planar images and thoraco-abdominal SPECT-CT obtained 24 h after the intravenous administration of 222 MBq of ^{111}In octreotide show a markedly increased uptake in the left pulmonary mass, with ipsilateral pleural, mediastinic and iliac bone involvement.

Teaching point

The total body scan performed with SRS allows the identification of unsuspected metastatic lesions, while SPECT-CT enables its precise anatomic localization.

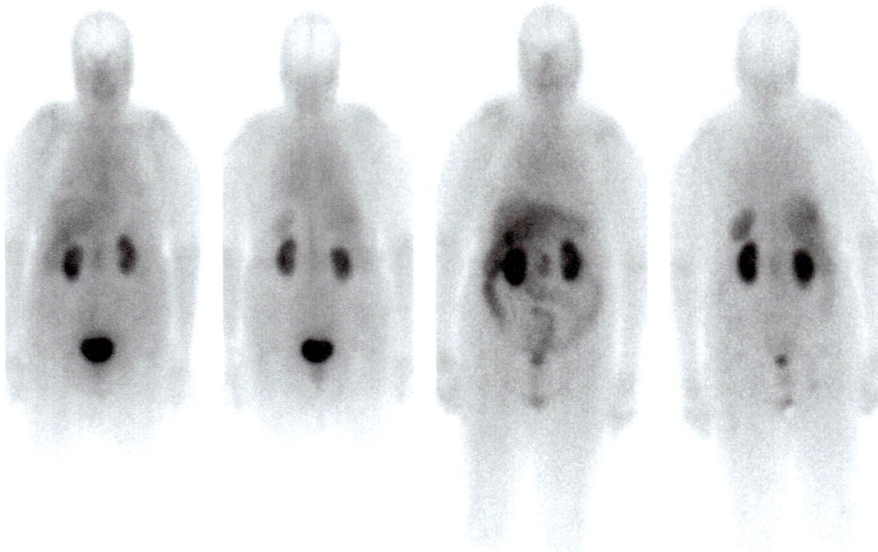

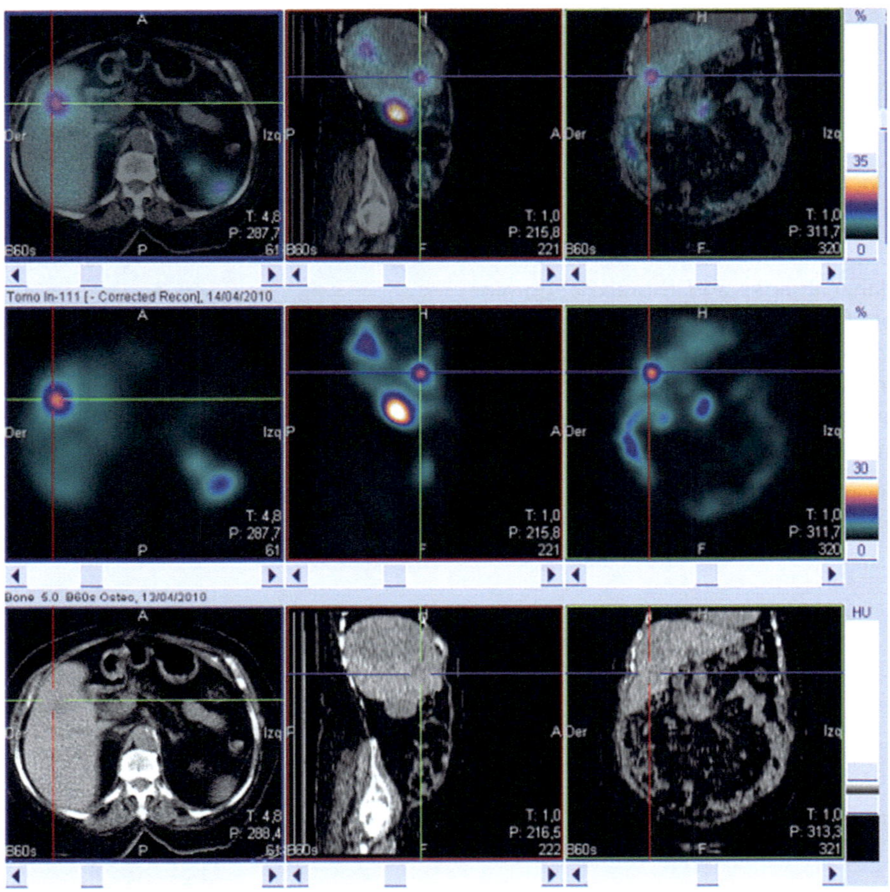

A patient diagnosed with neuroendocrine pancreatic tumor with hepatic metastases (stage IV). The patient is undergoing palliative treatment with lanreotide.

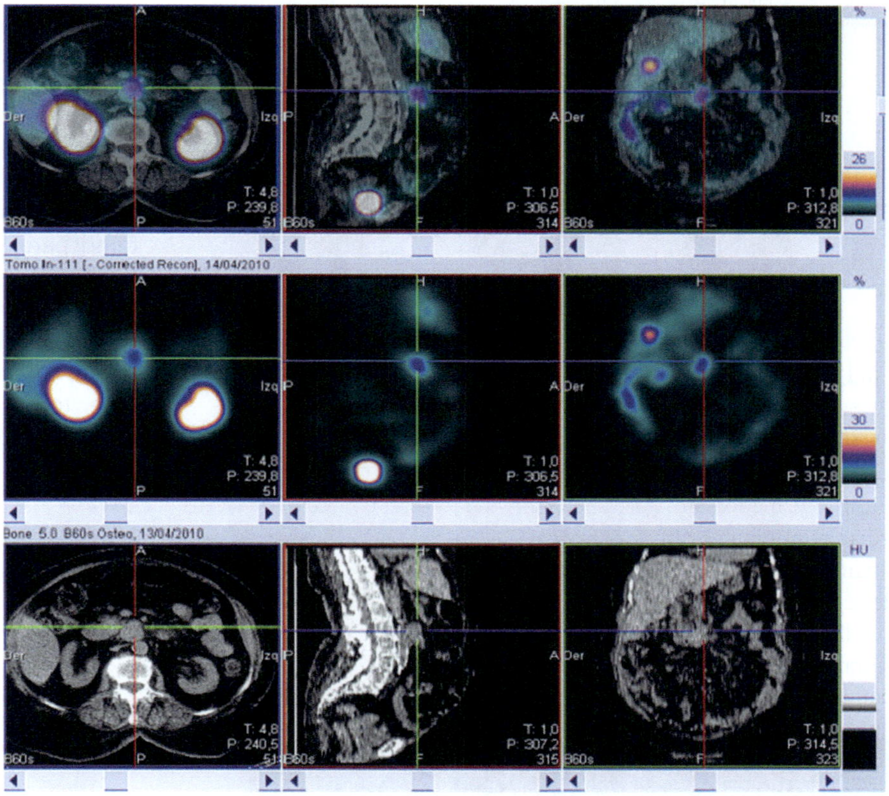

◘ ^{111}In octreotide findings

Total body planar images obtained 4 and 24 h after the intravenous administration of 222 MBq of ^{111}In octreotide and abdominal SPECT-CT performed 24 h after show pathological lesions with expression of somatostatine receptors in the liver (segments VI and VIII) and in a retropancreatic adenopathy.

Teaching point

^{111}In octreotide SPECT-CT is especially useful in the differential diagnosis between lymph node and organ involvement in the upper abdomen, as well as in the correct localization of liver lesions. Its use is not significantly affected by the simultaneous use of lanreotide, which may cause some degree of competition for the same receptors.

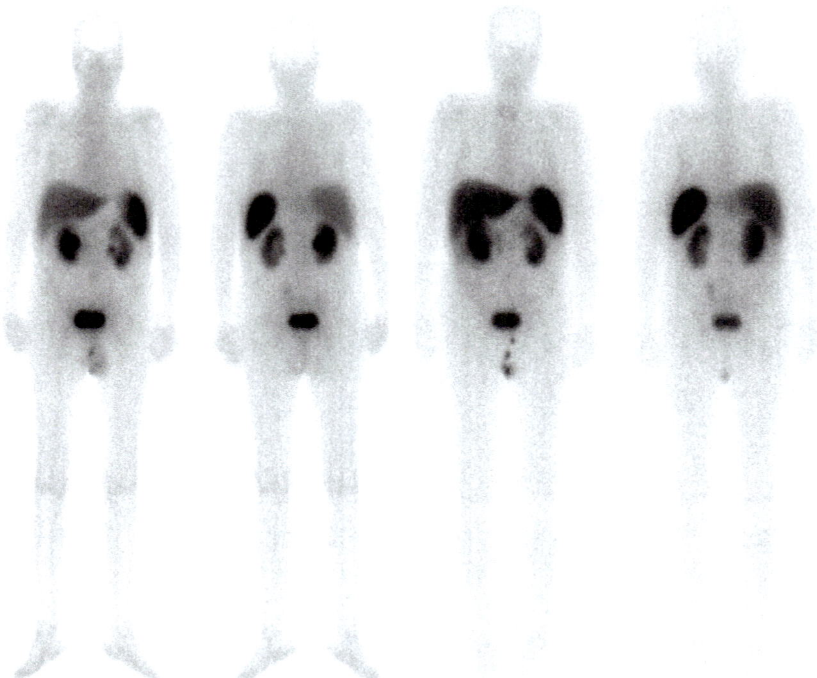

A patient with empiric diagnosis of prostate cancer (stage IV), blastic bone metastases in bone scintigraphy and elevated PSA. During the follow-up, the patient suffered paroxystical symptoms of perspiration and facial flushing. Analytical hydroxyindoleacetic acid (HIAA) in the 24-h urine rose to 11.5 mg/24 h (normal up to 8.2).

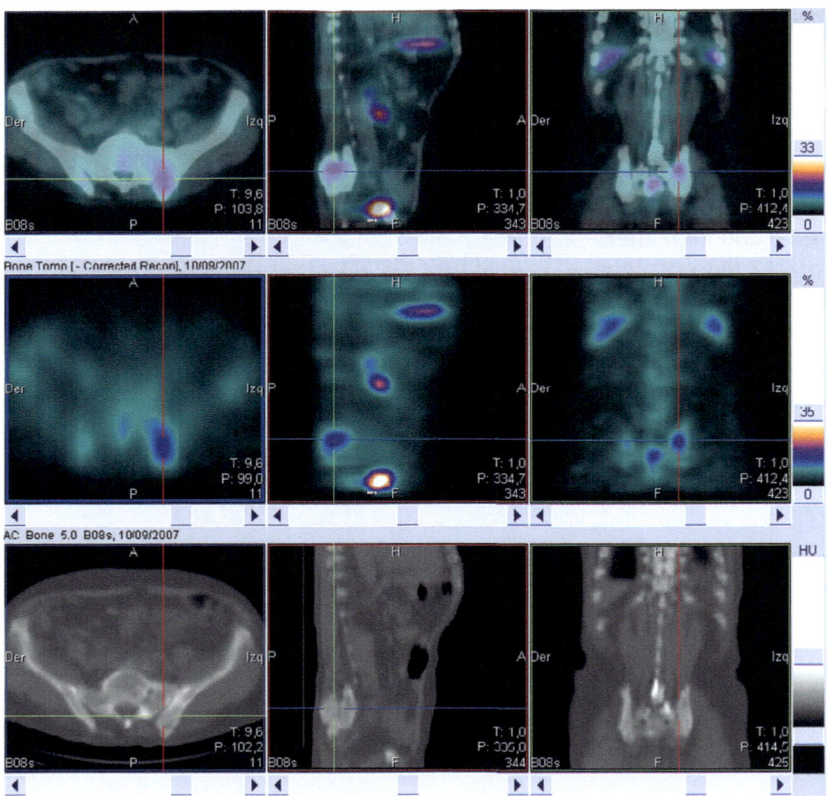

^{111}In octreotide findings

Total body planar images obtained 4 and 24 h after the intravenous administration of 222 MBq of ^{111}In octreotide and abdominal SPECT-CT performed at 24 h show a pathological increase in uptake in the left sacroiliac joint, in relation to bone metastases of prostate cancer detected in the previous bone scintigraphy.

Teaching point

Many others tumors, besides NETs, express SR. Their metastases can be detected in an ^{111}In octreotide scintigraphy. SPECT-CT is useful in the correct localization of these lesions.

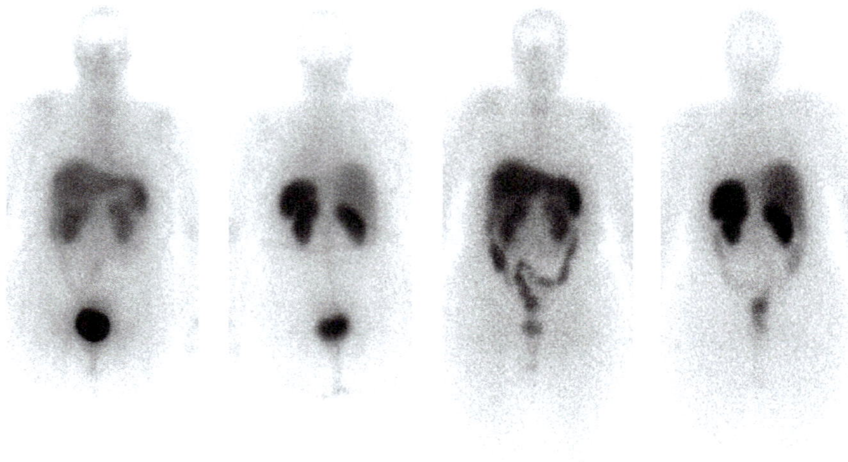

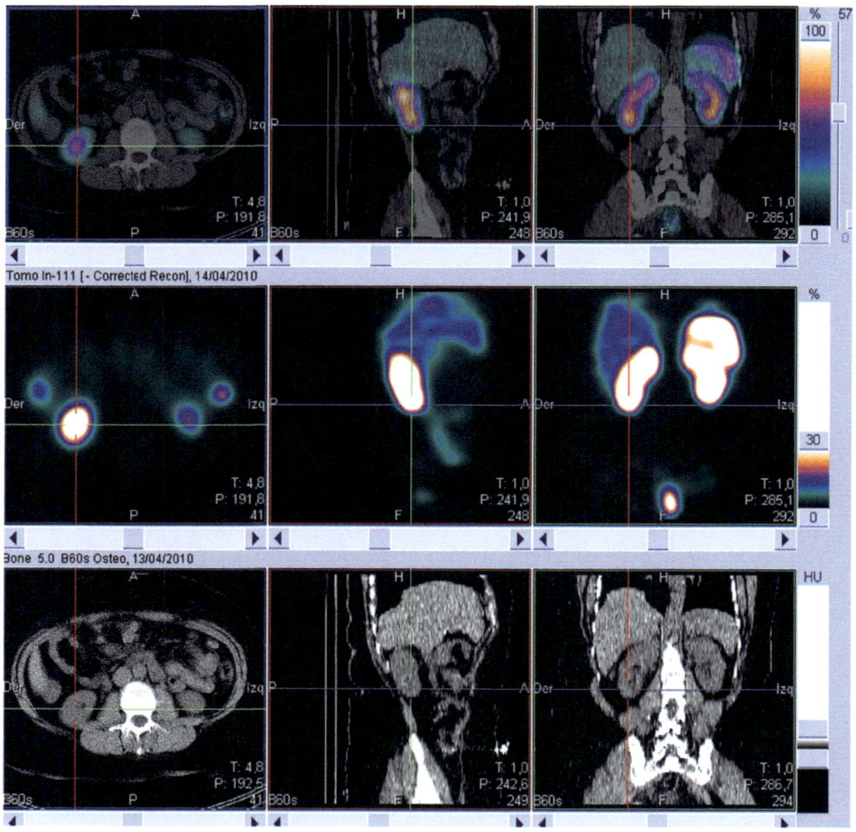

A patient studied because of cutaneous lesions (telangiectasias) in the neck and thorax, also presenting other signs and symptoms such as diarrhea and facial and neck flushing.

Mastocitosis was discarded as a diagnosis by skin biopsy. Blood analysis shows increased levels of urinary serotonin.

^{111}In octreotide findings

Total body planar images obtained 4 and 24 h after the intravenous administration of 222 MBq of ^{111}In octreotide and abdominal SPECT-CT performed at 24 h show no evidence of lesions with positive somatostatin receptors.

Teaching point

The high sensitivity of SRS and the increased specificity obtained by SPECT-CT are important tools for the exclusion of NET in cases of suspected disease.

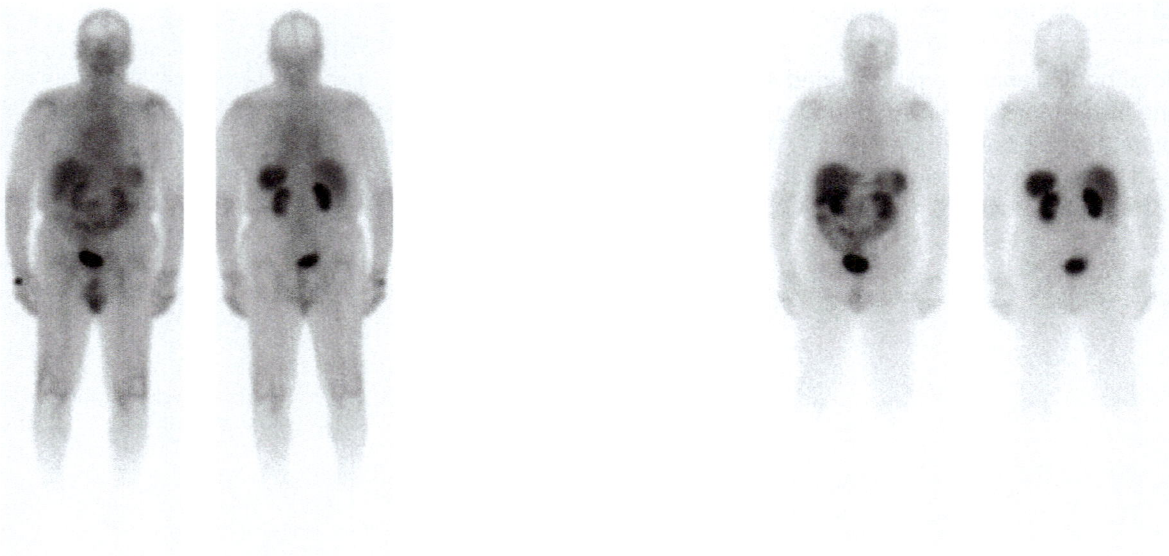

2006

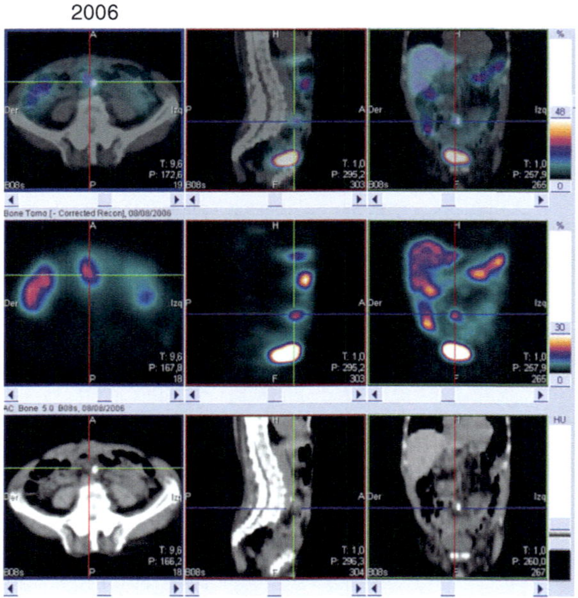

2010

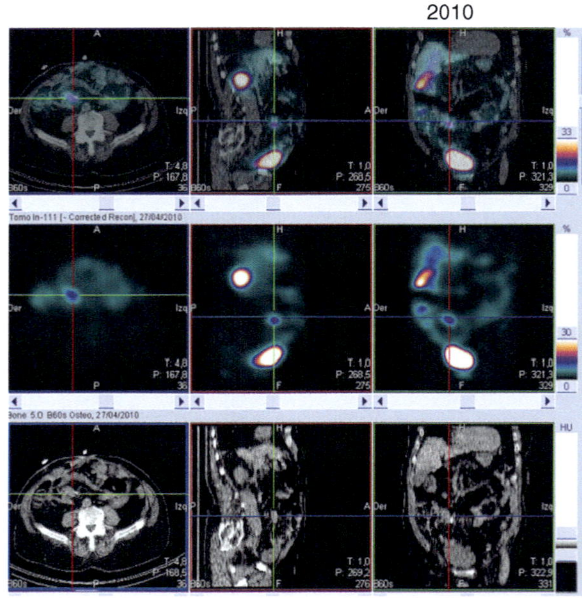

A patient who underwent palliative intestinal bypass surgery because of peritoneal carcinomatosis. Histopathological results show a carcinoid intestinal tumor. The patient is undergoing palliative treatment with lanreotide with suspicion of persistent disease. Blood analysis showed elevated chromogranin levels. Images show a comparison of the studies performed in 2006 (*left*) and 2010 (*right*).

^{111}In octreotide findings

Bottom images: Total body planar images and abdominal SPECT-CT obtained 24 h after the intravenous administration of 222 MBq of ^{111}In octreotide show persistence of mesenteric nodes with somatostatin receptor expression corresponding to stable disease.

Teaching point

The specificity of the ^{111}In octreotide scintigraphy is improved by SPECT-CT imaging, helping to differentiate between physiological and pathological uptake.

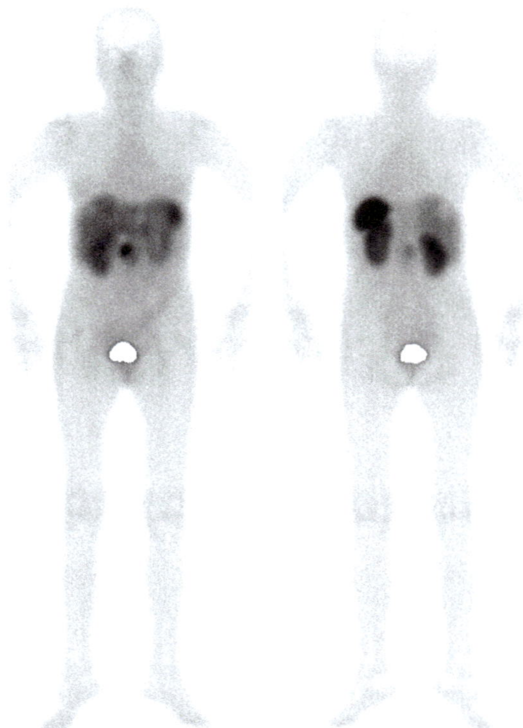

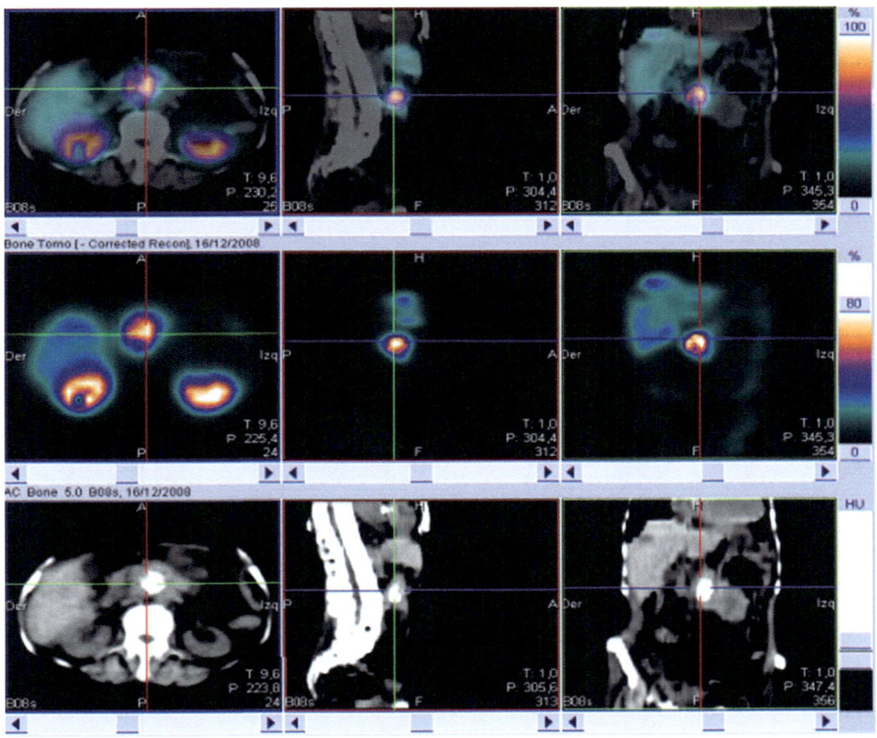

A patient diagnosed with low-grade pancreatic neuroendocrine carcinoma with hepatic metastasis.

The images in this page performed before treatment show increased expression of somatostatin receptors in the pancreatic primary lesion and diffuse liver involvement.

The images on page 29 were captured during lanreotide treatment.

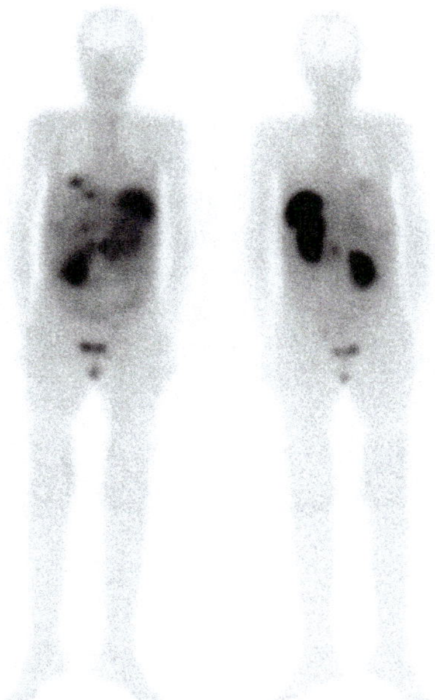

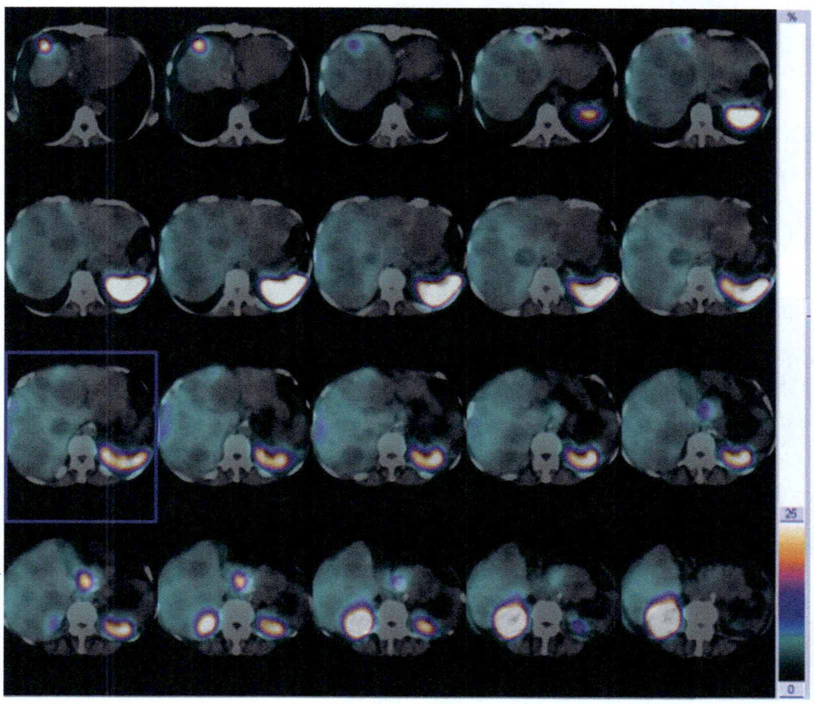

^{111}In octreotide findings

Images in this page Total body planar images and abdominal SPECT-CT obtained 24 h after the intravenous administration of 222 MBq of ^{111}In octreotide show the persistence of lesions with increased somatostatine receptors in the pancreatic area and liver that suggest a lack of treatment response.

Teaching point

^{111}In octreotide scintigraphy and especially SPECT-CT is useful to evaluate treatment response and for the follow-up of advanced disease.

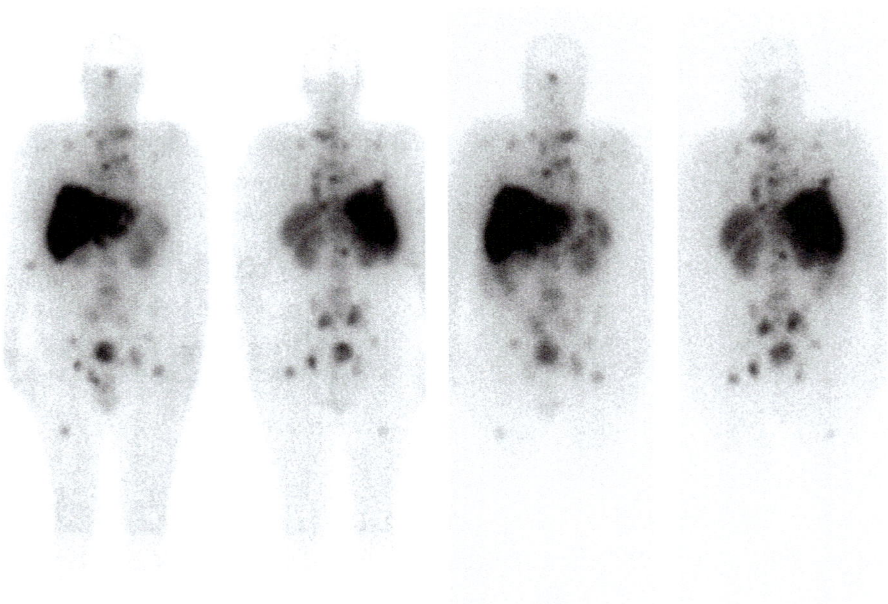

A patient diagnosed with carcinoid tumor with extension to the liver and bone. Previous CT showed diffuse metastatic infiltration of the liver and bone. Pulmonary nodule of unknown origin

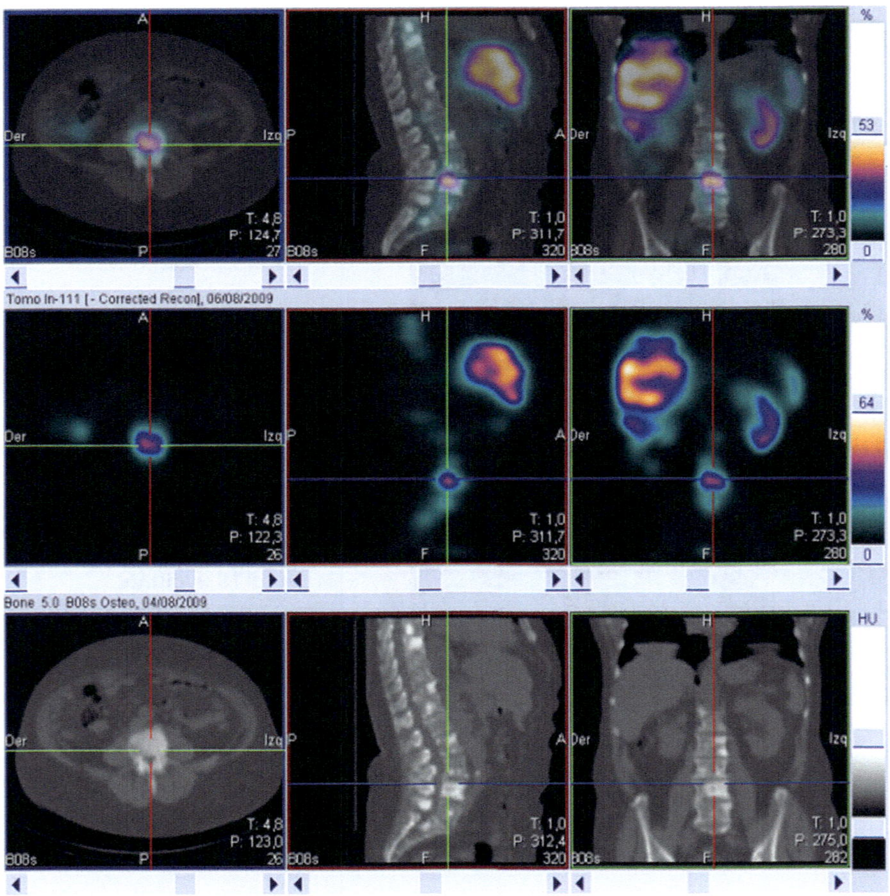

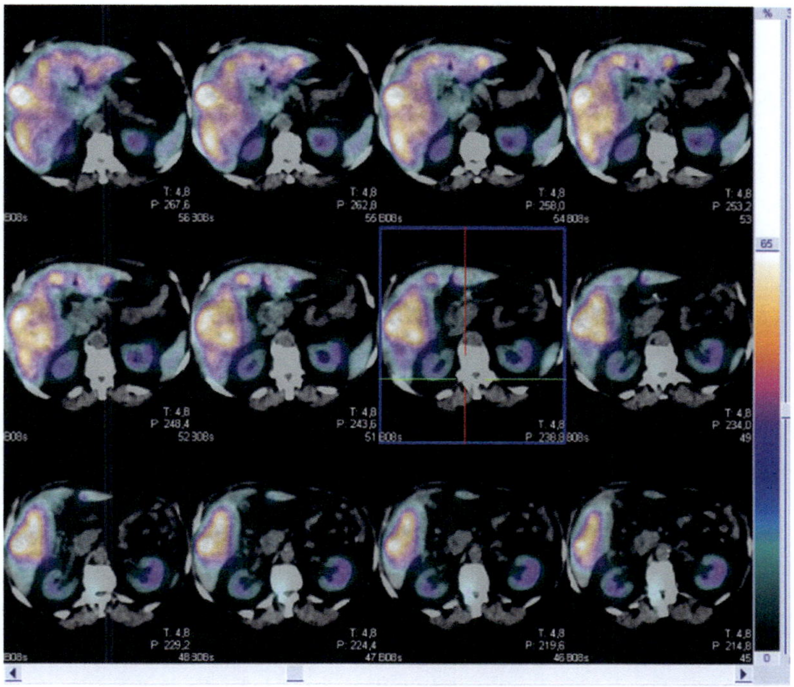

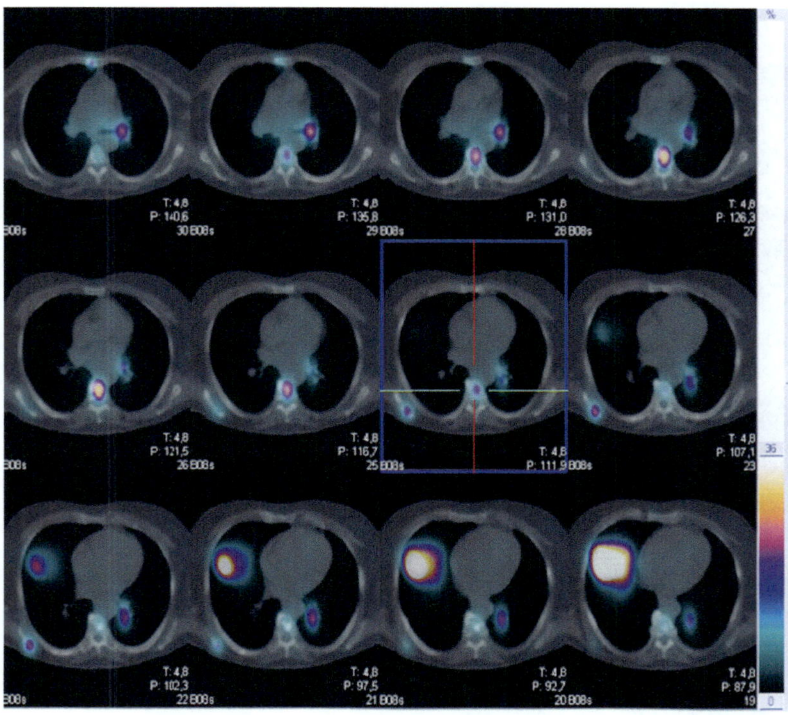

^{111}In octreotide findings

Total body planar images obtained 4 and 24 h after the intravenous administration of 222 MBq of ^{111}In octreotide and abdominal SPECT-CT performed at 24 h show an increased expression of somatostatine receptor in the liver, bone and lungs.

Teaching point

In advanced disease, SPECT-CT is very useful to correctly localize lesions, especially indeterminate lung nodes seen with conventional imaging.

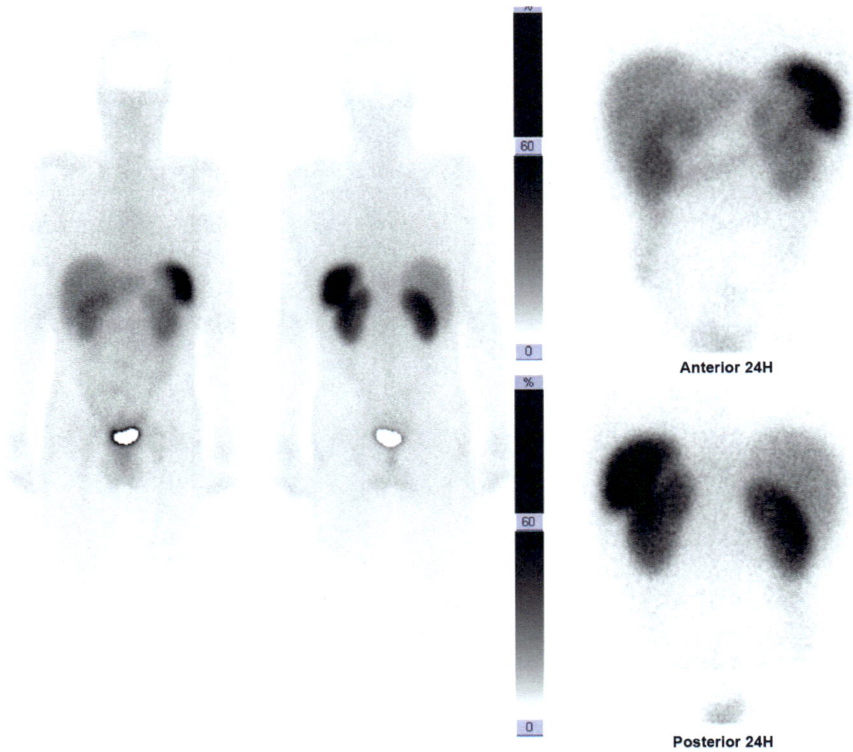

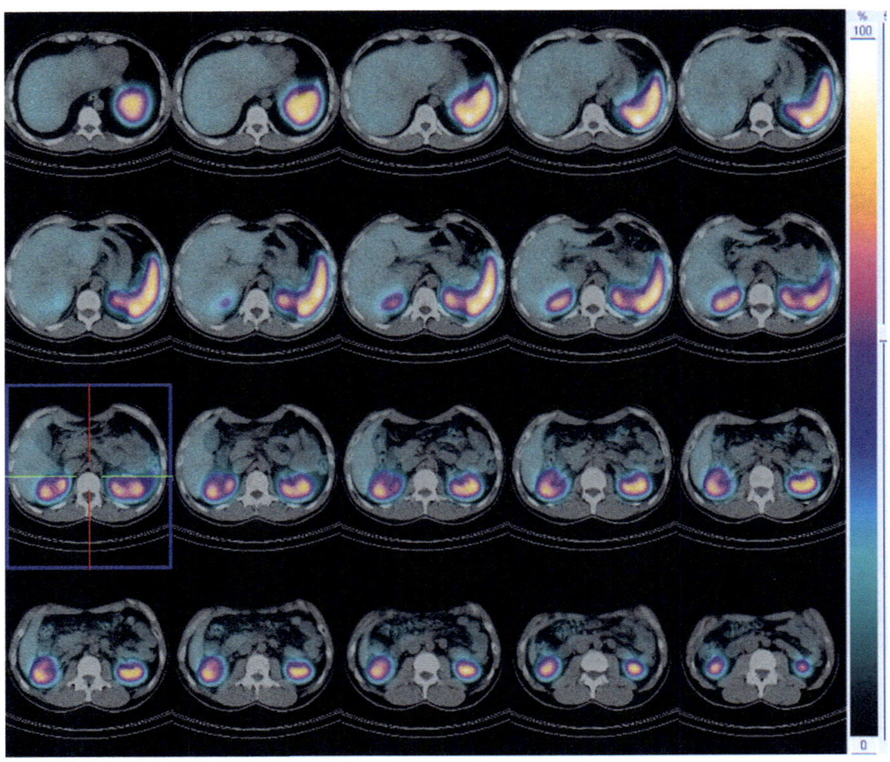

A patient with constantly increased gastrin levels. ^{111}In octreotide scintigraphy was requested to rule out gastrinoma.

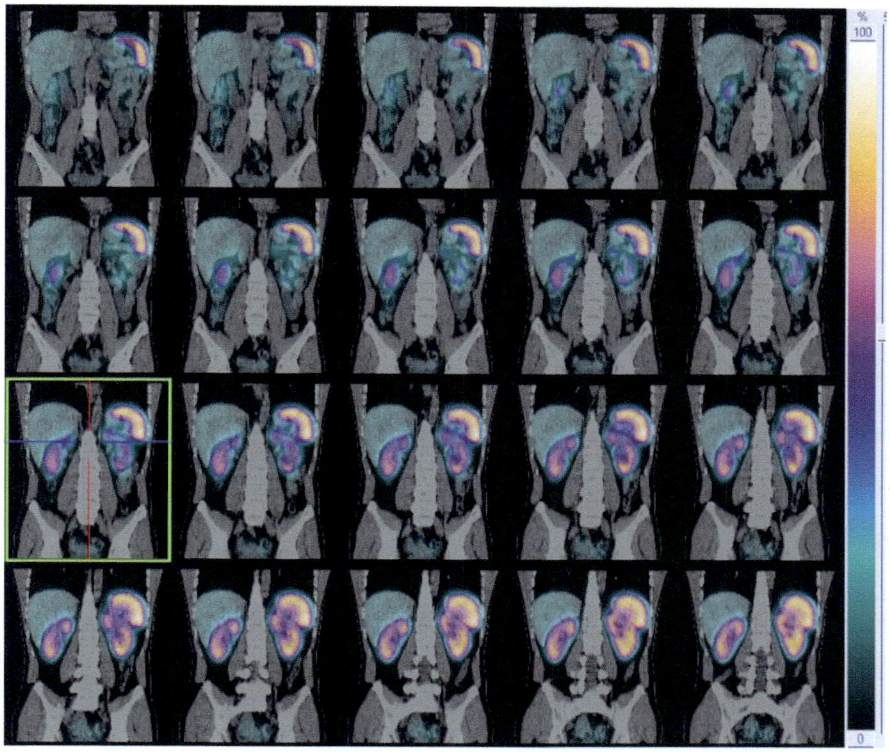

^{111}In octreotide findings

Total body planar images and abdominal SPECT-CT obtained 24 h after the intravenous administration of 222 MBq of ^{111}In octreotide show a normal distribution of the radiotracer without pathological uptakes.

Subsequently, other exams suggested inflammatory bowel disease.

Teaching point

^{111}In octreotide scintigraphy can be used in "selected cases" as screening in suspected neuroendocrine tumor.

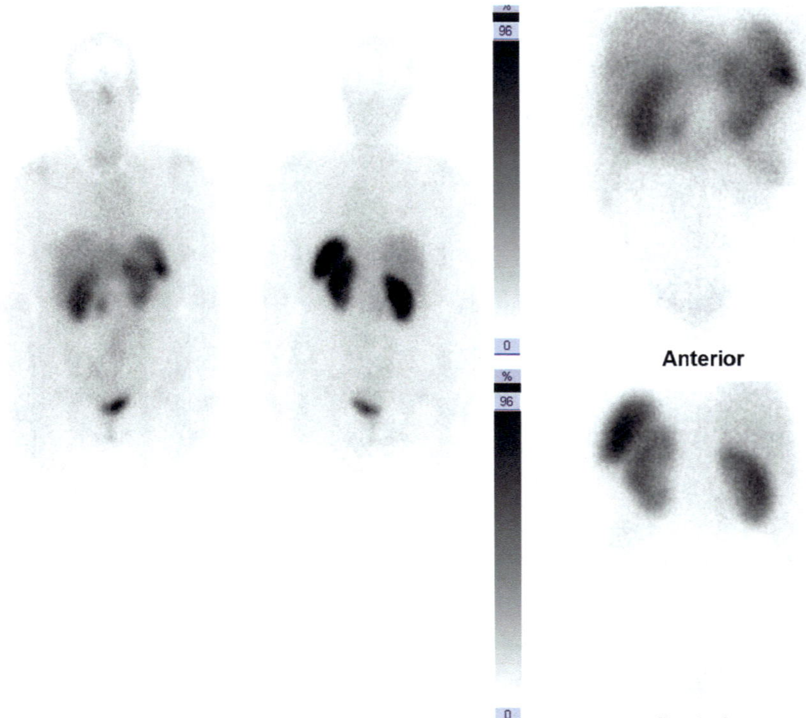

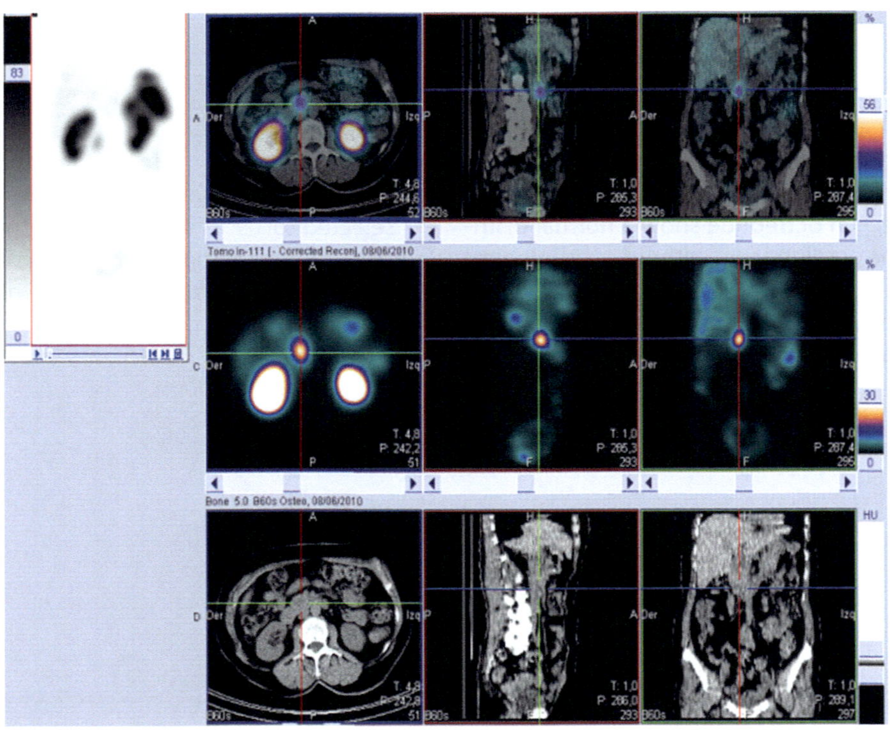

A patient with weight loss and postprandial epigastric pain.

Ultrasound Doppler and CT image shows a 23 × 20-mm solid nodule in the region of the uncinated process of the pancreas

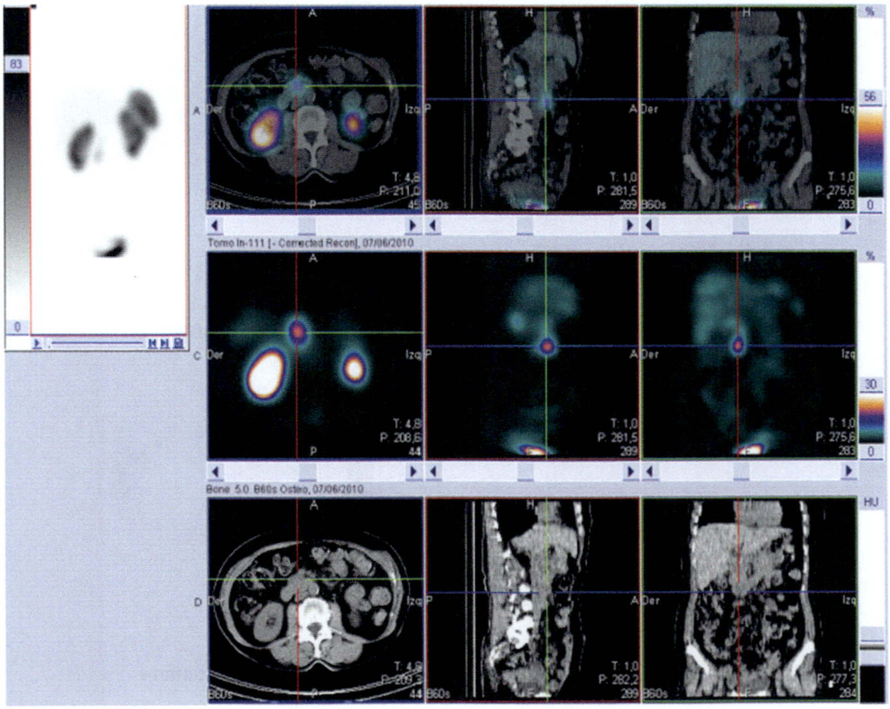

^{111}In octreotide findings

Total body planar images (4 h) and abdominal SPECT-CT obtained 24 h after the intravenous administration of 222 MBq of ^{111}In octreotide show focal uptake in the uncinate process of the pancreas. To date, no histopathological results are available.

Teaching point

SPECT-CT fusion images are useful for the correct localization of pancreatic lesions with somatostatine receptor expression and for differentiating them from, for example, physiological bowel uptake.

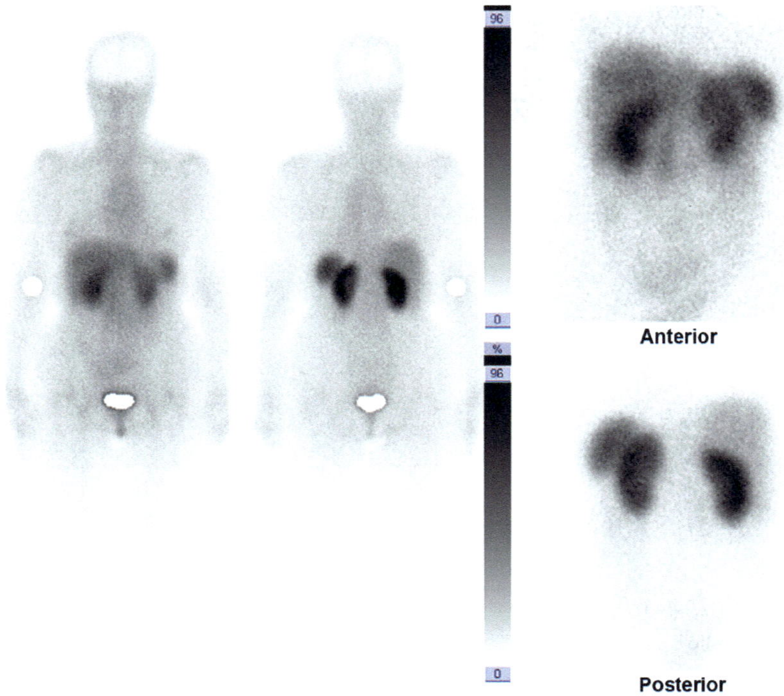

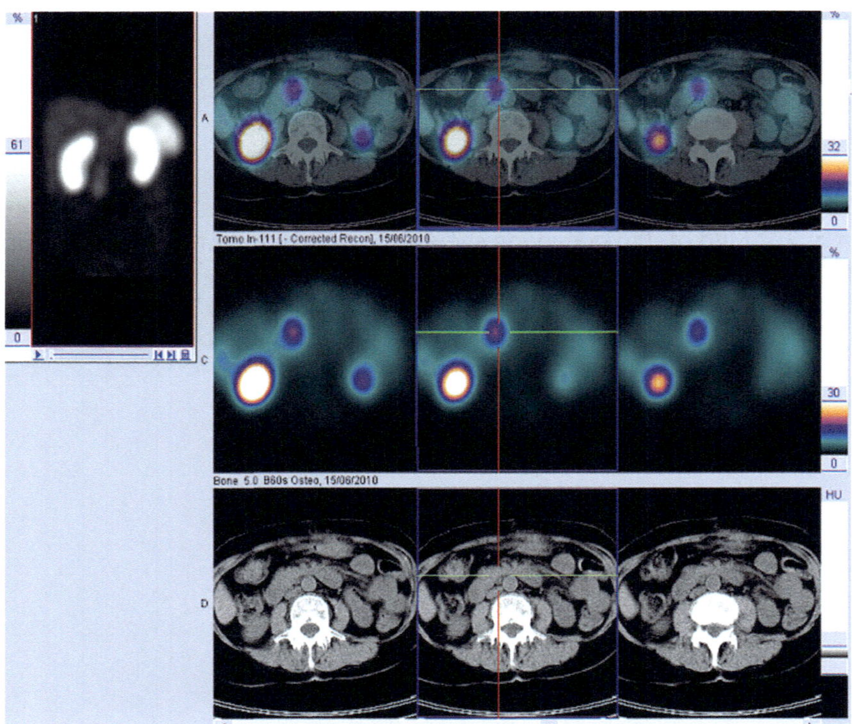

A 64-year-old woman surgically treated for an abdominal (jejunum) tumor with increased expression of somatostatine receptors. A post-surgical histopathological exam showed a well-differentiated (low-grade) endocrine carcinoma with extension to the lymphatic and vascular region (pT3N1Mx). In a control CT no pathological findings were visualized.

^{111}In octreotide findings

Total body planar images obtained 4 h after the intravenous administration of 222 MBq of ^{111}In octreotide with abdominal planar image and SPECT-CT at 24 h show increased expression of somatostatine receptors in the upper abdomen. In the SPECT-CT this finding corresponds to the head of the pancreas versus the jejunum. The final anatomopathological diagnosis was of a well differentiated endocrine carcinoma with infiltration of the jejunum wall and blood vessels. Lymph node metastasis.

Teaching point

The fusion of morphological and functional information improves the yield of each technique when compared with the separate use of both, providing a more complete evaluation and correct localization of the findings.

3.2 MIBG SPECT-CT

Angel Soriano Castrejón (✉), Ana María García Vicente, Prado Talavera Rubio, and John Patrick Pilkington Woll

Today MIBG scintigraphy is considered the best diagnostic technique for evaluation of the disease activity of tumors derived from the sympathetic nervous system, such as neuroblastomas, pheochromocytomas, ganglioneuroblastomas and paragangliomas [31]. These tumors originate from the adrenal gland and sympathetic ganglions anywhere from the neck to the pelvis. In the case of malignant tumors, metastases can be found in soft tissue, bone and bone marrow. Because of their neuroendocrine origin, these tumors are able to take up catecholamines and related substances. The diagnosis of these tumors is established biochemically by measuring the level of urinary and plasma catecholamines and their metabolites.

Neuroblastoma and pheochromocytoma are the two most common tumors of the adrenal medulla and the sympathetic and parasympathetic systems. Neuroblastoma is one of the most common childhood solid tumors. Up to 55% of neuroblastomas appear in the abdominal cavity; about 33% arise in the adrenal medulla, and the rest occur anywhere along the sympathetic chain, most often in the paravertebral region of the posterior mediastinum and the neck. Pheochromocytoma is an uncommon neoplasm that most often occurs in adults and rarely in children. About 85% of pheochromocytomas arise in the medulla of the adrenal glands; the rest come from any of the extraadrenal paraganglia, more often below the diaphragm. About 10% of intraadrenal pheochromocytomas are malignant. The risk of malignant development is higher in the extraadrenal tumors (20–40%).

Meta-iodobenzylguanidine (MIBG) is a structural and functional analog of norepinephrine and guanethidine that selectively accumulates in the noradrenergic neurosecretory granules of cytoplasmic vesicles found in the cells of organs with rich adrenergic innervation, such as the heart, salivary glands, spleen, adrenal medulla and tumors of medullary origin [32]. Uptake is proportional to granule density [33]. It can therefore serve as a biomarker that, appropriately labeled, helps in the detection of these tumors and that is also used as a carrier for targeted radionuclide therapy [34].

Iodine-labeled MIBG scintigraphy has good sensitivity for the diagnosis of neuroblastoma and pheochromocytoma, between 80% and 100%, and high specificity close to 100% for both [32, 35–37]. The uptake of radioiodinated MIBG in other neural crest cell-derived tumors, such as medullary thyroid carcinoma and carcinoid tumors, is more limited, resulting in lower sensitivity when used for these tumors. ^{131}I MIBG is a more stable and readily available isotope than ^{123}I, and has been widely used for the localization of neural crest tumors and the treatment of metastatic disease; however, ^{123}I is the preferred isotope for imaging because it is a pure gamma-emitter with a shorter half-life and greater avidity to neural crest tumors and, therefore, can be used at a higher dosage resulting in greater sensitivity and specificity for the detection of neural crest tumors [38, 39].

CT and MRI are the morphological imaging modalities of choice in localizing these tumors [40]. These techniques provide excellent anatomical details, but although their sensitivity is very high, both are lacking in specificity as difficulties may occur in distinguishing between tumors deriving from the sympathetic nervous system and other tumor entities [35, 41, 42]. Therefore, morphological imaging depicts only morphological abnormalities and cannot functionally characterize adrenal or extraadrenal masses.

The major advantages of radionuclide imaging are high sensitivity, very high specificity and the routinely performed whole-body scanning. Furthermore, in follow-up examinations, functional imaging is not affected by postoperative artifacts, such as scar tissue or metallic clips, and is extremely helpful in the detection of extra-adrenal tumor sites [35].

Widely applied whole-body ^{123}I-MIBG scintigraphy localizes neuroblastoma and pheochromocytoma with a high sensitivity. However, ^{123}I-MIBG scintigraphy comes with some disadvantages, such as limited spatial resolution; limited sensitivity in small lesions; the need for 2 or—in the case of SPECT—even more acquisition sessions with the consequent delay between the start of the examination and result; and the relatively high radiation exposure.

Today, MIBG scintigraphy is indeed considered the best diagnostic technique for evaluation of disease activity, both at presentation and at follow-up. In 5–7% of cases, however, MIBG scintigraphy is negative at presentation (there is no MIBG uptake by tumor cells) [43]. In such cases, PET using ^{18}F-FDG, ^{18}F-DOPA (dihydroxyphenylalanine) or ^{68}Ga-DOTATOC (DOTA-D-Phe[1]-Tyr[3]-octreotide) may be indicated [44, 45].

It has been established that MIBG rarely provides additional diagnostic information for patients who have a clear biochemical diagnosis of pheochromocytoma and a solitary tumor identified on cross-sectional imaging [46–50].

Therefore, it has been suggested that MIBG should be used selectively for patients with a high risk of recurrent, multifocal or malignant disease and for patients with a positive biochemical diagnosis who fail to demonstrate a lesion on CT or magnetic resonance imaging (MRI). However, few studies have investigated the use of MIBG SPECT or MIBG SPECT/CT as an imaging tool for pheochromocytoma, particularly in these situations [31, 51].

The diagnosis of the clinically occult pheochromocytoma remains a particular challenge to the clinician. Factors that may hinder diagnosis of the clinically occult or recurrent pheochromocytoma include non-functioning pheochromocytoma, the size and location of the tumor, the presence of multiple or metastatic lesions, recurrence at a site with distorted tissue planes or scarring from previous surgery, and the presence of an adrenal incidentaloma or other unrelated intra-abdominal lesions.

With the development of new tissue-specific radiopharmaceuticals, such as 11C-epinephrine, ^{11}C-hydroxyepinephrine,^{18}F-fluorodopamineand^{18}F-fluorodihydroxyp henylalanine, fusion PET/CT may become the new "gold standard" for pheochromocytoma imaging in the future [52, 53]. However, because of the current cost, limited availability and short half-life of many of the radioisotopes used, access to fusion PET/CT for most centers with these radiotracers will be limited. Therefore, radioiodinated MIBG remains the recommended initial agent of choice for the localization of pheochromocytoma [54].

In relation to the differences between planar and SPECT imaging in a multicenter prospective trial including 150 patients, SPECT had only a small effect on reader performance, producing a slight increase in sensitivity (82–86%) and a small drop in specificity (82–75%). Although SPECT increased reader confidence, this imaging only changed the consensus interpretation for ten patients (7%) [49].

With respect to SPECT/CT in cases of equivocal diagnostic CT (mainly distorted anatomy) or of suboptimal localization of MIBG-avid foci, SPECT/CT bridges the gap between MIBG scintigraphy and CT, helping to define the anatomic location of these foci and to characterize the benign or malignant significance of uncertain CT findings. However, some authors describe that low-resolution CT of SPECT/CT does not always allow an optimal interpretation of the CT images and should be supplemented—at least at presentation—by diagnostic contrast enhanced CT, providing superior anatomic resolution [31].

Rozovsky et al. [31] found that fused images enabled differentiation between the tumor's mass and surgically distorted anatomic structure, allowing the accurate anatomic localization of pathological MIBG uptake in the follow-up of patients with neuroblastoma and pheochromocytoma, whereas both contrast-enhanced CT and CT of SPECT/CT alone were equivocal. In their study, MIBG SPECT/CT greatly contributed to the diagnostic accuracy in 53% of all cases and 89% of discordant cases. These results are consistent with other published studies [55, 56].

Other situations in which MIBG SPECT/CT is beneficial is for the confirmation of a small extra-adrenal pheochromocytoma, small metastatic lesions or recurrence at a previous operative site, which may have a non-specific appearance on CT or MRI and are often poorly visible on conventional MIBG imaging [57].

References

31. Rozovsky K, Koplewitz BZ, Krausz Y, Revel-Vilk S, Weintraub M, Chisin R, et al. Added value of SPECT/CT for correlation of MIBG scintigraphy and diagnostic CT in neuroblastoma and pheochromocytoma. AJR. 2008;190: 1085–90.
32. Freitas JE. Adrenal cortical and medullary imaging. Semin Nucl Med. 1995;25:235–50.
33. Bomanji J, Levison DA, Flatman WD, et al. Uptake of iodine-123 MIBG by pheochromocytomas, paragangliomas, and neuroblastomas: a histopathological comparison. J Nucl Med. 1987;28:973–8.
34. Garaventa A, Guerra P, Arrighini A, et al. Treatment of advanced neuroblastoma with I-131 metaiodobenzylguanidine. Cancer 1991;67:992–8.
35. Kushner BH. Neuroblastoma: a disease requiring a multitude of imaging studies. J Nucl Med. 2004;45:1172–88.
36. Merrick MV. Essentials of nuclear medicine. 2nd ed. Berlin: Springer; 1998. p. 171–295.
37. Van Der Horst-Schrivers AN, Jager PL, Boezen HM, Schouten JP, Kema IP, Links TP. Iodine-123 metaiodobenzylguanidine scintigraphy in localizing phaeochromocytomas: experience and meta-analysis. Anticancer Res. 2006;26:1599–604.
38. Nakatani T, Hayama T, Uchida J, et al. Diagnostic localization of extra-adrenal pheochromocytoma: comparison of (123)I-MIBG imaging and (131)I-MIBG imaging. Oncol Rep. 2002;9:1225–7.
39. Anderson GS, Fish S, Nakhoda K, et al. Comparison of I-123 and I-131 for whole-body imaging after stimulation by recombinant human thyrotropin: a preliminary report. Clin Nucl Med. 2003;28:93–6.
40. Pfluger T, Schmied C, Porn U, et al. Integrated imaging using MRI and I-123- metaiodobenzylguanidine scintigraphy to improve sensitivity and specificity in the diagnosis of pediatric neuroblastoma. AJR. 2003;181:1115–24.
41. Lenders JW, Eisenhofer G, Mannelli M, Pacak K. Pheochromocytoma. Lancet. 2005;366:665–75.

42. Ilias I, Pacak K. Current approaches and recommended algorithm for the diagnostic localization of pheochromocytoma. J Clin Endocrinol Metab. 2004;89:479–91.
43. Pirson AS, Krug B, Tuerlinckx D. Additional value of I-123 MIBG SPECT in neuroblastoma. Clin Nucl Med. 2005;30:100–1.
44. Ilias I, Shulkin B, Pacak K. New functional imaging modalities for chromaffin tumors, neuroblastomas and ganglioneuromas. Trends Endocrinol Metab 2005;16:66–72.
45. Scanga DR, Martin WN, Delbeke D. Value of FDG PET imaging in the management of patients with thyroid, neuroendocrine, and neural crest tumors. Clin Nucl Med. 2004;29:86–90.
46. Greenblatt DY, Shenker Y, Chen H. The utility of metaiodobenzylguanidine (MIBG) scintigraphy in patients with pheochromocytoma. Ann Surg Oncol. 2008;15:900–5.
47. Miskulin J, Shulkin BL, Doherty GM, et al. Is preoperative iodine 123 meta-iodobenzylguanidine scintigraphy routinely necessary before initial adrenalectomy for pheochromocytoma? Surgery 2003;134:918–22; discussion 922–3.
48. Bhatia KS, Ismail MM, Sahdev A, et al. 123I-Metaiodobenzylguanidine (MIBG) scintigraphy for the detection of adrenal and extra-adrenal pheochromocytomas: CT and MRI correlation. Clin Endocrinol (Oxf). 2008;69:181–8.
49. Mihai R, Gleeson F, Roskell D, et al. Routine preoperative (123)I-MIBG scintigraphy for patients with pheochromocytoma is not necessary. Langenbecks Arch Surg. 2008;393:725–7.
50. Wiseman GA, Pacak K, O'Dorisio MS, Neumann DR, Waxman AD, Mankoff DA, et al. Usefulness of 123I-MIBG scintigraphy in the evaluation of patients with known or suspected primary or metastatic pheochromocytoma or paraganglioma: results from a prospective multicenter trial. J Nucl Med. 2009;50:1448–54.
51. Strobel K, Burger C, Schneider P, et al. MIBG-SPECT/CT angiography with 3-D reconstruction of an extra-adrenal pheochromocytoma with dissection of an aortic aneurysm. Eur J Nucl Med Mol Imaging. 2007;34:150.
52. Rufini V, Calcagni ML, Baum RP. Imaging of neuroendocrine tumors. Semin Nucl Med. 2006;36:228–47.
53. Ilias I, Pacak K. Anatomical and functional imaging of metastatic pheochromocytoma. Ann N Y Acad Sci. 2004; 1018: 495–504.
54. Gross MD, Gauger PG, Djekidel M, Rubello D. The role of PET in the surgical approach to adrenal disease. Eur J Surg Oncol. 2009;35(11):1137–45.
55. Ozer S, Dobrozemsky G, Kienast O. Value of combined XCT/SPECT technology for avoiding false positive planar (123) I-MIBG scintigraphy. Nuklearmedizin 2004;43:164–7.
56. Schillaci O, Danieli R, Manni C, Simonetti G. Is SPECT/CT with a hybrid camera useful to improve scintigraphic imaging interpretation? Nucl Med Commun. 2004;25:705–10.
57. Meyer-Rochow G-Y, Schembri GP, Benn DE, Sywak MS, Delbridge LW, Robinson BG, et al. The utility of metaiodobenzylguanidine single photon emission computed tomography/computed tomography (MIBG SPECT/CT) for the diagnosis of pheochromocytoma. Ann Surg Oncol. 2010;17:392–400.

Planar 4 hour images

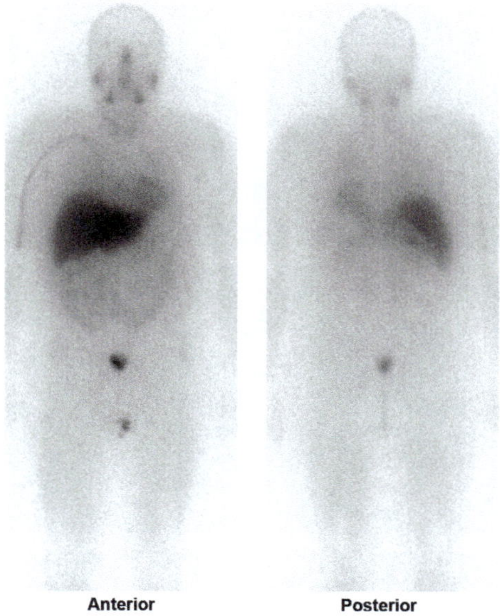

SPECT/ CT 4 hour images

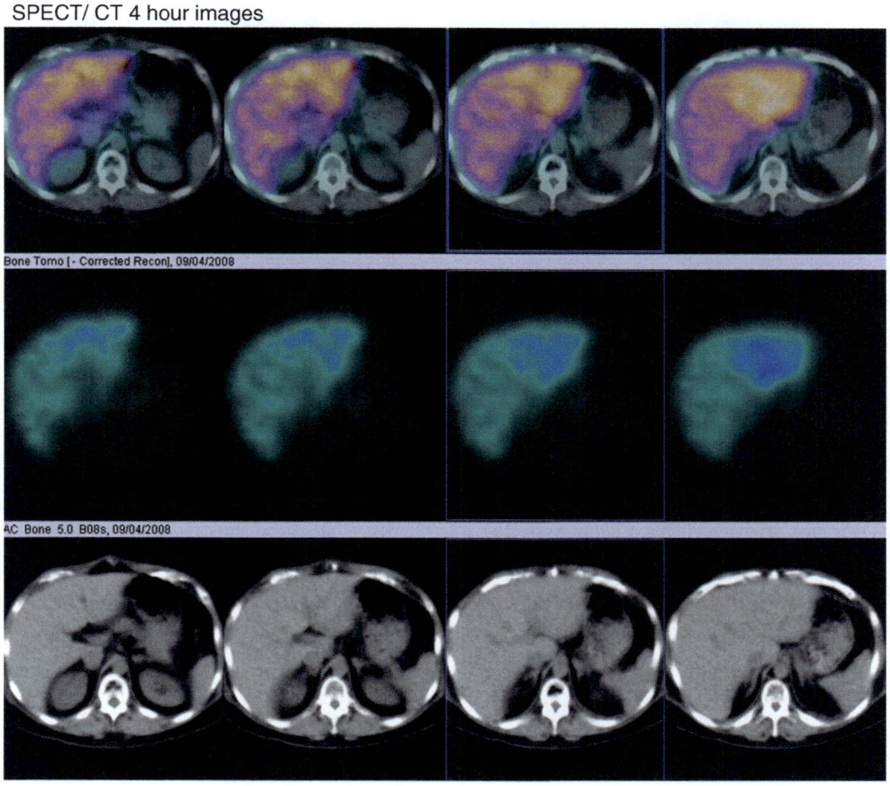

A patient with the suspected clinical diagnosis of Cushing syndrome that did not respond to treatment. Also, he had constant high pressure that did not respond to antihypertensive therapy.

Normal catecholamines.

Nevertheless, a MIBG SPECT/CT was required in order to discard other suprarenal aetiologies.

SPECT/CT 24 hour images

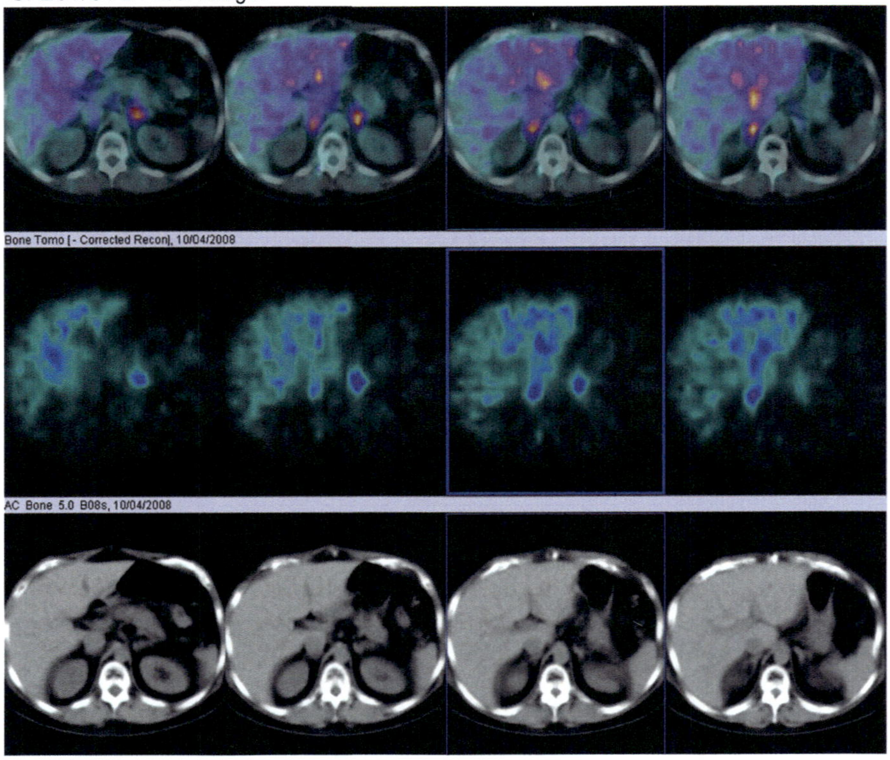

^{123}I-MIBG findings

Total body planar images and abdominal SPECT-CT obtained 4 and 24 h after the intravenous administration of 370 MBq of ^{123}I MIBG show, in the 24 h images, a slight increase of MIBG in both adrenal glands that was not seen in the early (4 h) SPECT/CT study and was interpreted as physiological uptake. Morphological images show a diffuse increase of the adrenal glands.

Post-surgical histopathological assessment showed bilateral diffuse cortical adrenal hyperplasia. He was treated with alternative Cushing medication and progressively responded.

Teaching point

In normal conditions, an absence or slight increase of uptake of the radiotracer in adrenal glands is observed.

MIBG SPECT/CT can facilitate correct anatomic localization and helps differentiate physiological variants from pathological uptake.

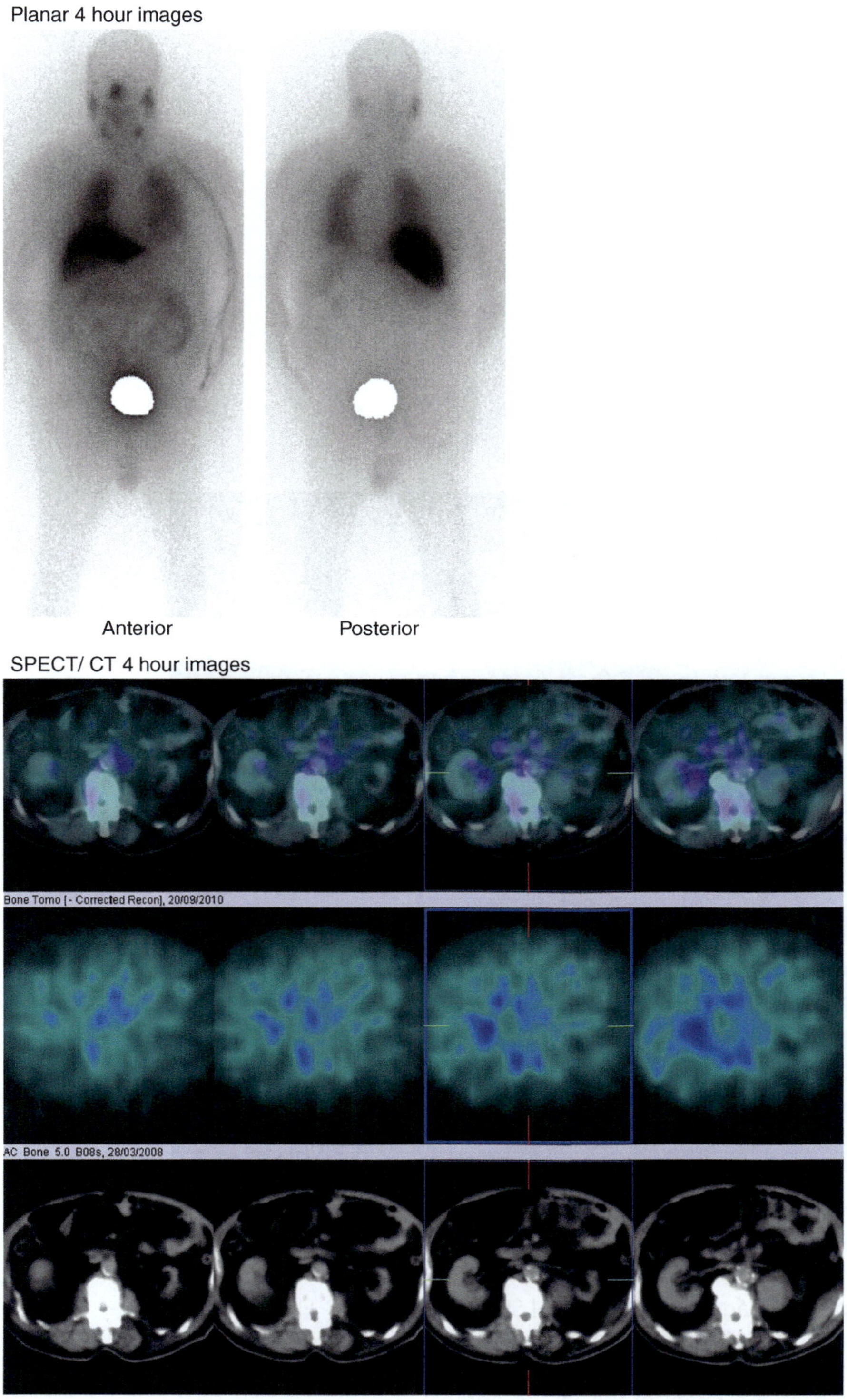

Patient with hypertension, DM of recent onset. Negative catecholamines.

Morphological images (abdominal CT) showed a left adrenal mass (incidentaloma).

A study with MIBG was required to rule out functional medullar adrenal involvement.

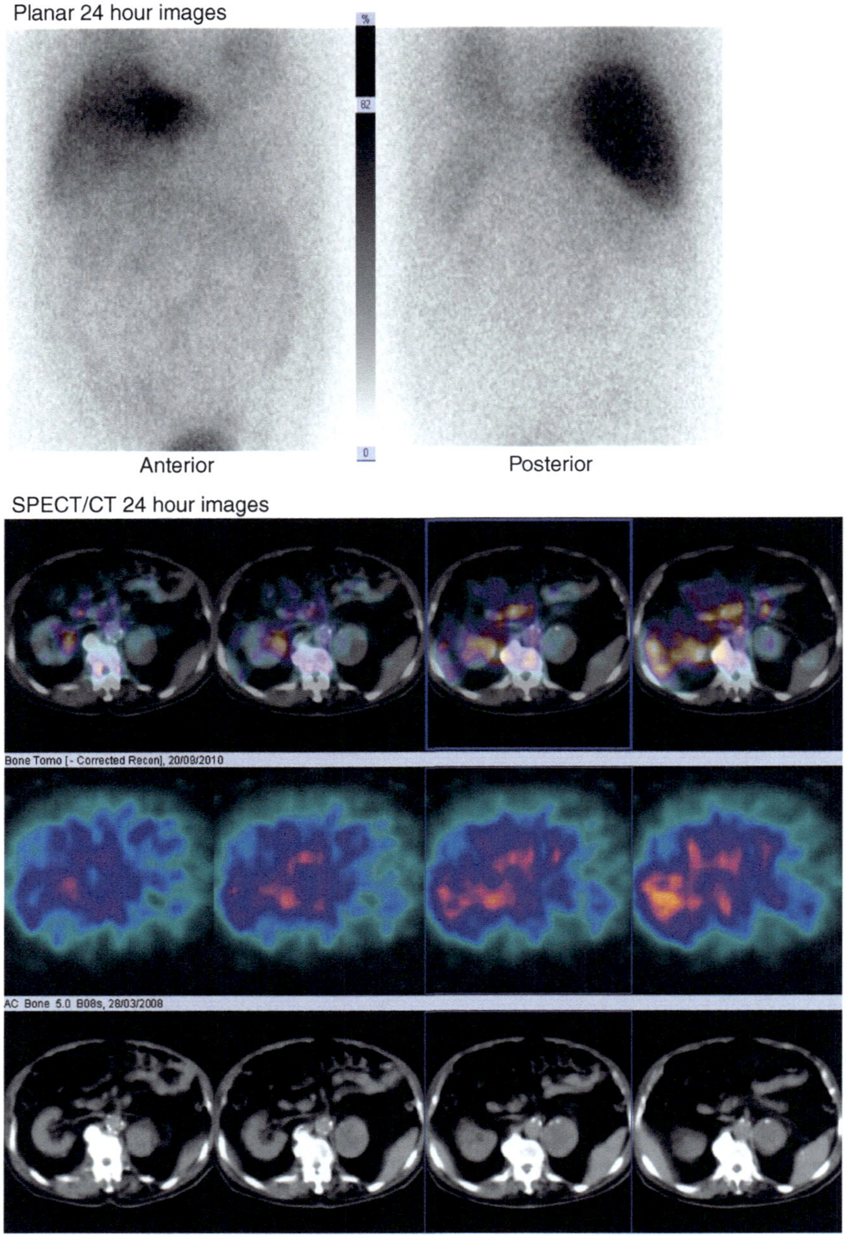

^{123}I-MIBG findings

Total body planar images and abdominal SPECT-CT obtained 4 and 24 h after the intravenous administration of 370 MBq of ^{123}I MIBG showed no pathological uptake of the radioisotope in the adrenal mass either in the early or in the late study. Morphological images confirmed the presence of an adrenal mass without affinity for MIBG.

Histopathological study showed a mass with necrosis and no viable cells.

Teaching point

MIBG SPECT/CT can be used to determine the functional state of an adrenal incidentaloma.

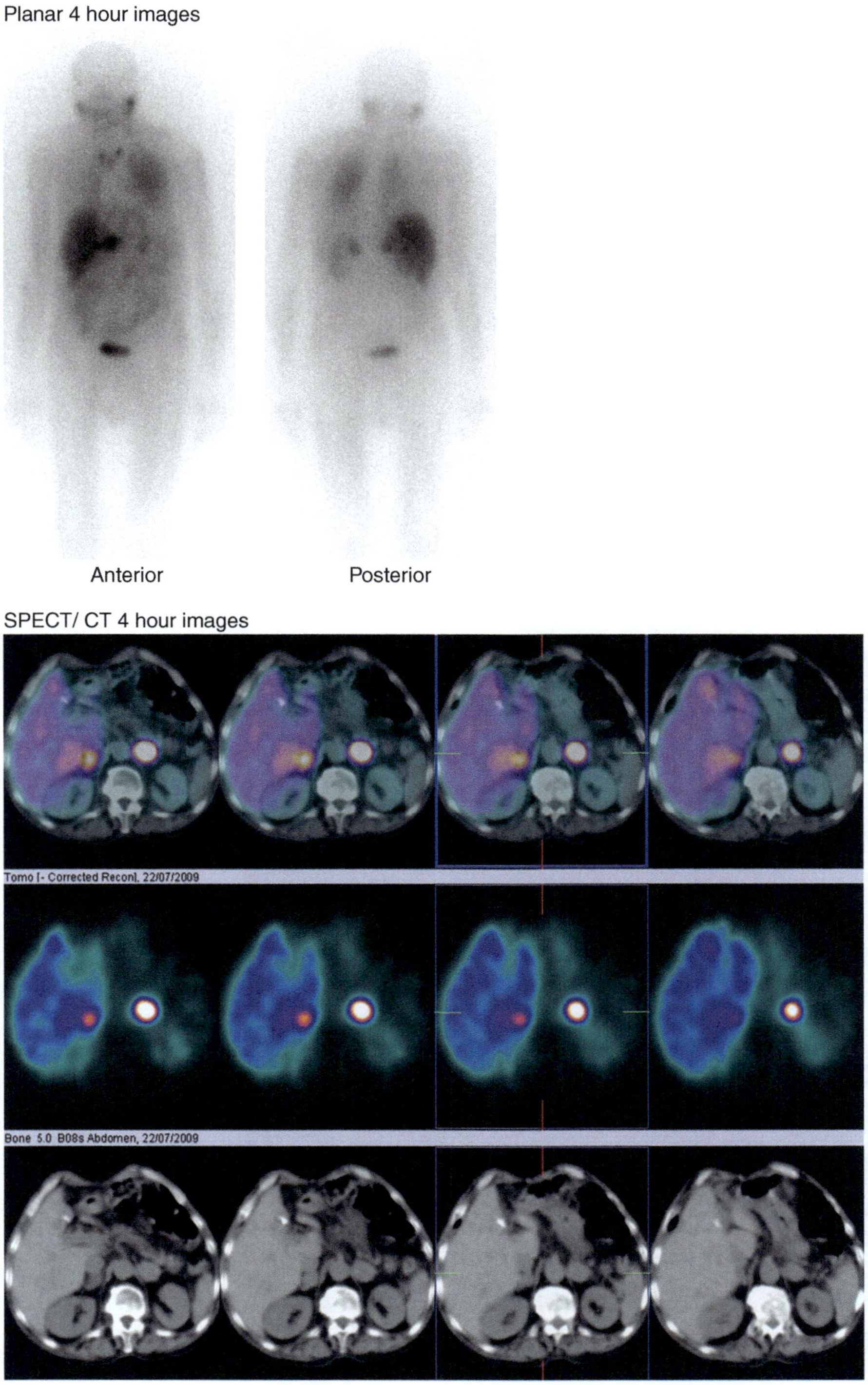

Patient with pancreatic adenocarcinoma, studied for hypertension and an increase of catecholamines.

MRI: bilateral adrenal masses (right: 3.3 cm/left: 5 cm) compatible with pheocromocitoma, but because of some characteristics of the lesions, metastasis from the pancreatic cancer cannot be ruled out.

The study was requested to establish the differential diagnosis.

Planar 24 hour images

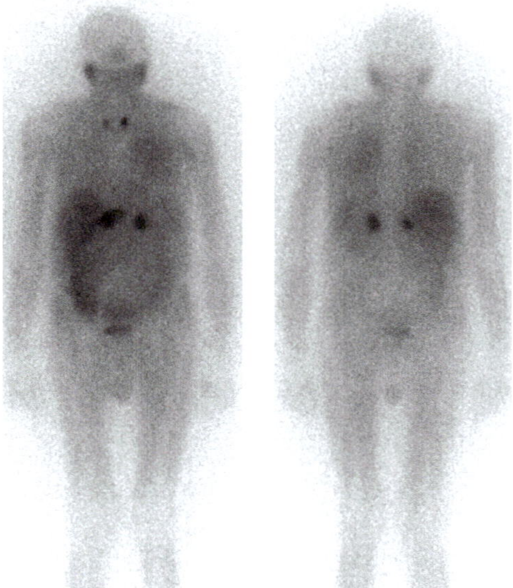

Anterior Posterior

SPECT/CT 24 hour images

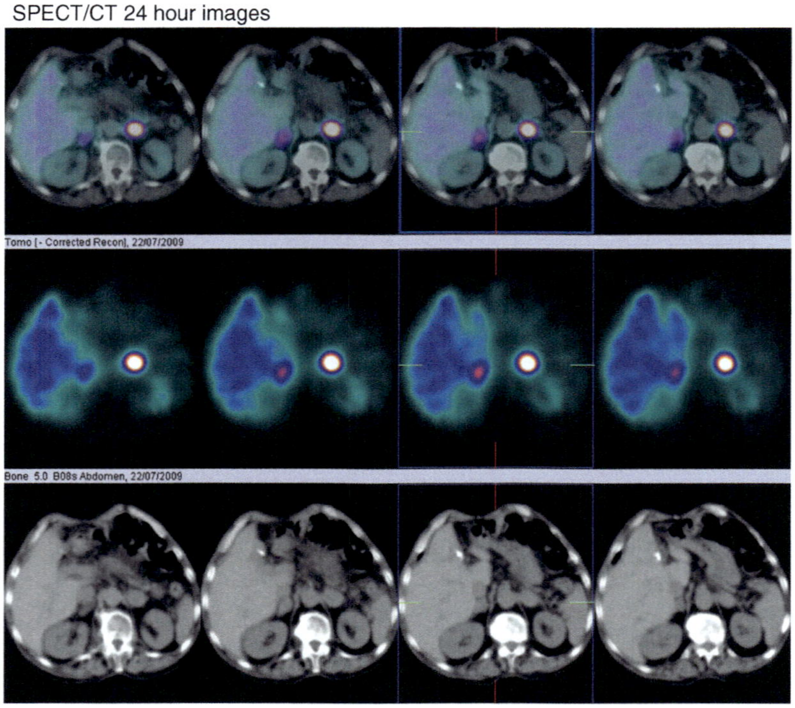

^{123}I-MIBG findings

Total body planar images and abdominal SPECT-CT obtained 4 and 24 h after the intravenous administration of 370 MBq of ^{123}I MIBG showed a great increase in the activity of the radioisotope in both adrenals masses.

Histopathological study confirmed bilateral pheochromocytoma.

Teaching point

This technique helps to establish a differential diagnosis between metastasis of non-neuroendocrine tumors from a medullar adrenal involvement. It is also an effective tool to anatomically locate the foci of increased activity, which is especially useful when planning surgery.

Planar 4 hour images

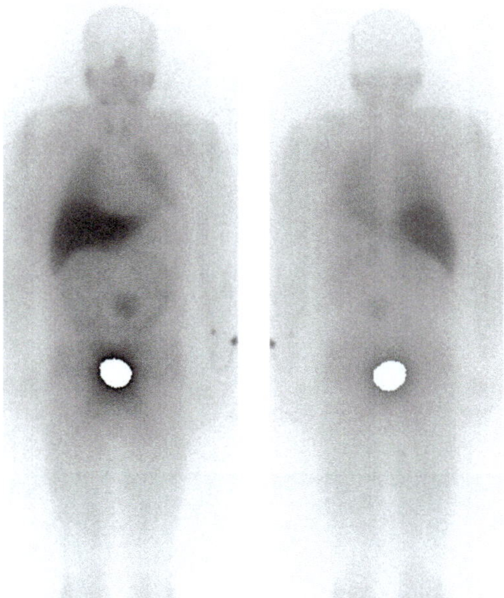

Anterior Posterior

SPECT/ CT 4 hour images

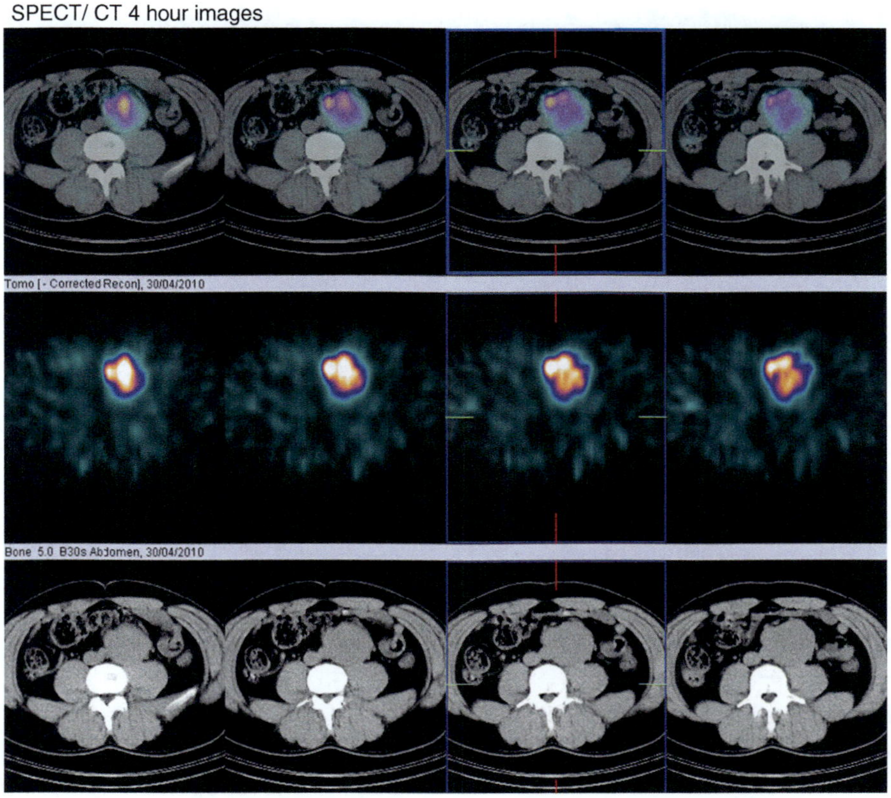

A patient with hypertension and increase of catecholamines in study for a possible pheochromocytoma/paraganglioma because of a retroperitoneal abdominal mass adjacent to the aorta of 6.8 × 5.3 × 6.3 cm detected by MRI.

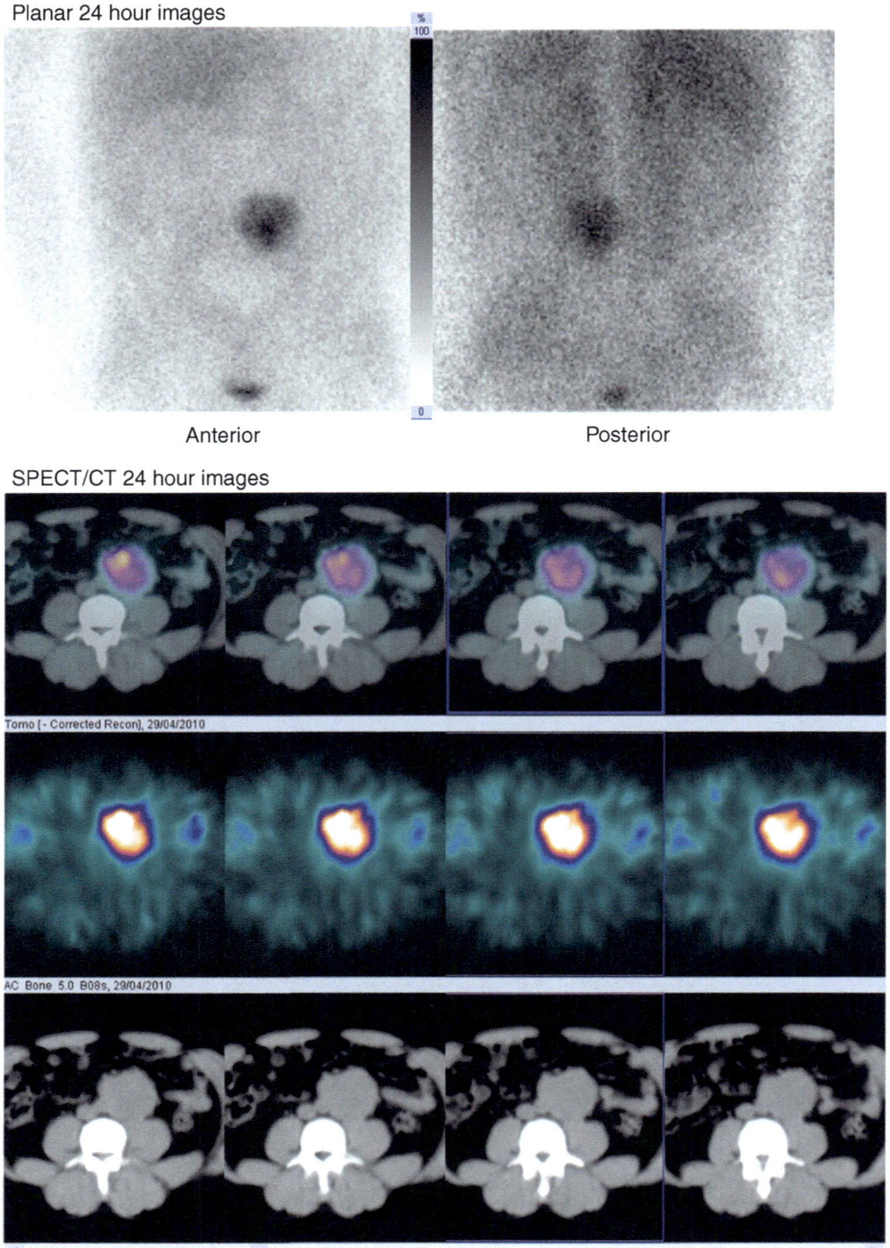

^{123}I-MIBG findings

Total body planar images and abdominal SPECT-CT obtained 4 and 24 h after the intravenous administration of 370 MBq of ^{123}I MIBG showed a mass in the previously described location with an intense uptake of MIBG that increased in the late study and was compatible with the suspected diagnosis.

The anatomopathology was positive for paraganglioma, without vascular invasion.

Teaching point

MIBG SPECT/CT helped to determine the origin of the retroperitoneal mass. SPECT/CT can facilitate correct anatomic localization.

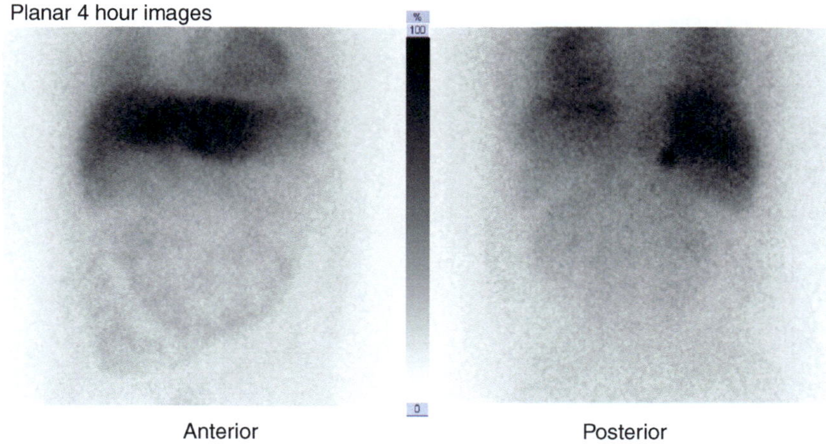

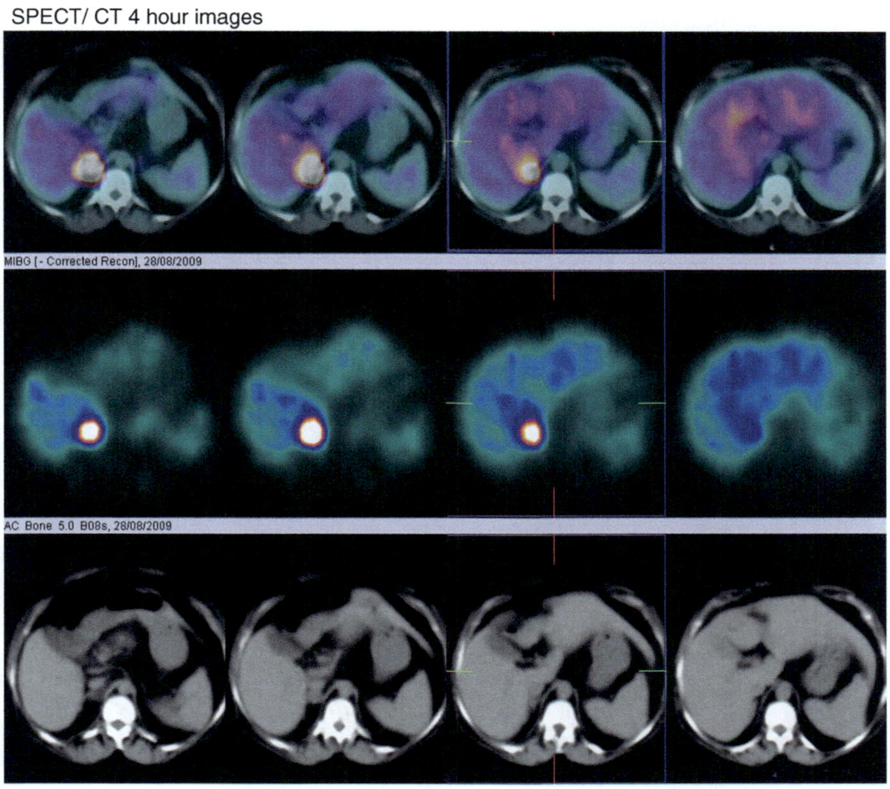

Patient in study for adrenal incidentaloma. Hypertension with a good response to antihypertensive therapy.

Slightly increased catecholamines.

In CT: node of 19 mm in the right adrenal gland. Possible adenoma.

MIBG study was required to complete the etiological diagnosis.

Planar 24 hour images

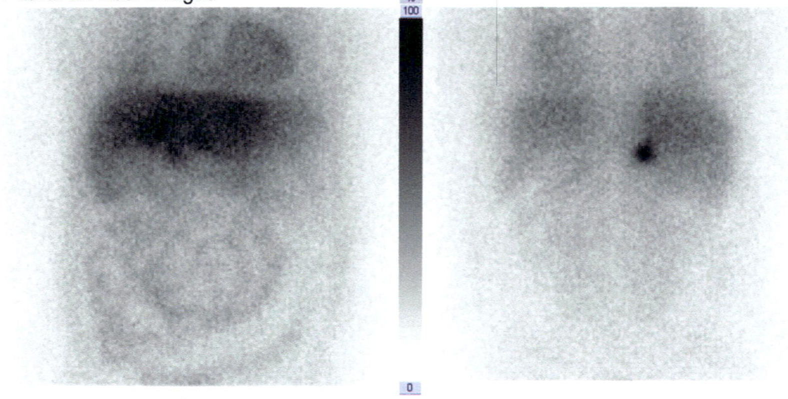

Anterior Posterior

SPECT/CT 24 hour images

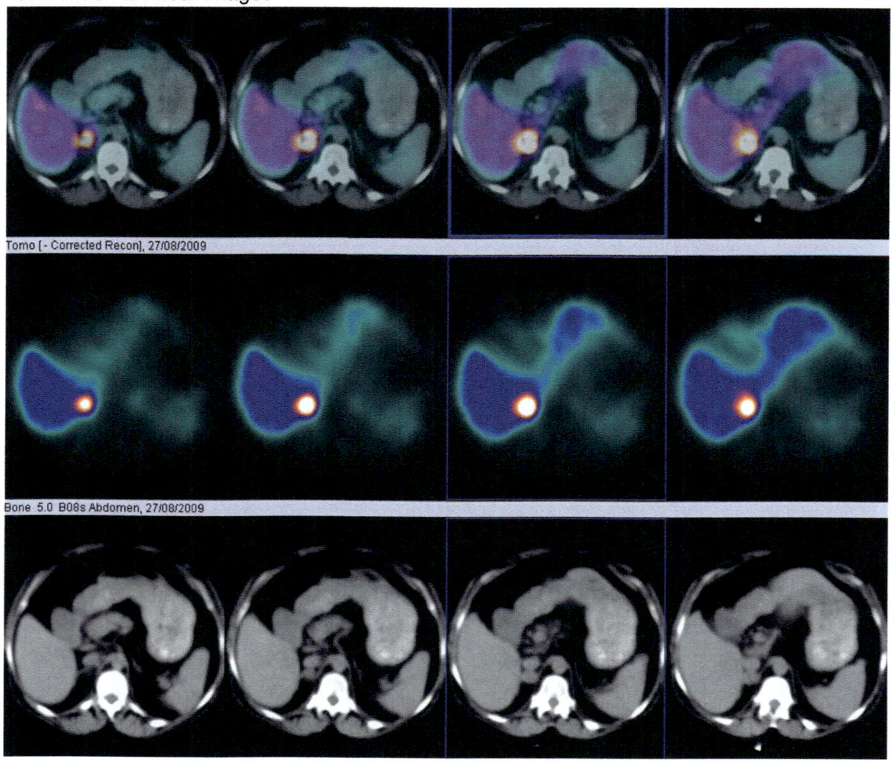

^{123}I-MIBG findings

Total body planar images and abdominal SPECT-CT obtained 4 and 24 h after the intravenous administration of 370 MBq of ^{123}I MIBG show an increase of MIBG in the right adrenal gland, both in the early (4 h) and the delayed study (24 h). Morphological images show the right adrenal incidentaloma.

Post-surgical anatomopathology confirmed pheochromocytoma in the right adrenal.

Teaching point

MIBG SPECT/CT is a useful tool to confirm/rule-out the involvement of the adrenal medulla when clinical symptoms point towards its probable involvement.

3.3 Iodine SPECT-CT

Ka Kit Wong (✉), Ryan A. Dvorak, and Anca M. Avram

3.3.1 Introduction

Thyroid carcinoma is the most common endocrine malignancy in adults with 37,200 (10,000M:27,200F) newly diagnosed cases in the United States in 2009 [58]. The incidence of thyroid carcinoma has been increasing over the last three decades partially due to earlier detection of small (<1.0 cm) tumors, although other factors may be involved [59–60]. This section focuses on the utility of hybrid SPECT-CT imaging performed with iodine scintigraphy for staging and management of well-differentiated thyroid cancers (WDTC), consisting of papillary and follicular types, and their variants, which have characteristic expression of the sodium iodide symporter. Medullary and anaplastic thyroid cancers do not concentrate iodine and are not discussed further.

The prognosis for the majority of patients with WDTC is excellent with a cancer-specific mortality of 1% at 20 years in low-risk groups (TNM stage I); however, this increases to between 25% to 45% at 10 years in high-risk patients (TNM stage III/IV) [61–63]. Risk stratification by tumor staging provides important prognostic information and guides management. Two examples of widely used staging systems are the AJCC TNM (7th edition) and MACIS classifications, both of which use patient age (<45 years) as a major determinant of low risk and better outcome. Radioisotopes of iodine have been used for over four decades for detection and treatment of WDTC. Usually following diagnosis of WDTC total or near-total thyroidectomy is performed, with or without cervical lymph node dissection, which removes the primary cancer, allows histopathological staging and removes normal thyroid tissue that concentrates radioiodine more avidly than thyroid carcinoma. Iodine-131 (I-131) with beta emission is then administered under endogenous or exogenous TSH stimulation with the goals of radioablation of remnant thyroid tissue, and to treat microscopic and macroscopic disease, although there is controversy regarding its role in very low risk patients [64–67]. Long-term surveillance uses a combination of thyroglobulin biomarker, neck ultrasound, whole body radioiodine scintigraphy and alternative imaging modalities including ^{18}F-fluorodeoxyglucose PET when there is non-iodine avid disease. Comprehensive guidelines have been published regarding management of WDTC [68, 69].

Hybrid SPECT-CT has been reported to be a powerful diagnostic tool when combined with iodine scintigraphy. Radionuclide imaging with I-131 has poor spatial resolution, and image quality is further degraded by septal penetration of energetic 364 keV gamma emissions. A paucity of anatomical information on radioiodine scans means interpretation of SPECT images is difficult and not used routinely. At the same time diagnostic CT has had a limited role in the evaluation of WDTC due to the need to avoid iodinated contrast and the frequency of nodal metastases in neck lymph nodes of normal size. Despite this, the synergistic combination of functional and anatomical information provided by SPECT-CT has been found to have many advantages over traditional planar imaging in different clinical settings. Optimal co-registration of tomographic volumes of data obtained by gamma cameras with inline CT, with the patient in the same bed position, allows precise localization of radioactivity foci. Additional benefits include CT-based attenuation correction and morphological information from a non-contrast CT with reduced mAs and kV. Several excellent reviews of the clinical applications of hybrid SPECT-CT provide context and outline the advantages of SPECT-CT imaging [70–74].

3.3.2 Utility of Iodine SPECT-CT

The use of iodine SPECT-CT in patients with thyroid cancer was first reported by Even-Sapir and colleagues in a subgroup of 4 patients out of 27 in whom SPECT-CT imaging was performed to evaluate endocrine neoplasms [75]. Subsequent studies reported the incremental diagnostic value of SPECT-CT in groups comprised entirely of patients with WDTC. In a study evaluating co-registration of separately acquired SPECT and CT data with the aid of external fiducial markers, combined SPECT-CT improved diagnostic evaluation compared to SPECT alone in 15/17 (88%) patients [76]. In 25 patients with post-therapy I-131 scans, it was reported that SPECT-CT improved diagnostic interpretation compared to planar images in 17/41

(41%) of radioactivity foci resulting in change to management in 6/24 (24%) patients [77]. In a large, bicenter study of 71 patients, of whom 54 had post-therapy and 17 had diagnostic I-131 imaging, Tharp and colleagues reported incremental diagnostic value of SPECT-CT over planar imaging in 41/71 (57%) of patients [78]. They observed that the anatomical information from low-resolution CT images allowed characterization of equivocal neck lesions on planar images. In 36 patients with SPECT-CT to evaluate foci distant from the neck, integrated SPECT-CT characterized equivocal foci as benign in 9/36 patients and precisely localized malignant lesions to the skeleton (12 patients) and lungs (5 patients). Information derived from SPECT-CT was found to alter patient management.

The utility of iodine SPECT-CT described in these early studies has been confirmed by investigators in a range of clinical settings [79–89]. Table 1 summarizes the published studies on iodine SPECT-CT to date. I-131 SPECT-CT has been performed with diagnostic scans using activities between 37 MBq–187 MBq (1 mCi–10 mCi) and post-therapy activities 1.1 GBq–8.1+ GBq (30 mCi–220+ mCi) with both endogenous and exogenous TSH stimulation. To date there has been only a single report on I-123 SPECT-CT [80]. Investigators have reported usefulness of iodine SPECT-CT for surveillance diagnostic imaging or following I-131 therapies [78, 80, 82, 86] and also in the post-surgical setting at the time of first radioiodine ablation either on diagnostic [88, 89] or post-therapy imaging [79, 81–85, 87].

Common to all studies in the literature is the ability of SPECT-CT to allow precise localization of radioactivity foci, which can then be characterized as benign, in remnant thyroid tissue or physiological distribution in normal structures, or as malignant in cervical nodal or distant metastases. In the neck region Wong and colleagues found an incremental value of SPECT-CT over planar imaging in 53/130 (41%) of neck foci, and described typical appearances of thyroglossal duct remnant and thyroid bed remnant, which have long been recognized on planar imaging but are often difficult to distinguish from neck nodal metastases with confidence [88, 90]. Indeed, one of the strengths of iodine SPECT-CT is to substantially reduce the number of equivocal foci on planar imaging alone. In 15 indeterminate planar neck lesions [86] and in 17 unclear neck foci [87], SPECT-CT was reported to reclassify all of them as thyroid remnant, lymph node metastases or contamination. Chen and colleagues reported that of 81 inconclusive planar foci (36 neck, 45 distant), SPECT-CT could clarify 69/81 (85%) of these [77]. Aide and colleagues reported that in 55 patients there were 29% indeterminate scans on planar imaging and only 7% with SPECT-CT. Of the 16 patients with indeterminate planar scans, reclassification with SPECT-CT as positive or negative for disease correlated more closely with success or failure of radioiodine treatment at follow-up [79].

Patterns of unusual radioiodine bio-distributions that could potentially mimic disease are well recognized and have been extensively reported [91–94]. Physiological radioiodine activity is seen in salivary glands, mucosa, breast, thymus, stomach, bowel, kidneys and bladder. Salivary and urinary contamination should be considered when unexpected bio-distribution occurs. SPECT-CT is a powerful diagnostic tool for rapid evaluation of suspected benign physiological radioactivity and can indicate distribution related to salivary glands, dental fillings, esophageal secretions, airway secretions, diverticuli, breast, thymus, hiatal hernia, bowel, skin contamination and benign uptake related to cysts. SPECT-CT is also useful for evaluation of distant metastatic disease [70–72, 76–79]. SPECT-CT can confirm osseous and pulmonary sites of metastases, providing additional anatomical diagnostic information to guide management decisions. In the thorax SPECT-CT can precisely localize malignancy to bone (ribs or spine), lung or mediastinal lymph nodes. There have been several reports of the value of SPECT-CT in difficult cases including unusual sites of metastases to the liver, kidney, muscle and trachea, and also benign uptake in the thymus, struma ovarii, menstruating uterus and simple renal cysts [96–103].

The sensitivity of diagnostic I-131 planar imaging ranges between 45% and 75% and the specificity between 90% and 100% [72, 78, 86]. Iodine SPECT-CT increases the accuracy of interpretation, although reports of sensitivity and specificity are currently lacking for I-131 SPECT-CT. This is because foci of radioactivity are usually treated with I-131 without biopsy confirmation, and when successful it is not possible to be sure if the uptake was due to thyroid carcinoma or normal residual thyroid tissue. Barwick and colleagues have reported on I-123 SPECT-CT test parameters and found sensitivity, specificity and accuracy for planar (41%, 68%, 61%), SPECT (45%, 89%, 78%) and SPECT-CT (50%, 100%, 87%) imaging [80]. Therefore, the value of I-123 SPECT-CT is to increase the specificity to imaging, and this may be

Table 1 Studies reporting utility of iodine SPECT-CT for evaluation of differentiated thyroid cancer[a]

Author Journal	No. pts/scans Design	Setting Indication	Radioiodine Activity	Camera CT setting	Site of radioactivity foci Findings/comments
Wong et al. 2010 AJR	48/48 Retro	First RA Selected	Diagnostic I-131 37 MBq	Symbia T6 140 kV, 100 mAs	Neck/distant SPECT-CT changed TNM stage in 10/48 (21%) patients SPECT-CT changed proposed I-131 dose selection in 28/48 (58%) patients SPECT-CT identified unsuspected metastases in 4/8 patients with M1
Mustafa et al. 2010 EJNMMI	151/151 Retro	First RA Routine	Post-Rx I-131 1.8–5.3 GBq	Symbia T2, T6 140 kV, 20–40 mAs	Neck Accuracy SPECT-CT > planar in 24.5% patients SPECT-CT revised N score in 24.5% patients LNM occurs in 26% of T1 patients, 22% with microcarcinoma (<1 cm)
Schmidt et al. 2010 EJNMMI	81/81 Retro	First RA Routine	Post-Rx I-131 1.5–5.3 GBq	Symbia T2, T6 140 kV, 40 mAs	Neck 60/61 patients with negative SPECT-CT were disease free at 5 months 17/20 patients with positive SPECT-CT were disease free at 5 months LN size < 0.9 ml predicted higher treatment success
Barwick et al. 2010 EJE	79/85 Retro	FU Routine	Diagnostic I-123 350–400 MBq	Millenium VG Hawkeye 140 kV, 2.5 mAs	Neck/distant Planar: sensitivity 41%, specificity 68%, accuracy 61% SPECT: sensitivity, 45% specificity 89%, accuracy 78% SPECT-CT: sensitivity, 50% specificity 100%, accuracy 87% SPECT-CT increased specificity
Aide et al. 2009 JCEM	55/55 Pros	First RA Routine	Post-Rx I-131 2.9–4.0 GBq	Symbia T2 ? kV, 60 mAs	Neck In 16 patients with indeterminate planar scans: 9/9 patients without disease had negative SPECT-CT 4/5 patients with disease had positive SPECT-CT
Kohlfuerst et al. 2009 EJNMMI	41/53 Pros	First RA (23 patients) FU (18 patients) Selected	Post-Rx I-131 2.9–7.5 GBq	Symbia T 130 kV, 25 mAs	Neck/distant SPECT-CT impact 21/33 (63.6%) patients, changed N score 12/33 (36.4%) SPECT-CT impact 14/19 (73.7%) patients, change in M score 4/19 (21.1%) Changed treatment in 10/41 (24.4%) patients 8/33 (24.2%) changed treatment due to N score 2/19 (10.5%) changed treatment due to M score

(continued)

Table 1 (continued)

Author Journal	No. pts/scans Design	Setting Indication	Radioiodine Activity	Camera CT setting	Site of radioactivity foci Findings/comments
Spanu et al. 2009 JNM	117/117 Pros	First RA (9/108) FU (99/108) Routine	Diagnostic I-123 185 MBq (108 pts) Post-Rx I-131 3.7 GBq (9 patients)	Millenium VG Hawkeye Infinia Hawkeye 140 kV, 2.5 mAs	Neck/distant Changed treatment in 35.6% patients with disease SPECT-CT led to avoidance of I-131 in 20% of patients without disease SPECT-CT identified 158 foci compared to only 116 foci on planar
Wang et al. 2009 Clin Imag	94/94 Retro	First RA Routine	Post-Rx I-131 3.7–7.4 GBq	Infinia Hawkeye 140 kV, 2.5 mAs	Neck/distant Accuracy SPECT-CT > planar in 20/94 (21%) patients Changed treatment in 22/94 (23%) patients SPECT-CT identified unsuspected metastases in 7/94 (7%) patients
Schmidt et al. 2009 EJNMMI	57/57 Retro	First RA Routine	Post-Rx I-131 1.5–5.3 GBq	Symbia T2, T6 140 kV, 40 mAs	Neck SPECT-CT completes N staging SPECT-CT changed N score in 20/57 (35%) patients SPECT-CT changed stage in 14/57 (24.5%) patients, both up and down
Wong et al. 2008 AJR	53/56 Retro	First RA (47 patients) FU (6 patients) Selected	Diagnostic I-131 37 MBq 150 MBq	Symbia T6 140 kV, 100 mAs	Neck/distant Diagnostic value SPECT-CT > planar in 53/130 (41%) neck foci Diagnostic value SPECT-CT > planar in 17/17 (100%) distant foci Allows adjustment of the first radioiodine activity selection
Chen et al. 2008 JNM	23/37 Pros	First RA Selected	Post-Rx I-131 3.7–7.4 GBq	Millenium VG Hawkeye 140 kV, 2.5 mAs	Neck/distant Diagnostic value SPECT-CT > planar in 17/23 (74%) patients SPECT-CT clarified 69/81 (85%) inconclusive planar foci Changed treatment in 8/17 (47%) patients
Tharp et al. 2004 EJNMMI	71/71 Retro	First RA (28/54) FU (26/54) Selected	Post-Rx I-131 1.4–9.7 GBq (54 patients) Diagnostic I-131 143–187 MBq (17 patients)	Millenium VG Hawkeye 140 kV, 2.5 mAs	Neck/distant SPECT-CT impact 41/71 (57%) patients Changed treatment in 7/17 (41%) patients with diagnostic SPECT-CT
Ruf et al. 2004 NMC	25/25 Pros	First RA Selected	Post-Rx I-131 3.7 GBq	Millenium VG Hawkeye 140 kV, 2.5 mAs	Neck/distant SPECT-CT impact in 17/41 (41%) foci Changed treatment in 6/24 (25%) patients
Yamamoto et al. 2003 JNM	17/17 Retro	First RA Routine	Post-Rx I-131 3.7–7.4 GBq	Aquilon CT Picker Prism	Neck/distant Accuracy SPECT-CT > SPECT 15/17 (88%) patients Co-registration with external fiducial markers feasible

Retro retrospective, *Pros* prospective, *First RA* post-surgery at time of first radioablation with I-131, *FU* follow-up from post-surgery 6 months onward, *Routine* SPECT-CT performed on consecutive patients, *Selected* SPECT-CT performed on selected patient group, *Post-Rx* post-therapy scan, *LNM* lymph node metastases, *Sen* sensitivity, *Spec* specificity

[a]PubMed search to June 1, 2010 using terms: SPECT-CT; SPECT/CT

expected to apply to I-131, although the authors acknowledge that biopsy proof was not possible in the majority of patients and that SPECT-CT was an integral component of the 'gold standard.' This limitation is inherent to all studies reported in the literature.

The use of iodine SPECT-CT has been reported to change clinical management in significant numbers of patients, both when utilized routinely on all consecutive patients and on selected patients with inconclusive planar images. Proposed changes in management include the decision to give or withhold radioiodine treatment, indicating and guiding the extent of surgery, selecting patients for external beam radiation therapy and indicating the need for alternative imaging strategies such as FDG PET. Change in management has been reported in 25% [77], 41% [79], 47% [82], 23% [88], 36% [87], 24% [82], 58% [89]and 11% of patients [80]. Risk stratification of patients following surgery is important to determine the prognosis and to guide decisions regarding management and surveillance. SPECT-CT has been found useful in staging of WDTC particularly using the AJCC TNM staging system. Precise localization with characterization of radioactivity foci using SPECT-CT lends itself well to N and M scoring. Schmidt and colleagues first reported the utility of post-therapy SPECT-CT at the first radioiodine ablation to complete N staging, changing the N score in 20/57 (35%) patients and the TNM stage in 14/57 (24.5%) patients, both upstaging and downstaging [85]. Kohlfuerst and colleagues found post-therapy SPECT-CT changed N scores in 12/33 (36.4%) patients and M scores in 4/19 (21.1%) patients [82]. Wong and colleagues found the use of iodine SPECT-CT with diagnostic scans prior to the first radioiodine ablation changed TNM staging in 10/48 (21%) patients, and changed selection of proposed I-131 activity in 28/48 (58%), to allow confident prescription of lower activities 1.1 GBq (30 mCi) for radioablation in low-risk patients and higher doses 3.7 GBq – 7.7+ GBq (100 mCi–200+ mCi) for therapeutic purposes [89]. They reported that SPECT-CT revealed unsuspected metastatic disease in 4/48 (8%) patients, similar to Wang and colleagues in 7/94 (7%) patients [87].

Iodine SPECT-CT also provides prognostic information regarding the success of radioiodine treatment as determined by clinical follow-up and surveillance I-131 whole-body imaging. Schmidt and colleagues using short-term follow-up reported that almost all patients with negative post-therapy SPECT-CT (60/61 patients) had negative 5-month diagnostic I-131 scan, and even the majority with positive post-therapy SPECT-CT (17/20 patients) still had negative diagnostic scan [84]. The authors identified a neck nodal volume of <0.9 ml on SPECT-CT to be highly likely to respond to I-131 therapy and commented that surgical resection of these lymph nodes would be excessive management. The positivity or negativity for disease as determined by post-therapy SPECT-CT correlated more closely to success or failure of radioiodine treatment than the planar imaging findings [79]. The use of post-therapy SPECT-CT at the first radioablation has also extended our knowledge regarding incidence of nodal metastases for patients with T1 tumors. Using a combination of pN1 (surgical neck dissection) and sN1 (SPECT-CT), a large, bicentric study of 151 patients found that lymph node metastases occurred in 26% of T1 (≤2.0 cm) tumors and 22% of microcarcinomas (≤1.0 cm), with implications for patient risk stratification and management [83].

3.3.3 Limitations of Iodine SPECT-CT

Iodine SPECT-CT is a powerful addition to the diagnostic armamentarium; however, limitations of the modality have been recognized. The spatial resolution of SPECT is limited by a partial volume effect in small lesions, and although intense activity in normal size neck lymph nodes is frequently detected, the modality could not be expected to resolve radioactivity related to micrometastases in the central compartment or even lateral neck lymph nodes. Similarly, SPECT-CT is insensitive to residual local invasive thyroid cancer after surgery unless there is gross residual tumor volume or anatomical findings of invasion. Staging therefore relies on the histopathological description of extra-thyroidal extension and the presence of positive surgical margins for the assignment of T score and central lymph node dissection for N score. SPECT-CT may also have limited sensitivity for pulmonary micronodular disease, although it is more sensitive than chest radiographs and more specific than diagnostic CT.

Patient preparation with a low iodine diet prior to imaging and avoidance of iodine sources such as iodinated contrast remains important prior to iodine SPECT-CT. Faint radioiodine uptake seen on planar and pinhole imaging using diagnostic I-131 activities may occasionally be unresolved on SPECT using 3D OSEM reconstruction parameters, and filtered back projection may be required [88]. Post-therapy images often have intense activity with septal penetration causing a star artifact that may interfere with evaluation of nearby tissues, making SPECT-CT interpretation more difficult; however, the availability of anatomical localization can mitigate this effect. Therefore, planar images remain valuable for providing an overview of radioiodine distribution throughout the body and identifying radioactive foci requiring anatomical correlation through the use of SPECT-CT. Misregistration between functional and anatomical datasets may still occur because of patient movement or even related to viewing software (when SPECT and CT volumes of coverage differ). Therefore, plausibility assessment of the fused images is required as a quality control step such as ensuring good co-registration of radioactivity to salivary glands in the head and neck region.

Non-iodine avid disease due to lack or subsequent loss of sodium iodide symporter expression may be a cause of reduced sensitivity of iodine SPECT-CT. This has been reported to occur in 30% of WDTC at time of diagnosis [48] and occurs more frequently with Hurthle cell thyroid cancer, papillary subtypes with unfavourable features (e.g., tall cell, columnar, cribiform) and with poorly differentiated (insular) thyroid cancer. Barwick and colleagues reported false-negative I-123 SPECT-CT in 11 patients with non-iodine avid disease [80]; however, their study used a Millenium VG Hawkeye, GE Amersham, UK, which is a first generation hybrid SPECT-CT camera with non-diagnostic quality CT images. Modern hybrid gamma cameras can detect non-iodine avid lymph node metastases in enlarged lymph nodes, which would otherwise require neck ultrasound to identify. Detection of non-iodine avid residual or recurrent disease on diagnostic 131-I significantly impacts clinical management directing treatment to surgical excision or external beam radiation therapy for patients who will no longer benefit from therapeutic 131-I administration. It may also indicate the need for alternative imaging strategies such as FDG PET.

SPECT-CT has an axial field of view limited to 40 cm in the current imaging systems; therefore, evaluation of both neck and distant radioactivity foci may require two SPECT-CT acquisitions. Although the CT component is usually deployed in low dose, non-diagnostic mode, there is an additional 1–4 mSv radiation exposure to the patient with each acquisition [71]. Analysis of benefit and potential risk should be performed on an individual basis in the young female and particularly the pediatric population [106].

3.3.4 Future Directions

There is interest in the value of diagnostic I-131 SPECT-CT being used to perform lesion-specific dosimetry. Information regarding lesion uptake and retention, and also tumor volume derived from the CT component could be used to calculate individualized I-131 activities and also determine therapeutic responses. An example of this approach in a patient with a large skull metastasis causing infringement of the brain has been reported [107]. It is worthwhile to briefly discuss I-124 scintigraphy using hybrid PET/CT technology. Several papers have been published reporting the use of I-124 PET/CT in patients with WDTC [108–111]. I-124 has a half-life of 4.2 days and a complex decay scheme including a high energy (602 keV) cascade gamma with 60% abundance that requires corrective modeling for dosimetry purposes and 23% positron emission allowing PET imaging. Preliminary data show that I-124 PET/CT has equivalent sensitivity to post-therapy I-131 scans, and to date thyroid stunning has not been reported. Therefore, 124-I PET-CT imaging, considered an 'older cousin' to I-131/123 SPECT-CT, has the advantages of hybrid imaging with superior spatial resolution, permits true whole body tomographic image acquisition and allows quantitative evaluation of radioiodine distribution over many days for dosimetry calculations.

In summary, iodine SPECT-CT is a powerful diagnostic tool that allows precise localization of radioiodine foci, superior characterization of benign and malignant radioactivity distributions compared to planar imaging, completion of TNM staging impacting on management in significant numbers of patients and providing prognostic information that may lead to reassessment of current WDTC management protocols.

Acknowledgements The authors would like to thank Carol Kruise for her assistance with assembling the figures for this chapter.

References

58. Jemal A, Siegel R, Ward E, Hao Y, Xu J, Thun MJ. Cancer statistics, 2009. CA Cancer J Clin. 2009;59(4):225–49.
59. Davies L, Welch HG. Increasing incidence of thyroid cancer in the United States, 1973–2002. JAMA. 2006;295(18):2164–7.
60. Chen AY, Jemal A, Ward EM. Increasing incidence of differentiated thyroid cancer in the United States, 1988–2005. Cancer. 2009;115(16):3801–7.
61. Hay ID, McConahey WM, Goellner JR. Managing patients with papillary thyroid carcinoma: insights gained from the Mayo Clinic's experience of treating 2,512 consecutive patients during 1940 through 2000. Trans Am Clin Climatol Assoc. 2002;113:241–60.
62. Jonklaas J, Sarlis NJ, Litofsky D, et al. Outcomes of patients with differentiated thyroid carcinoma following initial therapy. Thyroid 2006;16(12):1229–42.
63. Mazzaferri EL, Jhiang SM. Long-term impact of initial surgical and medical therapy on papillary and follicular thyroid cancer. Am J Med. 1994;97(5):418–28.
64. Hay ID. Management of patients with low-risk papillary thyroid carcinoma. Endocr Pract. 2007;13(5):521–33.
65. Hay ID, McDougall IR, Sisson JC. A proposition for the use of radioiodine in WDTC management. J Nucl Med. 2009;50(2):328–9; author reply 329–30. Epub Jan 21, 2009.
66. Mazzaferri EL. Management of low-risk differentiated thyroid cancer. Endocr Pract. 2007;13(5):498–512.
67. McDougall IR, Hay ID. ATA Guidelines: do patients with stage I thyroid cancer benefit from (131)I? Thyroid 2007;17(6):595–6; author reply 596–7.
68. Cooper DS, Doherty GM, Haugen BR, et al. Revised American Thyroid Association management guidelines for patients with thyroid nodules and differentiated thyroid cancer. Thyroid 2009;19(11):1167–214.
69. British Thyroid Association RCOP. Guidelines for the management of thyroid cancer. 2nd ed. 2007. http://www.britishthyroidassociation.org/Guidelines/. Accessed 24 Mar 2009.
70. Bockisch A, Freudenberg LS, Schmidt D, Kuwert T. Hybrid imaging by SPECT/CT and PET/CT: proven outcomes in cancer imaging. Semin Nucl Med. 2009;39(4):276–89.
71. Buck AK, Nekolla SG, Ziegler SI, Drzezga A. SPECT/CT. J Nucl Med. 2009;50(6):1009–10. Epub May 14,2009.
72. Delbeke D, Schoder H, Martin WH, Wahl RL. Hybrid imaging (SPECT/CT and PET/CT): improving therapeutic decisions. Semin Nucl Med. 2009;39(5):308–40.
73. Even-Sapir E, Keidar Z, Bar-Shalom R. Hybrid imaging (SPECT/CT and PET/CT)—improving the diagnostic accuracy of functional/metabolic and anatomic imaging. Semin Nucl Med 2009;39(4):264–75.
74. Mariani G, Bruselli L, Kuwert T, et al. A review on the clinical uses of SPECT/CT. Eur J Nucl Med Mol Imaging. 2010;37(10):1959–85. Epub Feb 25, 2010.
75. Even-Sapir E, Keidar Z, Sachs J, et al. The new technology of combined transmission and emission tomography in evaluation of endocrine neoplasms. J Nucl Med. 2001; 42(7): 998–1004.
76. Yamamoto Y, Nishiyama Y, Monden T, Matsumura Y, Satoh K, Ohkawa M. Clinical usefulness of fusion of 131I SPECT and CT images in patients with differentiated thyroid carcinoma. J Nucl Med. 2003;44(12):1905–10.
77. Ruf J, Lehmkuhl L, Bertram H, et al. Impact of SPECT and integrated low-dose CT after radioiodine therapy on the management of patients with thyroid carcinoma. Nucl Med Commun. 2004;25(12):1177–82.
78. Tharp K, Israel O, Hausmann J, et al. Impact of 131I-SPECT/CT images obtained with an integrated system in the follow-up of patients with thyroid carcinoma. Eur J Nucl Med Mol Imaging. 2004;31(10):1435–42.
79. Aide N, Heutte N, Rame JP, et al. Clinical relevance of single-photon emission computed tomography/computed tomography of the neck and thorax in postablation (131)I scintigraphy for thyroid cancer. J Clin Endocrinol Metab. 2009;94(6):2075–84.
80. Barwick T, Murray I, Megadmi H, et al. SPECT/CT using Iodine-123 in patients with differentiated thyroid cancer—additional value over whole body planar imaging and SPECT. Eur J Endocrinol. 2010;162(6):1131–9. Epub Mar 8, 2010.
81. Chen L, Luo Q, Shen Y, et al. Incremental value of 131I SPECT/CT in the management of patients with differentiated thyroid carcinoma. J Nucl Med. 2008;49(12): 1952–57.
82. Kohlfuerst S, Igerc I, Lobnig M, et al. Posttherapeutic (131)I SPECT-CT offers high diagnostic accuracy when the findings on conventional planar imaging are inconclusive and allows a tailored patient treatment regimen. Eur J Nucl Med Mol Imaging. 2009;36(6):886–93.
83. Mustafa M, Kuwert T, Weber K, et al. Regional lymph node involvement in T1 papillary thyroid carcinoma: a bicentric prospective SPECT/CT study. Eur J Nucl Med Mol Imaging. 2010;37(8):1462–6. Epub Apr 1, 2010.
84. Schmidt D, Linke R, Uder M, Kuwert T. Five months' follow-up of patients with and without iodine-positive lymph node metastases of thyroid carcinoma as disclosed by (131) I-SPECT/CT at the first radioablation. Eur J Nucl Med Mol Imaging. 2010;37(4):699–705.
85. Schmidt D, Szikszai A, Linke R, Bautz W, Kuwert T. Impact of 131I SPECT/spiral CT on nodal staging of differentiated thyroid carcinoma at the first radioablation. J Nucl Med. 2009;50(1):18–23.
86. Spanu A, Solinas ME, Chessa F, Sanna D, Nuvoli S, Madeddu G. 131I SPECT/CT in the follow-up of differentiated thyroid carcinoma: incremental value versus planar imaging. J Nucl Med. 2009;50(2):184–90.
87. Wang H, Fu HL, Li JN, Zou RJ, Gu ZH, Wu JC. The role of single-photon emission computed tomography/computed tomography for precise localization of metastases in patients with differentiated thyroid cancer. Clin Imaging. 2009;33(1):49–54.
88. Wong KK, Zarzhevsky N, Cahill JM, Frey KA, Avram AM. Incremental value of diagnostic 131I SPECT/CT fusion imaging in the evaluation of differentiated thyroid carcinoma. AJR Am J Roentgenol. 2008;191(6):1785–94.
89. Wong KK, Sisson JC, Koral KF, Frey KA, Avram AM. Staging of differentiated thyroid carcinoma using diagnostic 131-I SPECT-CT. AJR Am J Roentgenol. 2010;195(3):730–6.
90. Wong KK, Zarzhevsky N, Cahill JM, Frey KA, Avram AM. Hybrid SPECT-CT and PET-CT imaging of differentiated thyroid carcinoma. Br J Radiol. 2009;82(982):860–76.

91. Carlisle MR, Lu C, McDougall IR. The interpretation of 131I scans in the evaluation of thyroid cancer, with an emphasis on false positive findings. Nucl Med Commun. 2003; 24(6):715–35.
92. Leitha T, Staudenherz A. Frequency of diagnostic dilemmas in 131I whole body scanning. Nuklearmedizin. 2003; 42(2):55–62.
93. Mitchell G, Pratt BE, Vini L, McCready VR, Harmer CL. False positive 131I whole body scans in thyroid cancer. Br J Radiol. 2000;73(870):627–35.
94. Shapiro B, Rufini V, Jarwan A, et al. Artifacts, anatomical and physiological variants, and unrelated diseases that might cause false-positive whole-body 131-I scans in patients with thyroid cancer. Semin Nucl Med. 2000;30(2):115–32.
95. Agriantonis DJ, Hall L, Wilson MA. Utility of SPECT/CT as an adjunct to planar whole body I-131 imaging: liver metastasis from papillary thyroid cancer. Clin Nucl Med. 2009;34(4):247–8.
96. Aide N, Lehembre E, Gervais R, Bardet S. Unusual intratracheal metastasis of differentiated thyroid cancer accurately depicted by SPECT/CT acquisition after radioiodine ablation. Thyroid 2007;17(12):1305–6.
97. Dumcke CW, Madsen JL. Usefulness of SPECT/CT in the diagnosis of intrathoracic goiter versus metastases from cancer of the breast. Clin Nucl Med. 2007;32(2):156–9.
98. Macdonald W, Armstrong J. Benign struma ovarii in a patient with invasive papillary thyroid cancer: detection with I-131 SPECT-CT. Clin Nucl Med. 2007;32(5): 380–2.
99. Qiu ZL, Luo QY. Erector spinae metastases from differentiated thyroid cancer identified by I-131 SPECT/CT. Clin Nucl Med. 2009;34(3): 137–40.
100. Rachinsky I, Driedger A. Iodine-131 uptake in a menstruating uterus: value of SPECT/CT in distinguishing benign and metastatic iodine-positive lesions. Thyroid 2007; 17(9):901–2.
101. Thust S, Fernando R, Barwick T, Mohan H, Clarke SE. SPECT/CT identification of post-radioactive iodine treatment false-positive uptake in a simple renal cyst. Thyroid 2009;19(1):75–6.
102. von Falck C, Beer G, Gratz KF, Galanski M. Renal metastases from follicular thyroid cancer on SPECT/CT. Clin Nucl Med. 2007;32(9):751–2.
103. Wong KK, Avram AM. Posttherapy I-131 thymic uptake demonstrated with SPECT/CT in a young girl with papillary thyroid carcinoma. Thyroid 2008;18(8):919–20.
104. Zhao LX, Li L, Li FL, Zhao Z. Rectus abdominis muscle metastasis from papillary thyroid cancer identified by I-131 SPECT/CT. Clin Nucl Med. 2010;35(5):360–1.
105. Mian C, Barollo S, Pennelli G, et al. Molecular characteristics in papillary thyroid cancers (PTCs) with no 131I uptake. Clin Endocrinol (Oxf). 2008;68(1): 108–16.
106. Gelfand MJ, Lemen LC. PET/CT and SPECT/CT dosimetry in children: the challenge to the pediatric imager. Semin Nucl Med. 2007;37(5):391–8.
107. Sisson JC, Dewaraja YK, Wizauer EJ, Giordano TJ, Avram AM. Thyroid carcinoma metastasis to skull with infringement of brain: treatment with radioiodine. Thyroid 2009;19(3):297–303.
108. Capoccetti F, Criscuoli B, Rossi G, Ferretti F, Manni C, Brianzoni E. The effectiveness of 124I PET/CT in patients with differentiated thyroid cancer. Q J Nucl Med Mol Imaging. 2009;53(5):536–45.
109. Eschmann SM, Reischl G, Bilger K, et al. Evaluation of dosimetry of radioiodine therapy in benign and malignant thyroid disorders by means of iodine-124 and PET. Eur J Nucl Med Mol Imaging. 2002;29(6):760–7.
110. Freudenberg LS, Antoch G, Gorges R, et al. Combined PET/CT with iodine-124 in diagnosis of spread metastatic thyroid carcinoma: a case report. Eur Radiol. 2003;13 Suppl 4:L19–23.
111. Phan HT, Jager PL, Paans AM, et al. The diagnostic value of 124I-PET in patients with differentiated thyroid cancer. Eur J Nucl Med Mol Imaging. 2008;35(5):958–965.

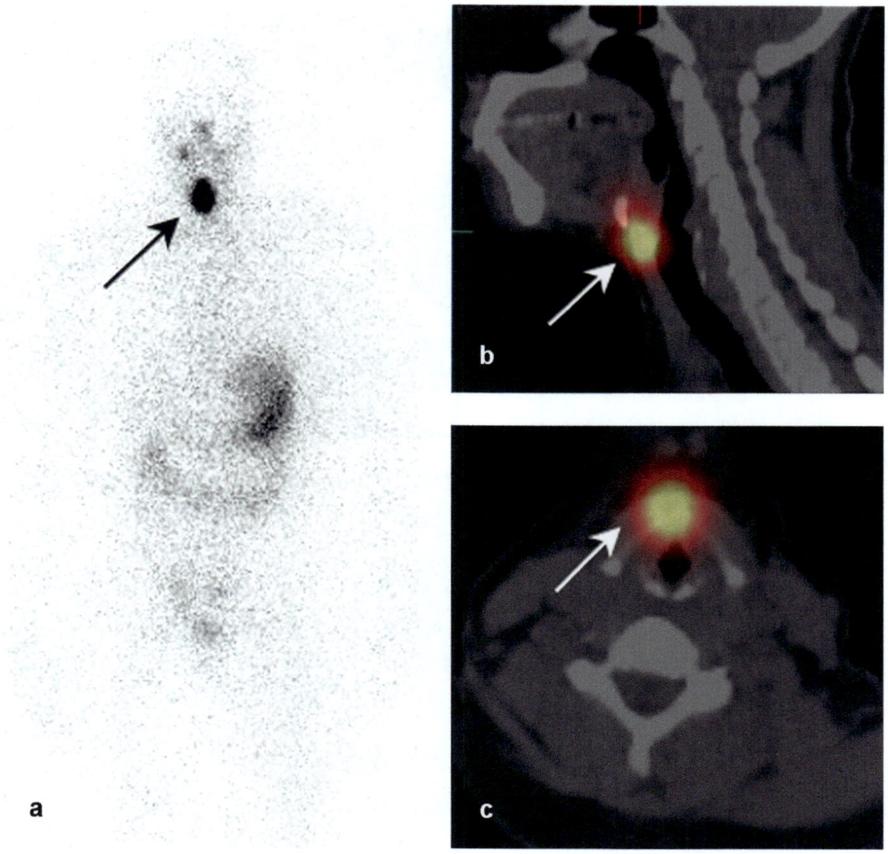

131-I scan in a 58-year-old woman status post-total thyroidectomy with resection of a 1.9-cm papillary thyroid cancer in the right lobe, without capsular invasion or extra-thyroidal extension and negative surgical margins; 0+/4 lymph nodes resected in the central neck.

^{131}Iodine findings

Planar anterior view (**a**) and SPECT-CT saggital (**b**) and transaxial (**c**) images show intensely focal central midline neck activity, which on SPECT-CT corresponds to residual functional thyroid tissue in thyroglossal duct remnant (*arrow*)

Teaching point

Following total or near-total thyroidectomy, a small amount of normal thyroid tissue often remains, termed remnant thyroid tissue. SPECT-CT is useful to characterize focal uptake in the neck, as either thyroid bed or thyroglossal duct remnant.

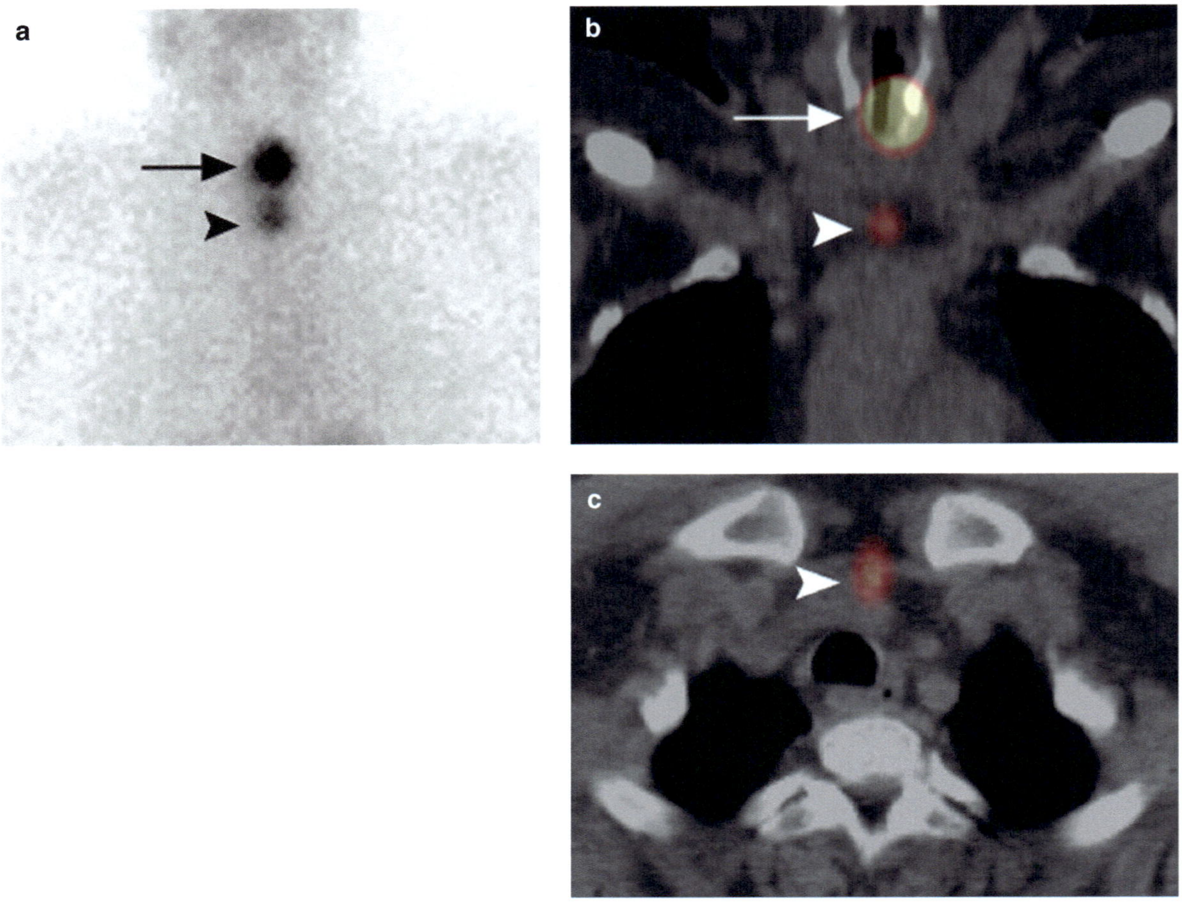

131-I scan in a 54-year-old woman status post-total thyroidectomy with resection of a 0.8-cm papillary thyroid cancer in the right lobe, without capsular or vascular invasion; the tumor displayed extra-thyroidal extension, but negative surgical margins; 2+/5 lymph nodes in the central neck contained metastasis with extra-nodal extension.

^{131}Iodine findings

Planar anterior view (**a**) and SPECT-CT coronal (**b**) and transaxial (**c**) images revealed midline focus of increased activity in the central neck superiorly consistent with thyroglossal duct remnant (*arrow*) and a fainter activity focus at the base of the neck (*arrowhead*), which on SPECT-CT corresponds to a 0.3-cm cervical level VII lymph node consistent with residual nodal metastasis (*arrowhead*)

Teaching point

Regional metastasis to neck lymph nodes may be detected more accurately with SPECT-CT localizing focal uptake in the neck to lymph nodes, which may be normal in size.

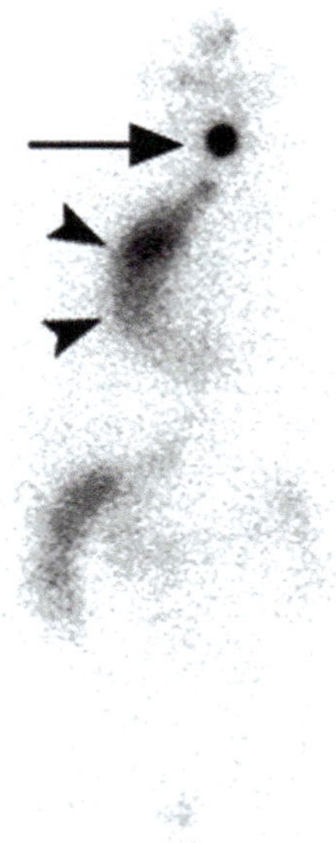

a

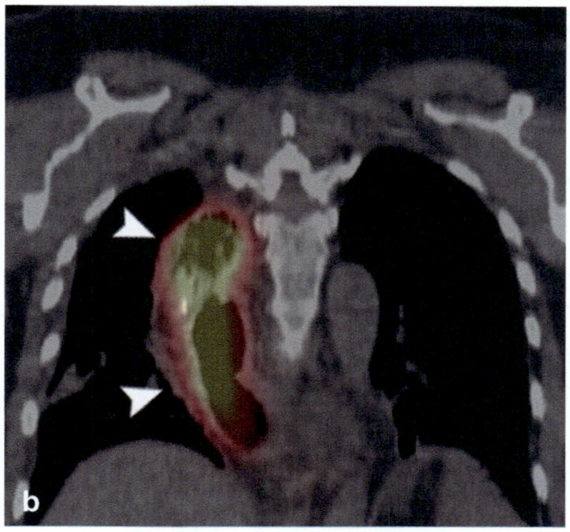

b

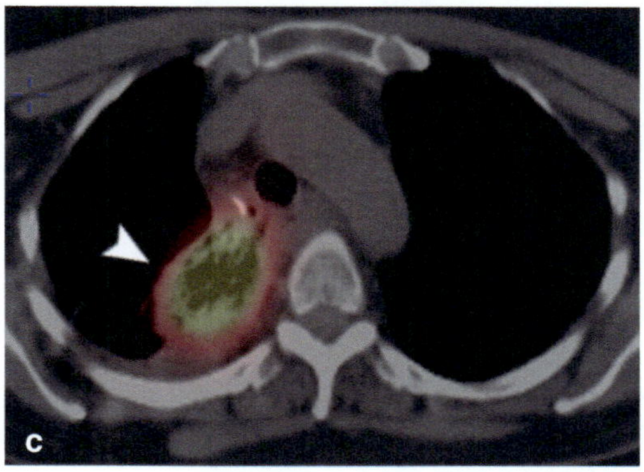

c

131-I scan in a 63-year-old woman status post-total thyroidectomy with resection of a 1.1-cm encapsulated papillary thyroid carcinoma in the right thyroid lobe with capsular invasion and focally present at the surgical margins. Medical record review reveals that the patient underwent transhiatal esophagectomy with cervical esophagogastric anastomosis for treatment of adenocarcinoma of the gastroesophageal junction.

^{131}Iodine Findings

Planar anterior view (**a**) and SPECT-CT coronal (**b**) and transaxial (**c**) images demonstrated focal central neck activity, which on SPECT-CT abuts the hyoid bone without a definite underlying anatomic correlate, consistent with thyroglossal duct remnant (*arrow*). There is diffuse physiological uptake throughout the intra-thoracic stomach (*arrowheads*)

Teaching point

A wide spectrum of physiological mimics of disease have been described on radioiodine scintigraphy. SPECT-CT is able to efficiently and rapidly confirm these patterns of uptake as benign.

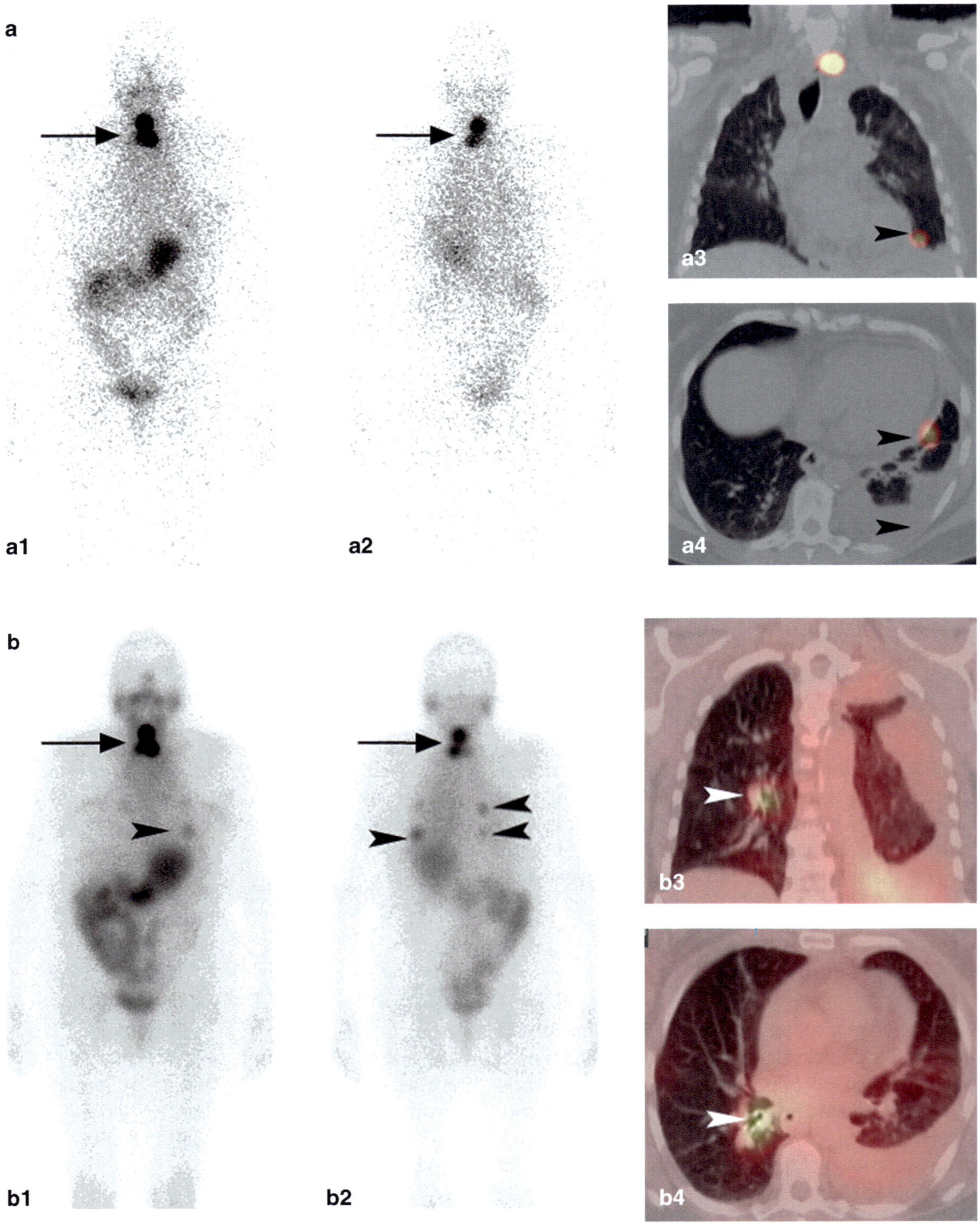

Diagnostic (**A**) and post-therapy (**B**) 131-I scans in a 70-year-old woman status post-total thyroidectomy with resection of a 7.2-cm minimally invasive, well-differentiated follicular carcinoma in the right lobe, displaying capsular and vascular invasion.

^{131}Iodine findings

Planar anterior (**a1**, **b1**) and posterior (**a2**, **b2**) views and SPECT-CT coronal (**a3**, **b3**) and transaxial (**a4**, **b4**) images demonstrate two foci of activity in the neck, corresponding on SPECT-CT to the thyroglossal duct remnant and the left thyroid bed (*arrow*). In addition, SPECT-CT reveals a pulmonary metastatic focus (*arrowhead*), which was not seen on planar imaging because of the presence of a left pleural effusion resulting in increased attenuation in the left hemithorax. This new finding resulted in prescription of high-dose 131-I activity for treatment of advanced (stage IV) disease, and the post-therapy 131-I scan demonstrates new metastatic foci in the lungs bilaterally (*arrowheads*), which were not evident on the diagnostic 131-I scan because of their small size and partial volume effect

Teaching point

Pulmonary metastases are a common site of distant metastatic spread. SPECT-CT localizes radioactivity to the lungs, due to either micronodular or macronodule disease, which may escape detection on chest x-ray.

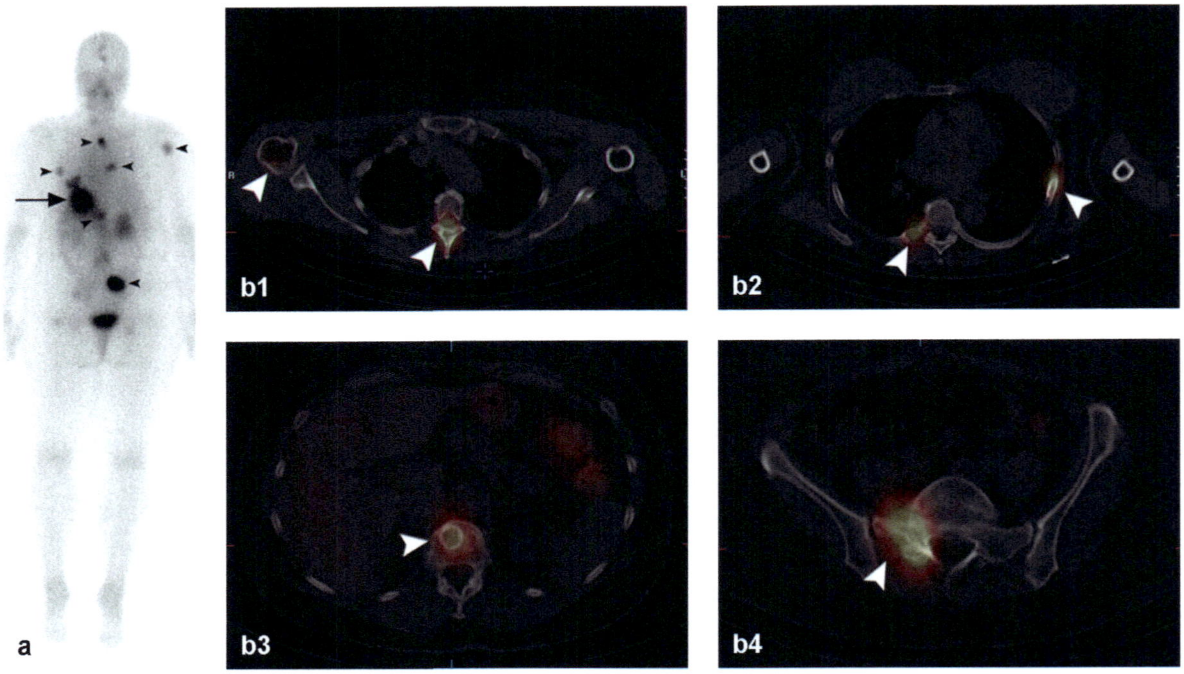

131-I scan in a 62-year-old woman who presented with widespread skeletal metastatic disease; total thyroidectomy specimen demonstrated a 3.0-cm macro-follicular variant papillary thyroid carcinoma in the left thyroid lobe with minimal extra-thyroidal extension and 3+/7 metastatic cervical lymph nodes.

^{131}Iodine findings

Planar posterior view (**a**) reveals intensely focal 131-I uptake in the left upper abdomen corresponding to physiological activity in the stomach (*arrow*) and multiple foci of abnormal uptake in the right shoulder, bilateral chest wall, midline back and right pelvis. SPECT-CT images (**b**) localize these foci to lytic osseous lesions in the proximal right humerus and T4 spinous process (**b1**), bilateral ribs (**b2**), T12 vertebral body (**b3**) and right iliac wing (**b4**)

Teaching point

Osseous metastases can be precisely localized on SPECT-CT and may guide management decisions regarding surgery, radioiodine, or external beam radiation therapy, eg. spinal metastases with impending cord compression.

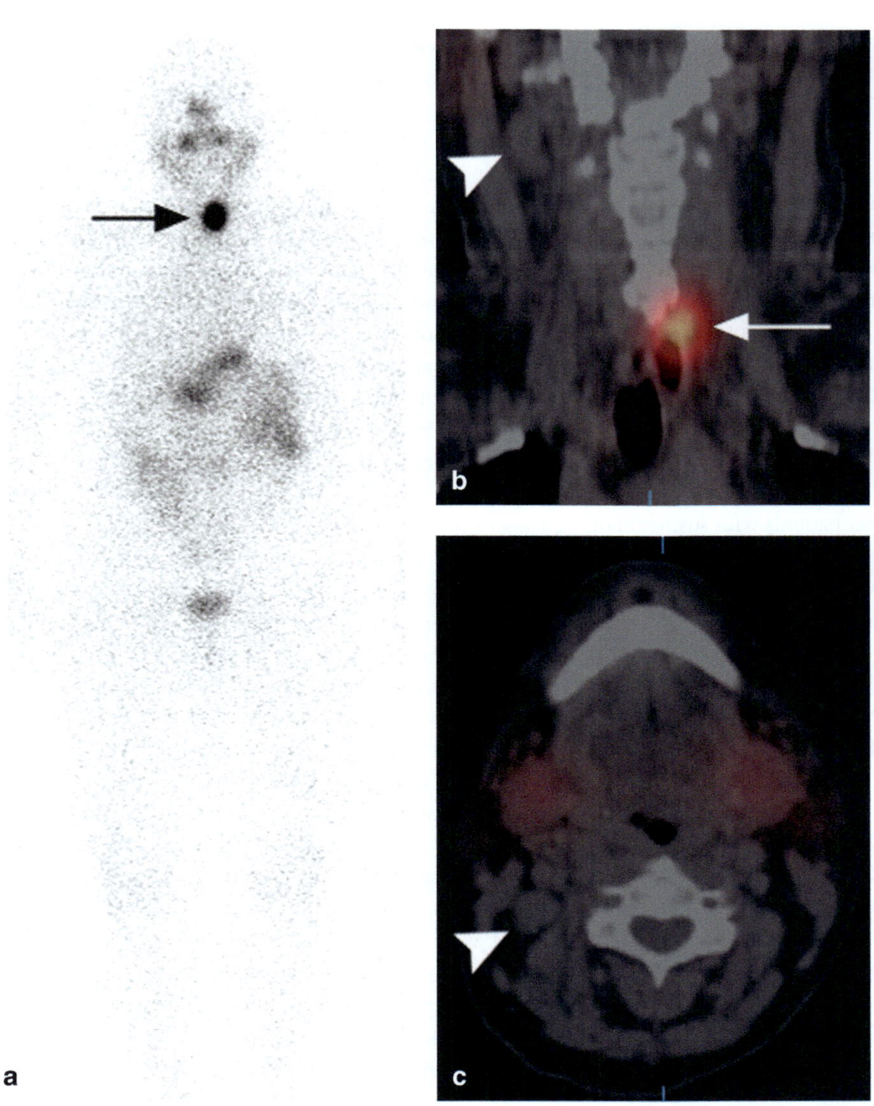

Teaching point

Non-iodine avid disease may be detected on the CT component of the SPECT-CT. Early detection may change management towards surgical or radiation therapy approach, or prompt use of FDG PET for staging.

131-I scan in a 48-year-old woman status post-total thyroidectomy with resection of multifocal, bilateral papillary thyroid carcinoma with tall cell features (1.2 and 2.3 cm tumors) with capsular and vascular invasion into the right internal jugular vein, displaying extra-thyroidal extension and positive surgical resection margins; 6+/13 metastatic lymph nodes with extra-nodal extension resected in bilateral neck and central neck compartments.

^{131}Iodine findings

Planar anterior view (**a**) demonstrates intensely focal activity in the left thyroidectomy bed consistent with thyroid remnant tissue in the left thyroid bed (*arrow*); given the positive surgical margins, a component of residual tumor at this site cannot be excluded. SPECT-CT coronal (**b**) and transaxial (**c**) images reveal the presence of an enlarged (1.4 × 1.4 cm.) non-iodine avid right cervical level IIB lymph node (*arrowhead*), which on US-guided FNA biopsy produced cells of papillary thyroid carcinoma

3.4 Prostascint SPECT-CT

Carina Mari Aparici, Randall Hawkins, and
Youngho Seo (✉),

^{111}In-Capromab pendetide, better known as ProstaScint, is a murine monoclonal antibody (7E11C5.3) radiolabeled with indium-111 that targets the intracellular epitope of prostate-specific membrane antigen (PSMA) and therefore can be used for staging and restaging of prostate cancer. Since full-length monoclonal antibody imaging requires at least 2–4 days for target accumulation and background clearance, ^{111}In-ProstaScint, with a physical half-life of 2.83 days, possesses a favorable pharmacokinetic behavior for diagnostic imaging. ^{111}In-ProstaScint scans are generally indicated for prostate cancer patients with suspicion of recurrent or residual disease following definitive treatment, or for patients with elevated prostate-specific antigen (PSA) levels and suspected metastatic disease outside the prostate gland. The most commonly used ^{111}In-ProstaScint imaging protocol is a combination of a 2-dimensional two-view (anterior-posterior) scintigraphy followed by a single photon emission computed tomography (SPECT) so that both the whole-body distribution of ^{111}In-ProstaScint and the tomographic cross-sectional views are reviewed for the diagnosis of prostate cancer spread.

Immunohistochemistry (IHC) studies using the 7E11C5.3 monoclonal antibody have shown that PSMA is expressed by all prostate cancers and that the level of PSMA expression in the primary tumor can be correlated with the tumor grade. Radiolabeled 7E11C5.3, ProstaScint, provides a noninvasive mapping of PSMA expression by using an in vivo imaging method that detects radioactive photons. Combined with a therapeutic radionuclide (e.g., 90Y or 177Lu), the antibody (7E11C5.3) itself is also a good candidate for targeted radioimmunotherapy, potentially effective in killing cancer cells that express high levels of PSMA.

In spite of that, the value of ^{111}In-ProstaScint scans in prostate cancer evaluation is currently somewhat limited. One of the reasons may be that no method to effectively use the information provided by ^{111}In-ProstaScint scans in the clinical management of prostate cancer has been found. However, a more compeling issue seems to be that ^{111}In-ProstaScint scans are difficult to interpret, even for specialized nuclear medicine physicians. The primary reason for this is widespread nonspecific uptake of ProstaScint in bowel and bone marrow, and the trace of ProstaScint that is not cleared completely from the blood stream. This nonspecific biodistribution obscures the specific areas of ProstaScint uptake, resulting in far from optimal target-to-background contrast. Thus, it has been recommended that ProstaScint scans be combined either with blood-pool imaging such as dual-isotope scans (99mTc-labeled red blood cells injected at the time of the 72–96 postinjection ^{111}In-ProstaScint scan) or with a structural imaging technique such as computed tomography (CT) or magnetic resonance imaging (MRI). Although the red blood cell scan is a practical solution performed simultaneously with the ^{111}In-ProstaScint scan, it only outlines the vasculature, therefore providing very limited anatomical information.

The advent of the combined dual-modality SPECT/CT scanner in the early 2000s led to a gain in popularity for the combined functional-structural imaging procedure as the imaging modality for ^{111}In-ProstaScint scans. The delivery of anatomical details from CT scans outperforms the blood pool images provided by 99mTc-labeled red blood cell scans. A hypothetical SPECT/MRI scanner could even provide better details of soft tissue contrast. Unlike SPECT/MRI as a whole-body imager, SPECT/CT does not need RF coils that must be placed close to the imaging object and provides a photon attenuation map that is a desirable feature to correct attenuation errors in SPECT reconstruction using a direct conversion method from CT images. For these reasons, SPECT/CT scanners are becoming more available as a dual-modality hybrid imaging system for oncological studies such as ^{111}In-ProstaScint.

Currently, SPECT/CT scanners are offered as either SPECT with low-mA (limited resolution) CT or SPECT with high-mA diagnostic multislice CT. Both of the SPECT/CT types have capabilities with regard to anatomical localization of SPECT uptake and CT-derived attenuation map generation for SPECT reconstruction. However, the SPECT with low-mA CT does not provide sufficiently high spatial resolution to localize small structures, such as <10-mm size lymph nodes, where ^{111}In-ProstaScint accumulates. In contrary, the high-mA diagnostic multislice CT provides greater anatomical details of most small lymph nodes in which ^{111}In-ProstaScint uptake—seen by SPECT—can be correlated. In the following pictorial examples of ^{111}In-ProstaScint SPECT/CT, we present SPECT, hybrid SPECT/CT and CT images from both types of scanners, and show distinguishable features with annotations corresponding to the specific examples.

A typical imaging protocol for ^{111}In-ProstaScint with SPECT/CT (without 99mTc-labeled red blood cell imaging) would be: (1) dose: 185 MBq of ^{111}In-ProstaScint, intravenously, (2) two-view anterior-posterior whole-body scintigraphy at 72–96 h postinjection and (3) SPECT/CT (CT followed by SPECT) scan of the abdomen-pelvis.

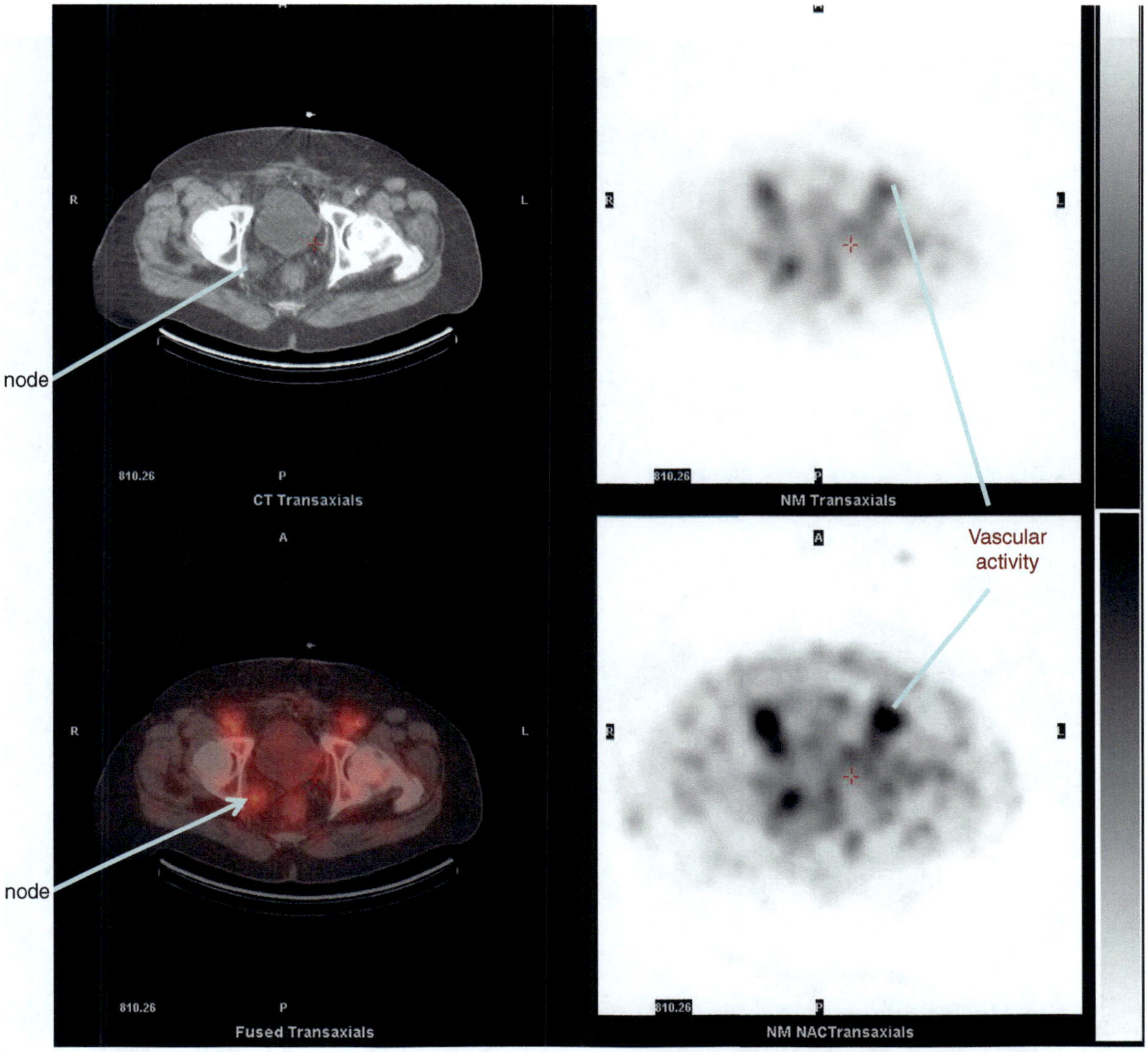

^{111}In-ProstaScint findings

A. 2.5-cm right pelvic sidewall node with moderately intense ProstaScint uptake, consistent with metastatic disease; patient has prostate cancer

Teaching point

SPECT-CT allows to differentiate between physiological vascular activity and pathological lymph nodes.

^{111}In-ProstaScint SPECT/CT

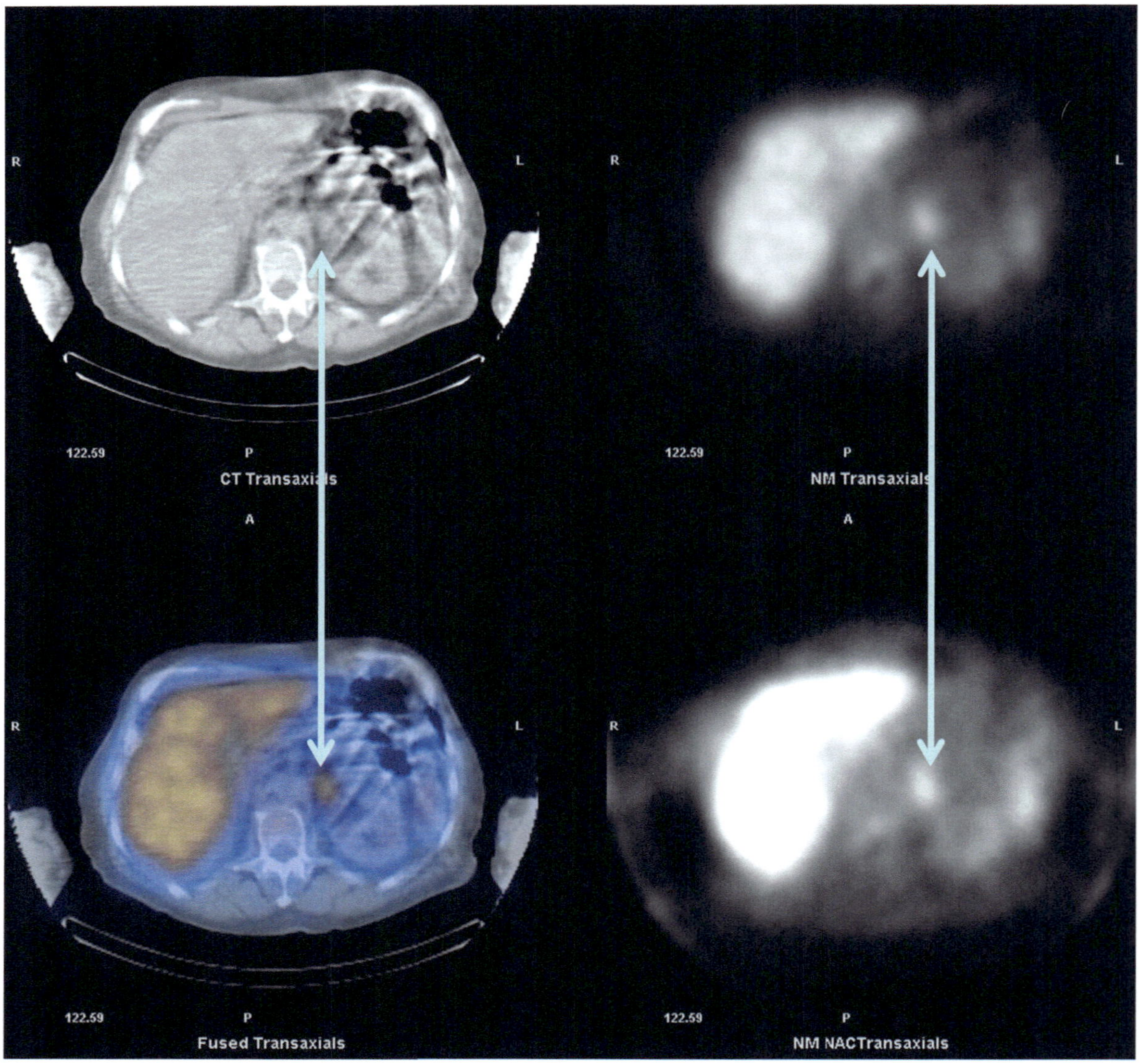

^{111}In-ProstaScint findings

ProstaScint demonstrating abnormal uptake in left adrenal gland.

Contrast-enhanced CT

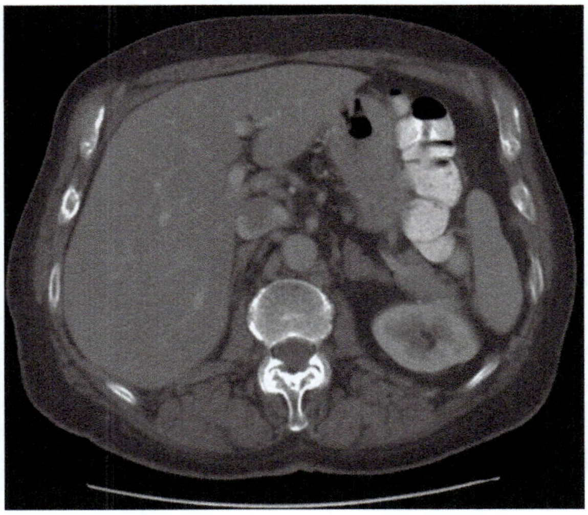

Contrast-enhanced CT finding

Separate standard CT (not low-mA) demonstrates enlarged left adrenal gland.

Teaching point

SPECT-CT allows confident anatomical localization of sites with increased uptake of tracer. Adrenal metastases from prostate cancer are unusual but have been reported.

^{111}In-ProstaScint SPECT/CT

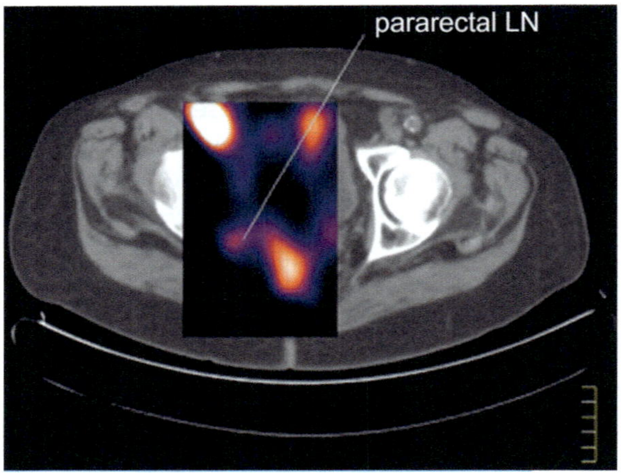

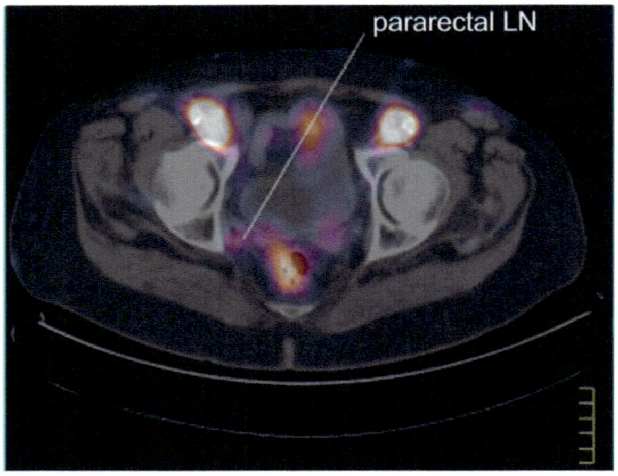

Noncontrast CT

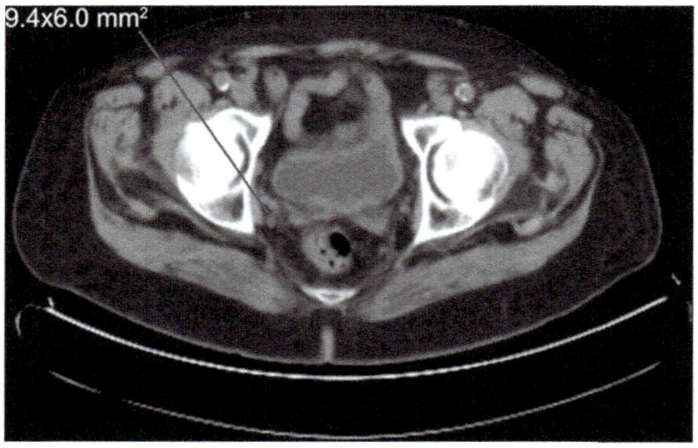

^{111}In-ProstaScint finding

ProstaScint SPECT uptake in right pararectal lymph node, correlated with CT (from the same SPECT-CT scan) measurement of (9.4 × 6.0 mm^2)

Teaching point

SPECT-CT allows a more confident diagnosis of pathological sites of disease.

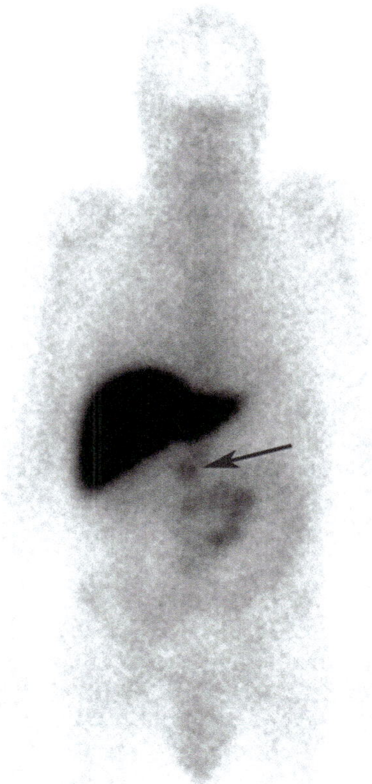

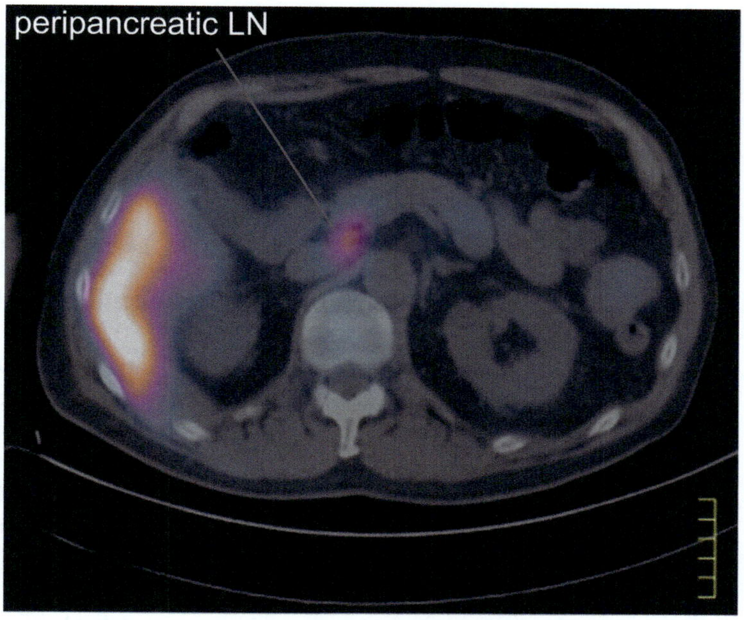

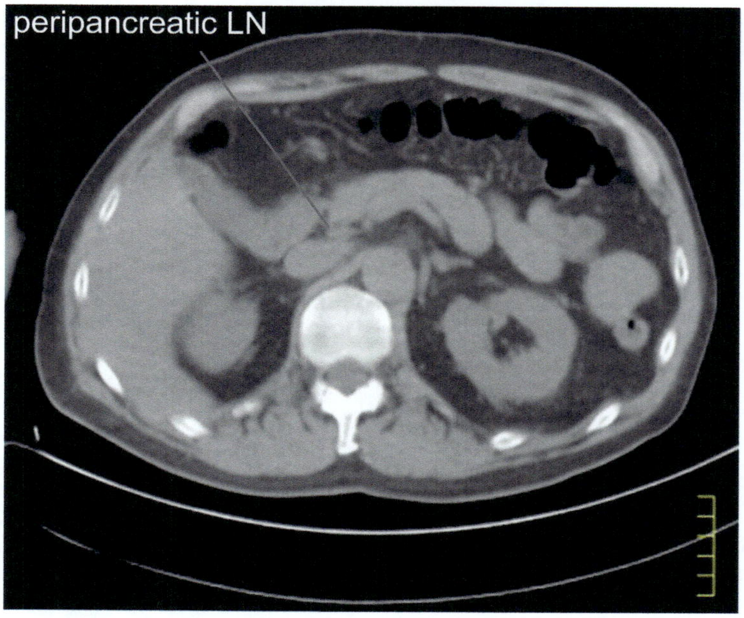

¹¹¹In-ProstaScint finding

ProstaScint WB scintigraphy indicates suspicious peripancreatic lymph node uptake. Corresponding SPECT/CT (*left images*) confirms the ProstaScint uptake localized in peripancreatic LN.

Teaching point

SPECT-CT allows localization and size determination of pathological lymphnodes.

3.5 Hynic SPECT-CT

Jure Fettich (✉), and Marina Hodolic

Scintigraphy with ^{111}In- or ^{99m}Tc-labeled somatostatin analogs has become the main imaging technique for neuroendocrine tumors (NET), particularly those expressing a high density of somatostatin receptors. Combined with SPECT, it is currently the first choice imaging technique for these tumors. Somatostatin receptor scintigraphy not only has a crucial role in the diagnosis and staging of NET, but also in assessing suitability for treatment with cold and radiolabeled somatostatin analogs as well as in monitoring response to treatment and detecting recurrent disease.

Somatostatin analogs can be radiolabeled not only with ^{111}In (e.g., Octreoscan®), but also with ^{99m}Tc, e.g., ^{99m}Tc-EDDA/HYNIC-TOC ([^{99m}Tc-EDDA/HYNIC-D-Phe 1, Tyr 3] octreotide).

3.5.1 Radiopharmaceutical Preparation

[^{99m}Tc-EDDA-HYNIC-D-Phe^1,Tyr^3]octreotide (^{99m}Tc-EDDA-HYNIC-TOC) can be used for imaging and gamma probe detection. It can be prepared via EDDA/tricine coligand exchange labeling [112]; 20 µg HYNIC-TOC is heated with 10 mg ethylenediamine N,N' diacetic acid (EDDA), 20 mg tricine, 10 µg stannous chloride dihydrate and 2 GBq of ^{99m}Tc-pertechnetate in 2 ml 0.05 M phosphate buffer at pH 6 at 100°C for 10 min. The solution is purified using a Sep-Pak Light C18 cartridge eluted with 70% ethanol and diluted with 5 ml saline. Radiochemical purity above 95% is determined in all cases using high-performance liquid chromatography. The purified radiopharmaceutical is sterilized by filtration, and 550–650 MBq of the resulting solution can be used for the patient study.

Because of the advantages of ^{99m}Tc-labeled radiopharmaceuticals, we examined the feasibility of producing ^{99m}Tc-octreotide in our laboratory, its quality and clinical utility following modification of the technique suggested by E. von Guggenberg et al. [112] and compared our results with those using ^{111}In-octreotide in the same patients (Figs. 1 and 2).

^{111}In-octreotide is commercially available and has a long half-life, which allows for repeated imaging up to 72 h post injection. Extensive experience with this radiopharmaceutical has been accumulated over the past

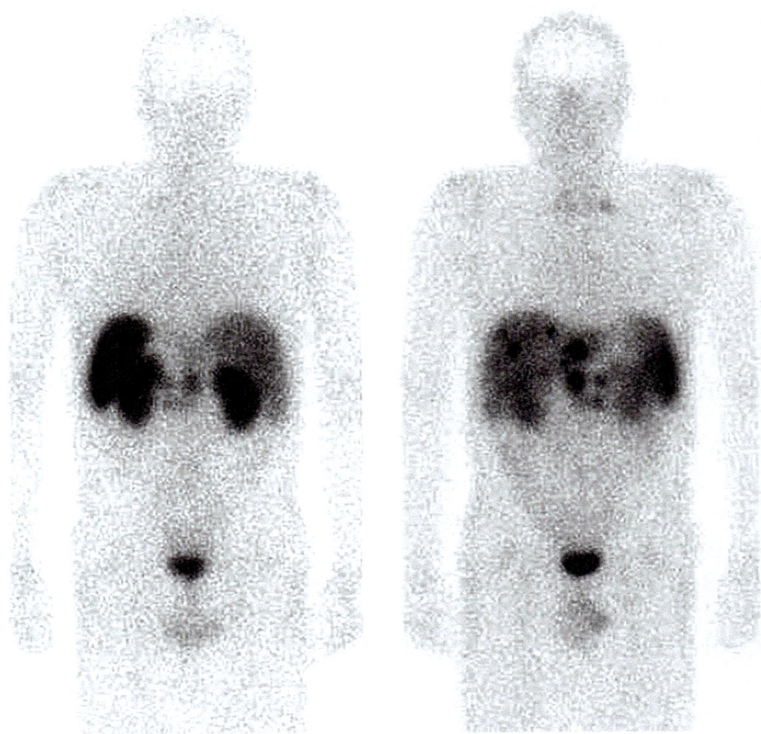

Fig. 1 Physiological ^{111}In octreotide uptake in spleen, liver, kidneys and thyroid. Pathological tracer uptake in primary and metastatic NET (carcinoid)

Fig. 2 99m-Tc octreotide uptake in the same patient as in Fig. 1

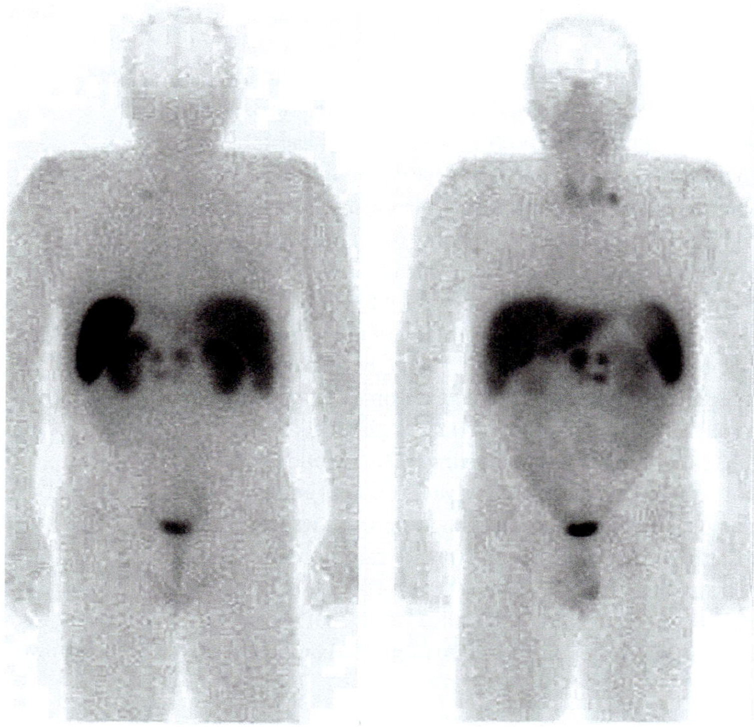

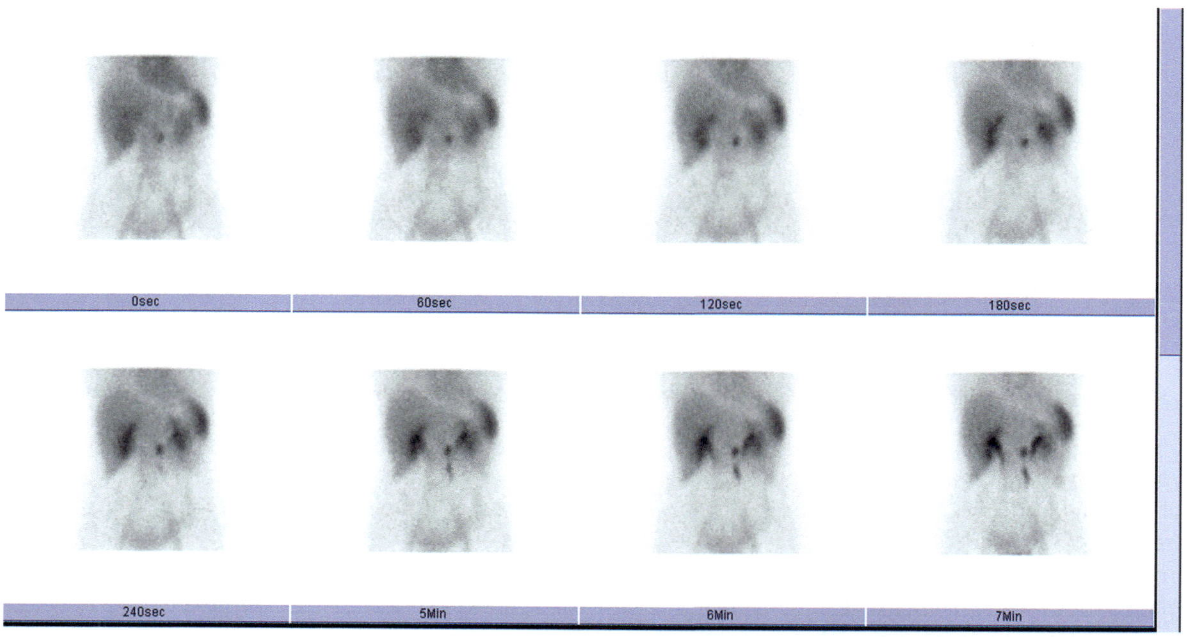

Fig. 3 Eight 1-min dynamic images of the abdomen immediately after tracer injection showing fast tracer uptake by the tumor

years. It has suboptimal energy for imaging, a high absorbed dose for the patients, is expensive and is not readily available. The three-dimensional structure of ^{99m}Tc-octreotide is not exactly the same as the ^{111}In-labeled one. ^{99m}Tc-octreotide profits from nearly ideal imaging characteristics of ^{99m}Tc, is inexpensive and always available if produced locally, but allows imaging maximally 24 h post-injection. This does not appear to be an important disadvantage since tracer uptake by NET is very rapid, seen already in the first minutes after injection (Fig. 3). An appropriate low amount of the octreotide can be labeled with high enough ^{99m}Tc activity to allow good image resolution, also using SPECT up to 24 h post injection. From the quality of the images obtained, 24 h post-injection it appears that labeling of the peptide is stable not only in vitro but also in vivo. Diagnosis and localization of somatostatine-expressing tumors as well as somatostatine-expressing tumor spread can be determined with higher sensitivity using ^{99m}Tc-EDDA/HYNIC-TOC than ^{111}In-octreotide [113]; also ^{99m}Tc-EDDA/HYNIC-TOC allows earlier diagnosis (10 min–4 h) compared with ^{111}In-DTPA-octreotide (4–24 h) [114]. Its advantages are availability, low cost, decreased absorbed dose for the patients and high quality of scintigraphic images [115].

References

112. Von Guggenberg, Sarg E, Lindtner H, et al. Preparation via coligand exchange and characterization of 99m-Tc-EDDA-HYNIC-D-Phe1, Tyr3-octreotide (99m-Tc-EDDA/HYNIC-TOC). J Label Compd Radiopharm. 2003;46:07–18.
113. Gabriel M, Decrisoforo C, Donnemiller E, et al. An intra-patient comparison of ^{99m}Tc-EDDA/HYNIC-TOC with ^{111}In-DTPA-octreotide for diagnosis of somatostatin receptor-expressing tumors. J Nucl Med. 2003;44:708–16.
114. Bangard M, Behe M, Guhlke S, et al. Detection of somatostatin receptor-positive tumors using the new ^{99m}Tc-tricine-HYNIC-D-Phe^{1}-Tyr^{3}-octreotide: first results in patients and comparison with ^{111}In-DTPA-D-Phe^{1}-octreotide. Eur J Nucl Med. 2000;27:628–37.
115. Kolenc P, Fettich J, Slodnjak I, et al. Comparison of ^{99m}Tc-EDDA/HYNIC-TOC and ^{111}In-DTPA-octreotide uptake in patients without know pathology. Eur J Nucl Med Mol Imaging. 2004;31 Suppl 2:358 (abs).

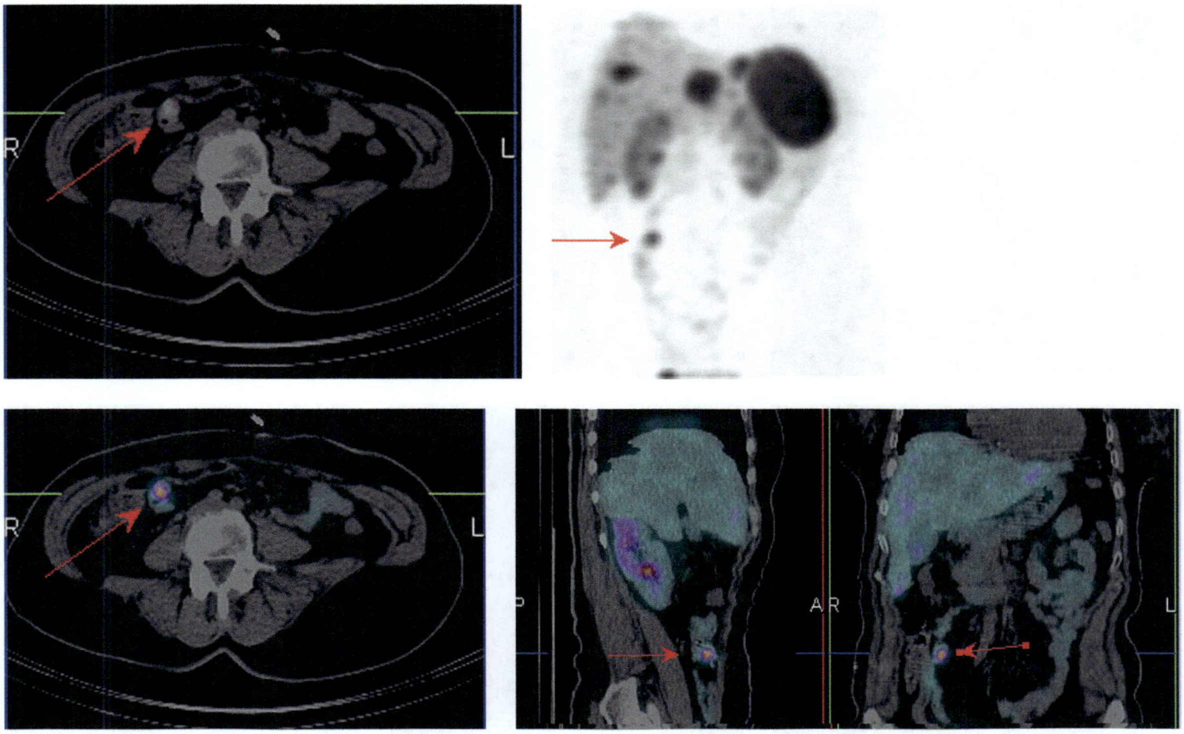

^{99m}Tc HYNIC-TOC finding

Increased tracer uptake in the terminal ileum and in the liver.

Teaching point

The terminal ileum is a typical localization for midgut NE carcinomas. Patients with midgut NET frequently present with clinical signs and symptoms of carcinoid syndrome only after liver metastases are present. In some hospitals surgeons tend to remove the primary tumor even when liver metastases are present to prevent development of mesenteric fibrosis and consequent problems with bowel passage, including ileus.

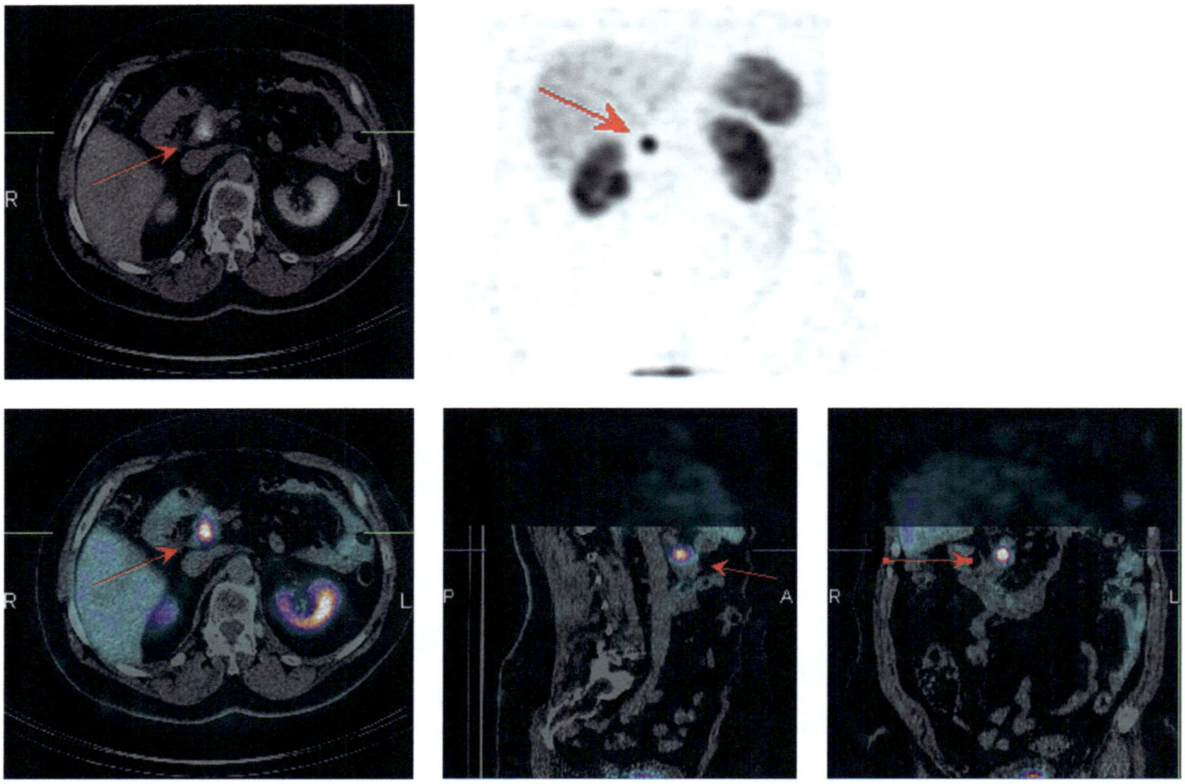

^{99m}Tc HYNIC-TOC finding

SPECT-CT images show increased tracer uptake in the head of the pancreas, biochemically insulinoma.

Teaching point

In case of a solitary lesion with expressed somatostatin receptors and good tracer uptake, radioguided surgery using a gamma probe may be used after injection of 99 m-Tc HYNIC-TOC a few hours before surgery.

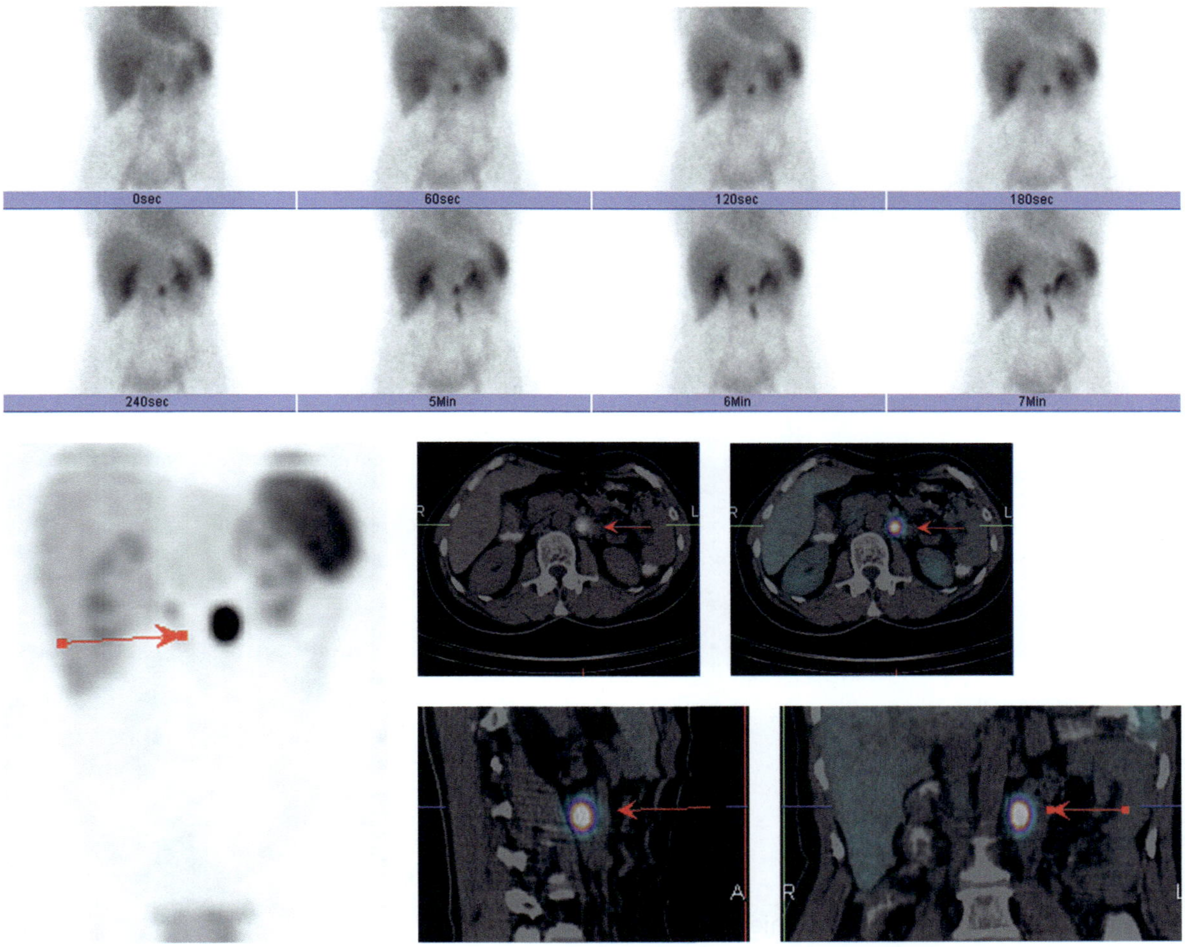

■ ^{99m}Tc HYNIC-TOC finding

Dynamic images of the abdomen immediately after tracer injection and SPECT-CT images 4 h post-injection revealing a solitary lesion in the abdomen located in the paraaortic lymph node.

Teaching point

CT allows exact localization of the lesion and therefore differentiation between primary tumor in the intestinal wall or pancreas (see case no. 1 and 2) vs. metastasis in the lymph node.

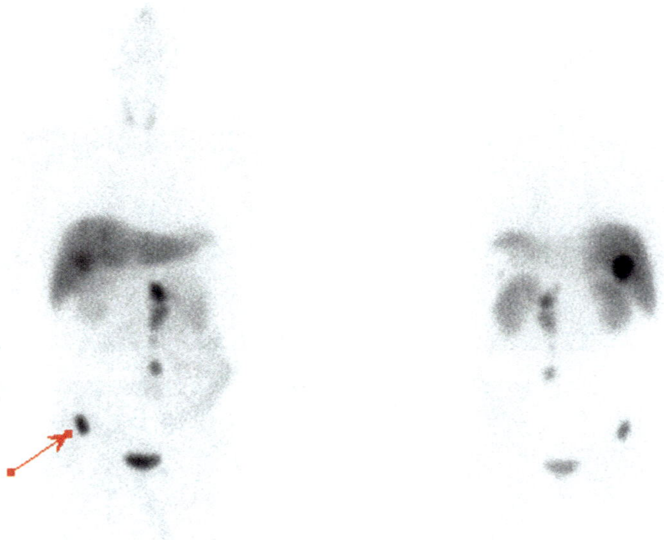

^{99m}Tc HYNIC-TOC findings

99 m-Tc HYNIC-TOC study 4 h post-injection reveals several metastases in the liver and abdomen.

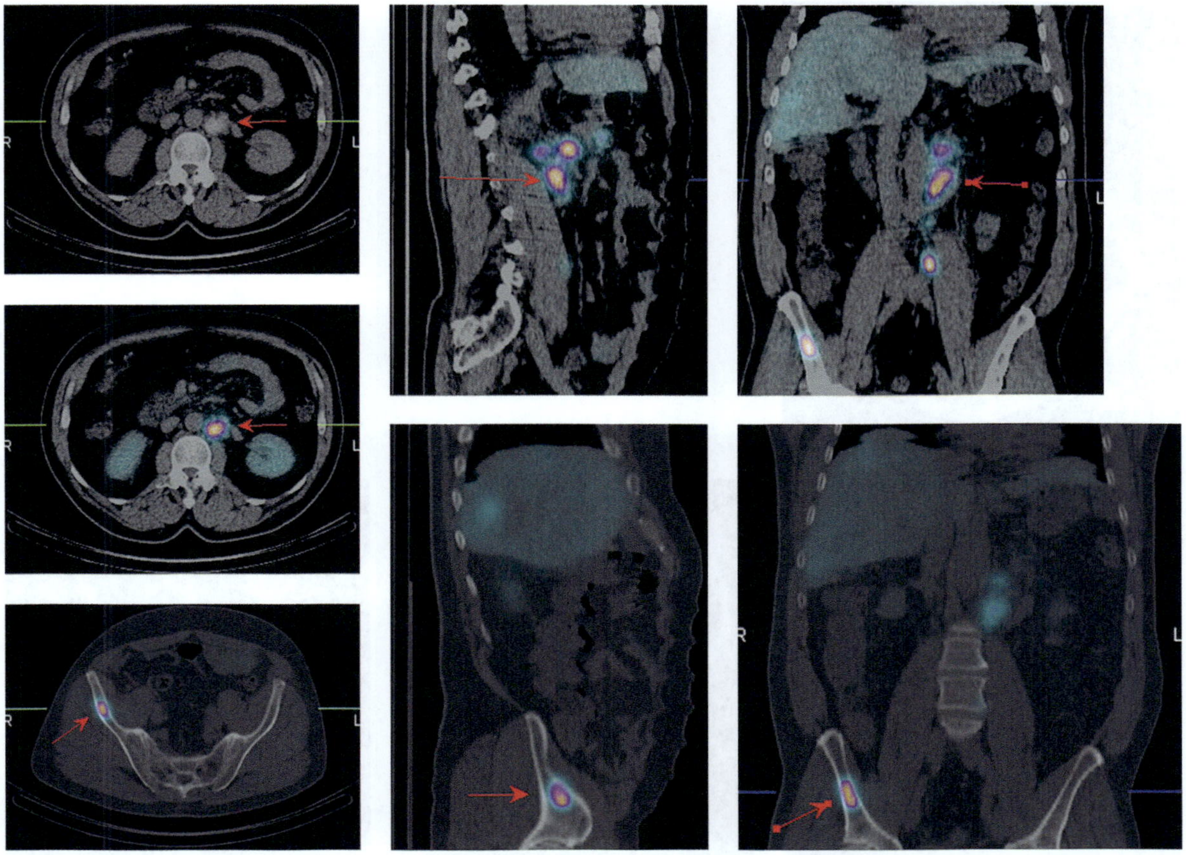

Teaching point

An important contribution of the CT component is localization of the abdominal metastases in paraaortic (*arrow*) lymph nodes and one located in the bone (*lower arrow*).

Presence of bony metastases is considered to be a contraindication for radiotherapy using 90-Y or 177-Lu octreotide in patients with metastatic spread of neuroendocrine carcinoma.

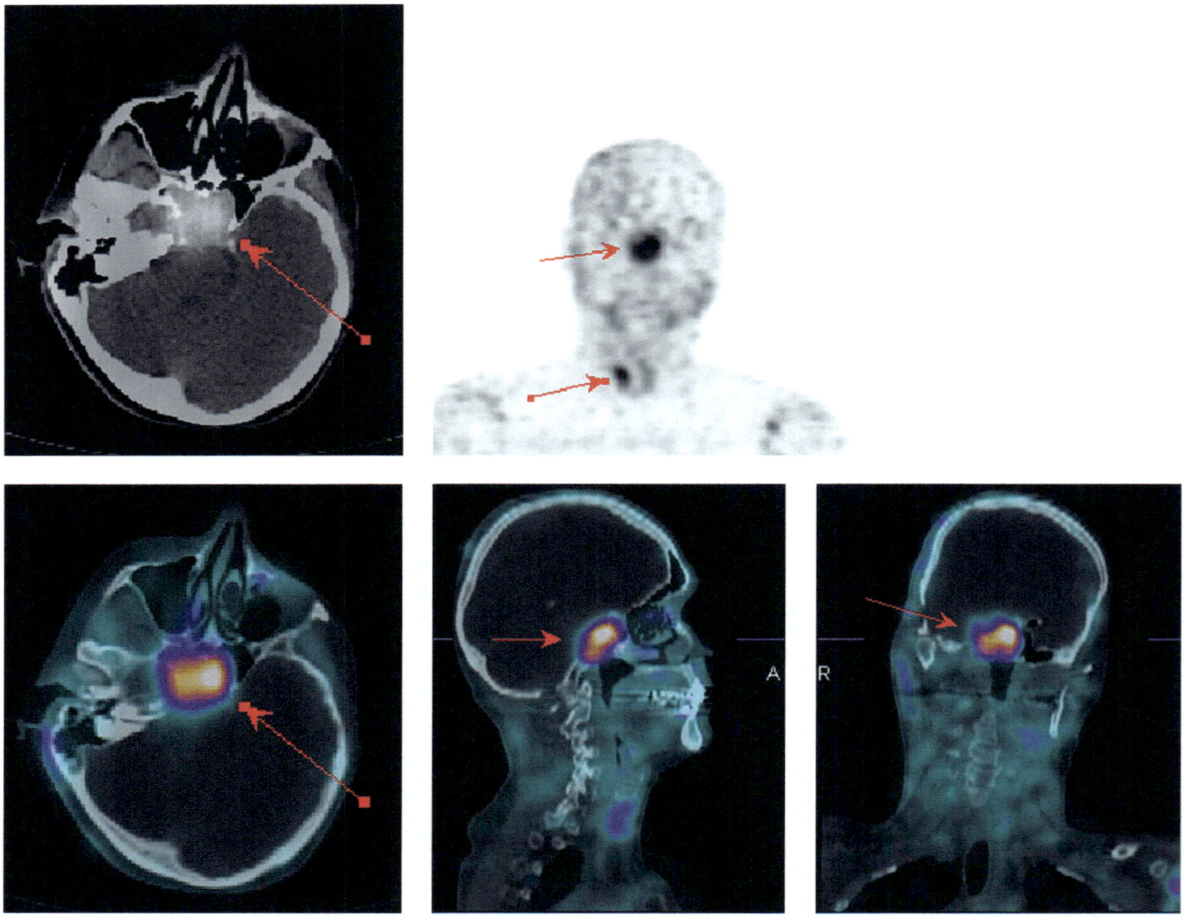

^{99m}Tc HYNIC-TOC finding

Images show invasive adenoma of the hypophysis pituitary gland invading after unsuccessful surgery (*upper arrow*).

Teaching point

Confirmation of expression of somatostatine receptors is necessary if the tumor is inoperable and octreotide (Somatostatin LAR@) therapy is planned.

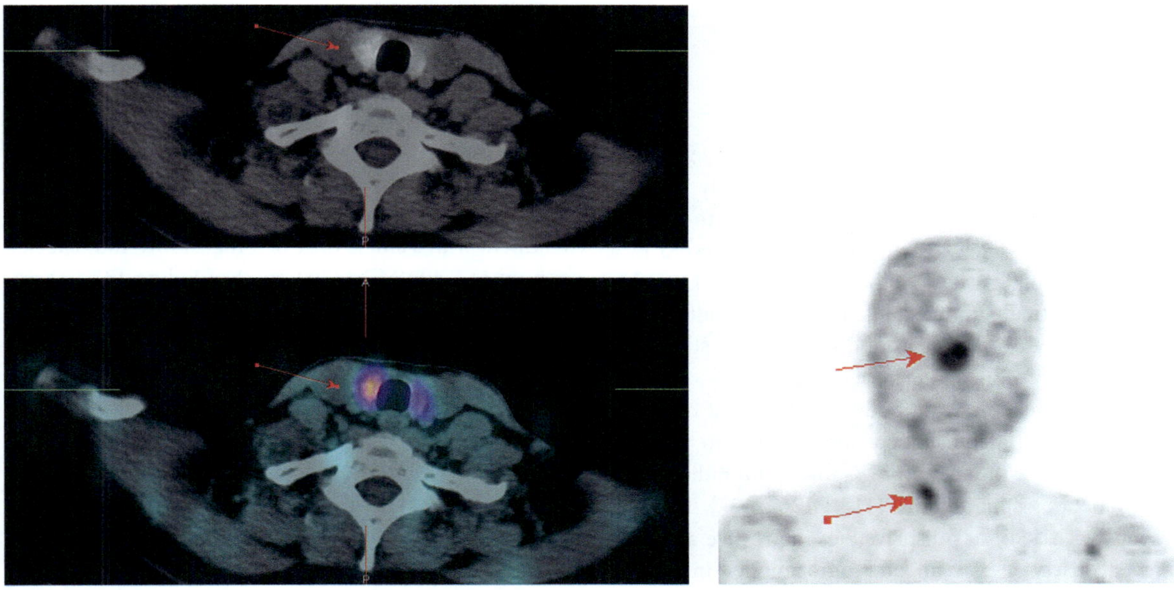

^{99m}Tc HYNIC-TOC finding

The same patient: incidental finding of increased tracer uptake in the thyroid (*lower arrow*). After appropriate clinical workup (serum calcitinine and fine-needle biopsy of the node), medullary carcinoma of the thyroid was diagnosed.

Teaching point

In case of NET tumors that can be part of multiple endocrine neoplasia (MEN) syndromes, the whole body needs to be imaged.

3.6 New Tracers

Paola A. Erba (✉)

The human recombinant mini-antibody L19 selectively binds the angiogenesis-related, alternatively spliced extra-domain B (ED-B) of fibronectin, one to three a tumor-stroma-associated antigen widely expressed in a variety of normal tissues and body fluids [116–123] This antigen is virtually undetectable in normal adult tissues, but is strongly expressed around neovascular structures in the majority of malignancies [124, 125].

The ^{131}I-labeled L19 antibody in SIP format has been shown in three different independent studies to be superior compared to the scFv and IgG format for radioimmunotherapeutic applications [118, 126, 127]. Indeed, ^{131}I-labeled L19SIP has displayed an impressive ability to target a variety of experimental tumor models in rodents and to stain a large variety of human tumor specimens, thus making it a potentially suitable candidate for radioimmunotherapeutic applications. The dosimetries displayed by ^{131}I-L19SIP in murine models of cancer are among the best reported so far in the field of radioimmunotherapy [128, 129]. Furthermore, ^{131}I-L19SIP has displayed a therapeutic benefit in rodent models of human cancer.

Thus, the mini-antibody L19 has been evaluated in a phase I and a subsequent phase I/II dose finding and efficacy study in patients with a variety of advanced cancers where ^{131}I-L19SIP has shown a selective uptake to tumor tissues and an excellent tolerability at radioactive doses as high as 7,400 MBq (200 mCi), and therapeutic benefit for some patients enrolled in the study [130–133]. At this stage, it is in a two-phase I/II trial in combination with external beam radiotherapy and concurrent chemotherapy in patients with inoperable, locally advanced (stage III) NSCLC and with whole brain radiation therapy in patients with multiple brain metastases from solid tumors.

All the studies are designed to obtain a first dose of ^{131}I-L19SIP radiolabeled with up to 185 MBq (5 mCi) for dosimetric purposes ("dosimetric phase"). Following i.v. administration, whole body, planar images and SPECT-CT are recorded at several time points (typically including 30 min, 2–6 h, 24 h, 48 h, 72 h and >90 h). Additionally, blood samples are collected for PK determination. The resulting images are used to calculate the radiation doses absorbed by the tumor lesions and all major organs. Whenever the radiation dose in at least one tumor lesion is found to be appropriate (at least ten-fold higher compared to the dose delivered to the bone marrow, the rate-limiting organ for phase I study, and four-fold higher compared to the dose delivered to normal muscle in the phase I/II dose finding), the patient became eligible for a treatment with a single dose of 5 mg L19SIP radiolabeled with up to 7,400 MBq (200 mCi) of iodine-131 ("therapeutic phase").

The following images demonstrate some examples of ^{131}I-L19SIP selective uptake in a series of patients with both hematological malignancies and solid cancers enrolled in the phase I and phase I/II trials and studied at the Regional Center of Nuclear Medicine of the University of Pisa Medical School, Italy (Figs. 1–5).

F16 antibody in the same SIP format has been introduced more recently to target the extra-domain A1 of tenascin-C, another very interesting component of the modified extracellular matrix, which is strongly overexpressed at tumor sites, with a prominent perivascular pattern of expression [116, 117]. The F16 antibody recognizes the alternatively spliced domain A1 of tenascin, one of the best characterized markers of angiogenesis [133]. Tenascin-C is an extracellular matrix component that is widely expressed in a variety of normal tissues and body fluids. Different Tenascin-C isoforms can be generated by alternative splicing of the Ten-C pre-mRNA, a process that is modulated by cytokines and extracellular pH. The domains A1 to D may be included or omitted in the Ten-C molecule. The Ten-C isoform containing the domain A1 is undetectable immunohistochemically in normal adult tissues, with the exception of tissues undergoing physiological remodeling (e.g., endometrium and ovary) and during wound healing. By contrast, its expression in tumors and fetal tissues is high; A1(+)-tenascin-C is strongly expressed in multiple cancers at levels as high as L19, but there are certain human tumors where its expression is predominant (i.e., breast cancer and some lung cancers) [126, 132, 134]. The possibility of selectively targeting tumoral vasculature using the human recombinant antibody fragment scFv (F16), specific to the domain A1 of Tenascin-C, has been reported in animal models of cancer, and a murine monoclonal antibody to the same antigen has been shown to be able to selectively accumulate at tumor sites in patients with cancer [135]. These investigations have paved the way for

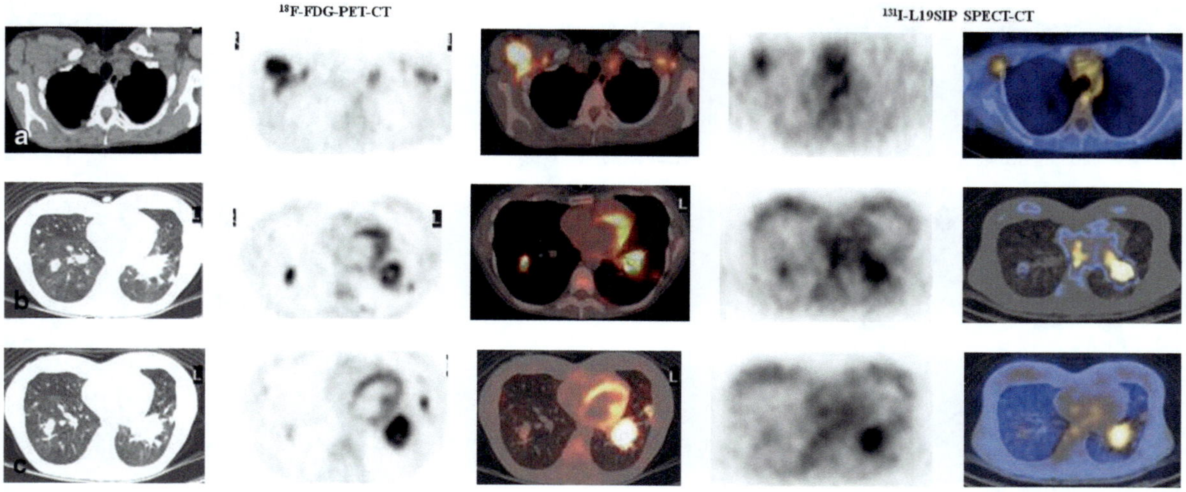

Fig. 1 Selective uptake of ^{131}I-L19SIP in a patient with HD. [^{18}F]FDG PET/CT scans on *left column* show intense glucose metabolism in multiple enlarged supraclavicular, axillary and mediastinal lymph-nodes (**a**) as well as in intrapulmonary lesions (**b**, **c**). The same patient received intravenous injection of ^{131}I-L19-SIP imaging for diagnostic (185 MBq) and therapeutic (5,550 MBq) purposes. SPECT/CT transaxial images of the thorax are shown, demonstrating selective uptake of ^{131}I-L19-SIP into the ^{18}F-FDG avid lymphomatous lesions (*right column*)

the construction of several therapeutic derivatives of scFv(F16), which have been extensively tested in animal models of cancer. Importantly, F16 fused to human interleukin-2 has entered multicenter clinical trials in Europe in combination with doxorubicin or taxol for the therapy of breast, lung and ovarian cancer.

Similarly to ^{131}I-L19, iodine-131 radiolabeled F16 has been recently evaluated in a phase I/II dose finding and efficacy study in patients with a variety of advanced cancers (same protocol design of L19).

Figure 6 reports an illustrative example of ^{131}I-F16 accumulation in a patient with MALT-B nHL.

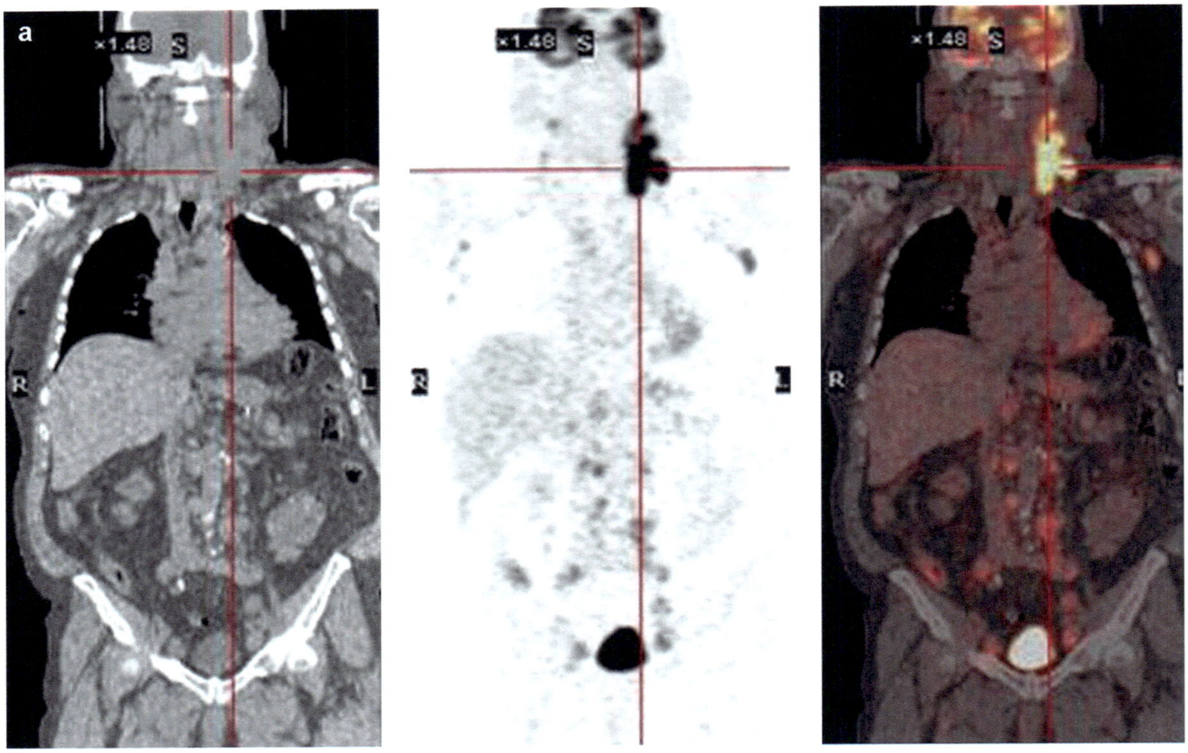

Fig. 2 ^{131}I-L19SIP uptake in lymphoma lesions in a patient with NHL SLL. (**a**) [^{18}F]FDG PET/CT scans demonstrate intense glucose metabolism in multiple enlarged lymph nodes, particularly in the left latero-cervical region. Coronal images are shown on the *left*, and transaxial images of the cervical regions are displayed on the *right side* panel. (**b**) The same patient received an intravenous infusion of ^{131}I-L19SIP: 185 and 5,550 MBq for diagnostic and therapeutic purposes, respectively. Transaxial, coronal and sagittal SPECT/CT images of the cervical regions (**b**–**d**, respectively) were acquired 8 days after the therapeutic dose of 5,550 MBq. *Left column* shows scintigraphic images, *central column* CT images and *right column* CT scintigraphy fused images

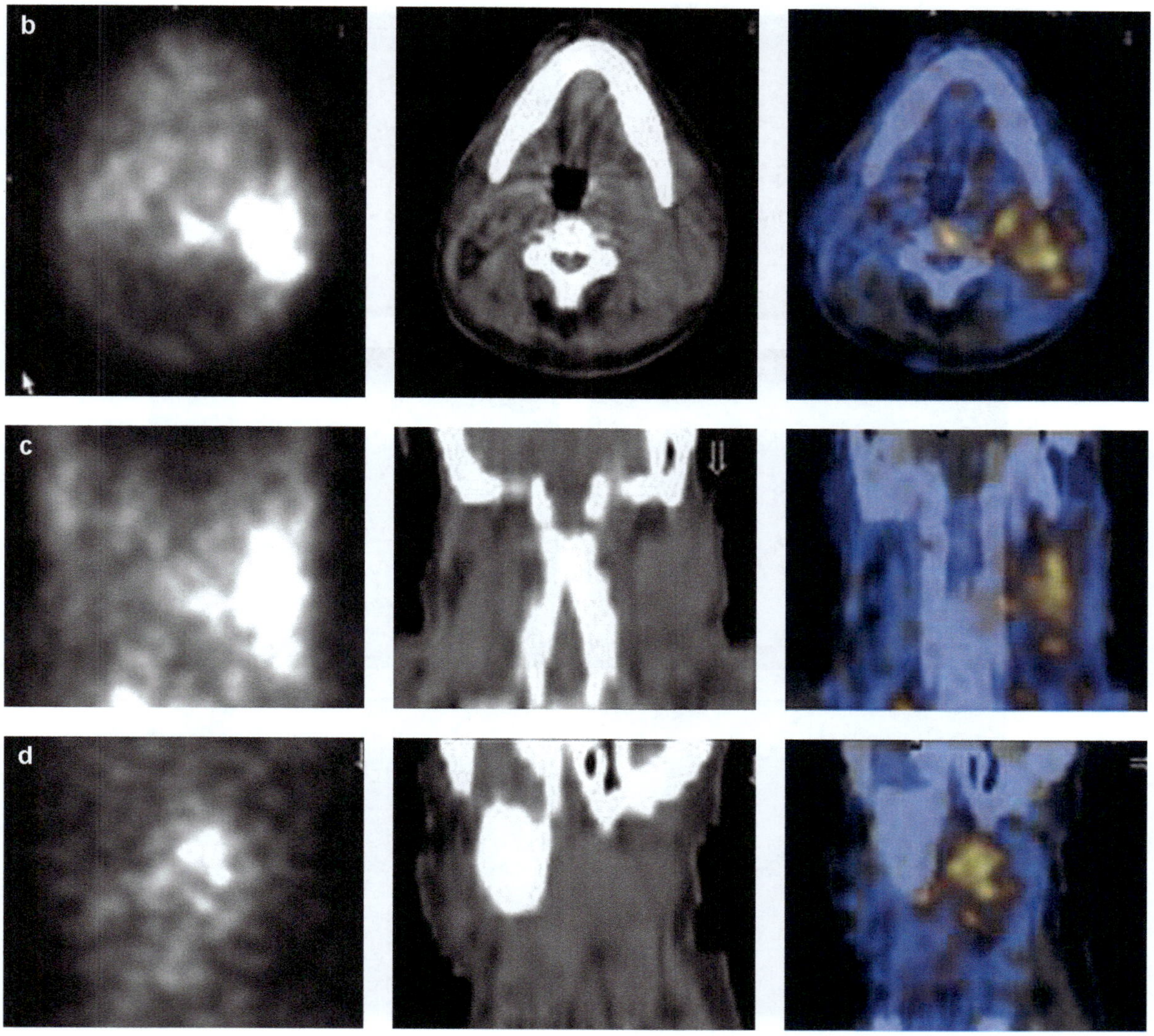

Fig. 2 (continued)

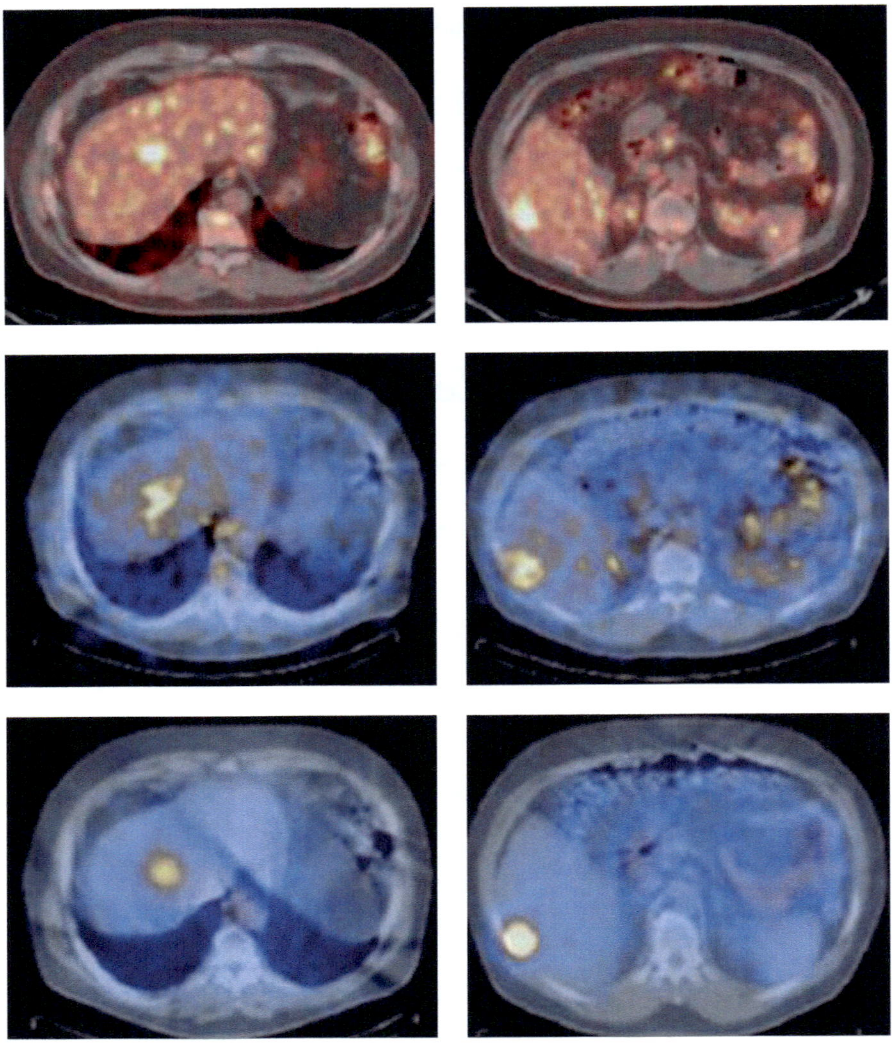

Fig. 3 ^{131}I-L19SIP uptake in patient with metastatic thymoma. Selective uptake of the radiopharmaceutical is clearly detectable in liver lesions as demonstrated in the diagnostic transaxial fused SPECT/CT images (*central panel*) (185 MBq) and further confirmed in post-radioimmunotherapy transaxial fused SPECT/CT images acquired 8 days after the therapeutic dose of 8,140 MBq (*lower panel*). [^{18}F]FDG PET/CT corresponding to transaxial fused images (*upper panel*) demonstrates intense glucose metabolism in the same lesions

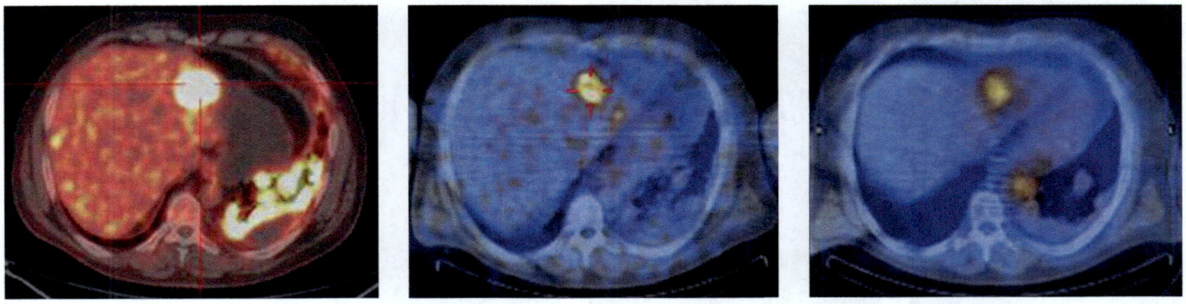

Fig. 4 ^{131}I-L19SIP uptake in a patient with lung SCLC and liver metastasis. Selective uptake of the radiopharmaceutical is clearly detectable in a single liver lesion as demonstrated in the diagnostic transaxial SPECT/CT fused images (185 MBq, *central column*) and post-radioimmunotherapy transaxial SPECT/CT fused images acquired 7 days after the therapeutic dose of 9,990 MBq (*right column*). [^{18}F]FDG-PET/CT corresponding to transaxial fused images (*left column*) demonstrates intense glucose metabolism in the same lesions

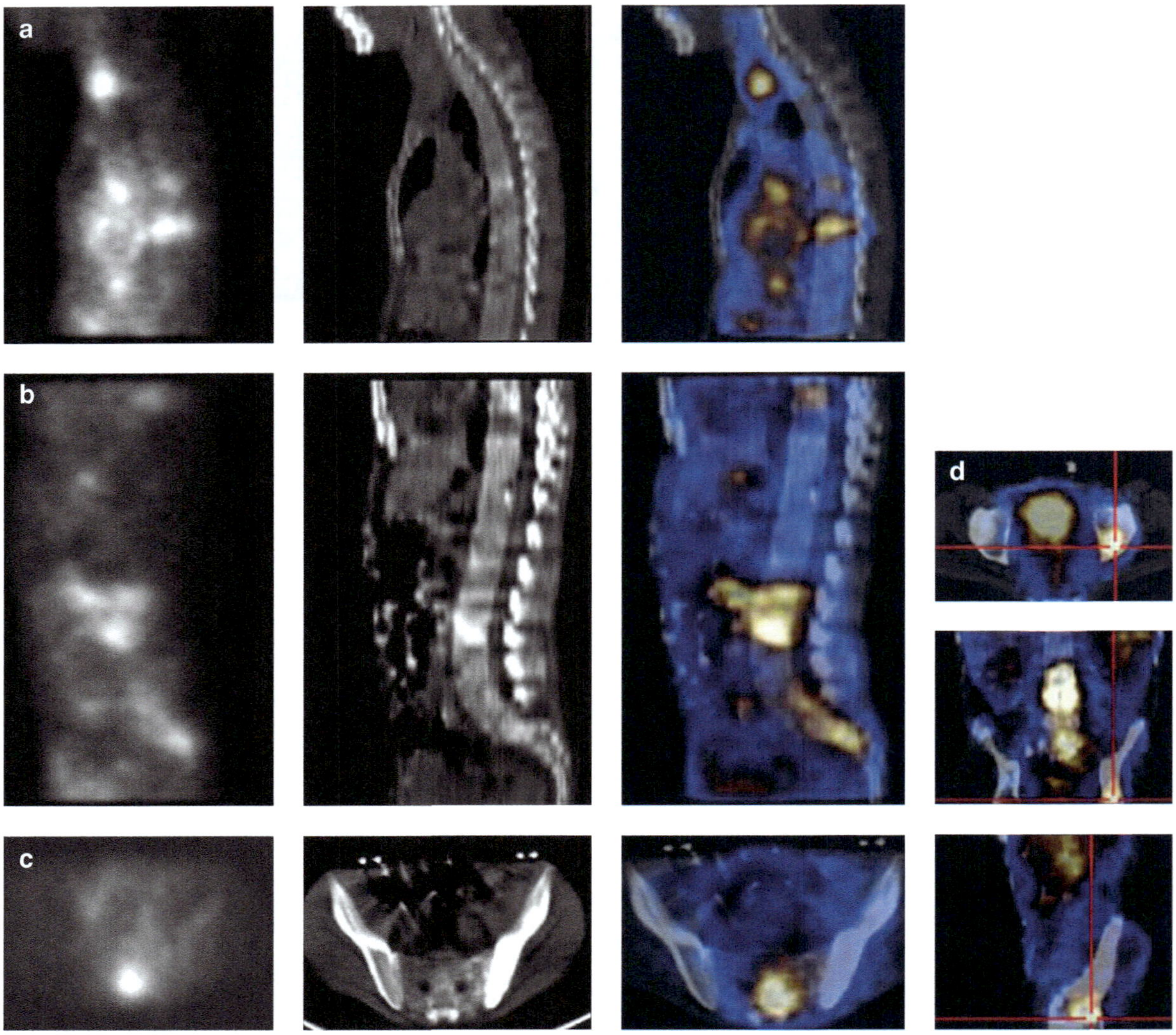

Fig. 5 ^{131}I-L19 uptake in a patient with metastatic thymoma. Intense radiopharmaceutical uptake is clearly detectable in multiple bone lesions at post-radioimmunotherapy transaxial SPECT/CT images acquired 10 days after the therapeutic dose of 1,850 MBq. Lesions are located in the spine (**a**, **b**, *left column* sagittal SPECT images, *central column* CT images and *right column* fused images), sacrum (**c**, *left column* transaxial SPECT images, *central column* CT images and *right column* fused images) and in the left femoral epiphysis (**d** transaxial, coronal and sagittal fused images)

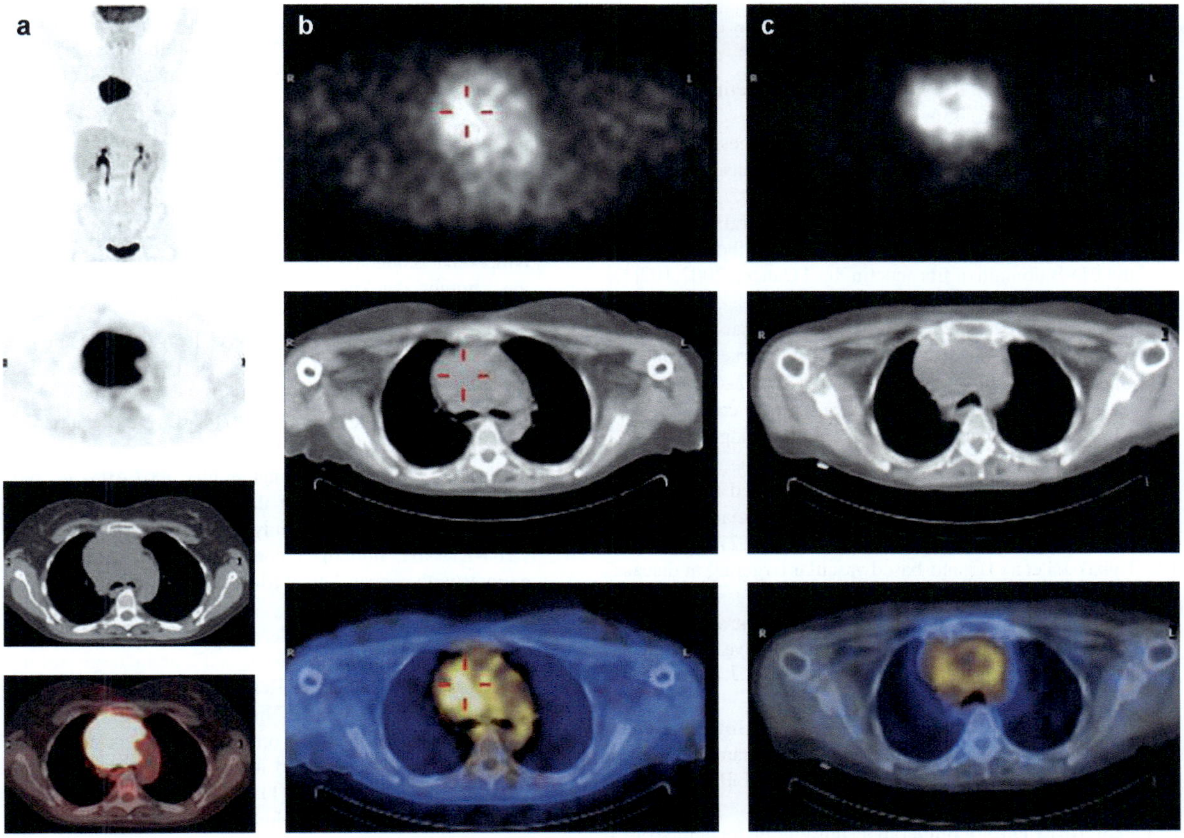

Fig. 6 Post-radioimmunotherapy transaxial SPECT/CT images (**b**, **c**, *upper line* transaxial SPECT images, *central line* CT images and *lower line* fused images) acquired 7 days after the therapeutic dose of 1,850 MBq of ^{131}I-F16 in a patient with MALT-B nHL. Intense radiopharmaceutical uptake is clearly detectable in the large mediastinal mass identified by [^{18}F] FDG-PET/CT (**a**, *upper line* MIP projection and corresponding transaxial emission, CT and fused images)

References

116. Neri D, Bicknell R. Tumor vascular targeting. Nat Rev Cancer. 2005;5(6):436–46.
117. Trachsel E, Neri D. Antibodies for angiogenesis inhibition, vascular targeting and endothelial cell transcytosis. Adv Drug Deliv Rev. 2006;58(5–6):735–54.
118. Borsi L et al. Selective targeting of tumoral vasculature: comparison of different formats of an antibody (L19) to the ED-B domain of fibronectin. Int J Cancer. 2002;102(1): 75–85.
119. Carnemolla B et al. Phage antibodies with pan-species recognition of the oncofetal angiogenesis marker fibronectin ED-B domain. Int J Cancer. 1996;68(3):397–405.
120. Castellani P et al. The fibronectin isoform containing the ED-B oncofetal domain: a marker of angiogenesis. Int J Cancer. 1994;59(5):612–8.
121. Neri D et al. Targeting by affinity-matured recombinant antibody fragments of an angiogenesis associated fibronectin isoform. Nat Biotechnol. 1997;15(12): 1271–5.
122. Rybak JN et al. Ligand-based vascular targeting of disease. Chem Med Chem. 2007;2(1):22–40.
123. Zardi L et al. Transformed human cells produce a new fibronectin isoform by preferential alternative splicing of a previously unobserved exon. EMBO J. 1987;6(8): 2337–42.
124. Castellani P et al. Differentiation between high- and low-grade astrocytoma using a human recombinant antibody to the extra domain-B of fibronectin. Am J Pathol. 2002; 161(5):1695–7003.
125. Pedretti M et al. Comparative immunohistochemistry of L19 and F16 in non-small cell lung cancer and mesothelioma: two human antibodies investigated in clinical trials in patients with cancer. Lung Cancer. 2009;64(1):28–33.
126. Berndorff D et al. Radioimmunotherapy of solid tumors by targeting extra domain B fibronectin: identification of the best-suited radioimmunoconjugate. Clin Cancer Res. 2005;11(19 Pt 2):7053s-63.
127. Tijink BM et al. Radioimmunotherapy of head and neck cancer xenografts using 131I-labeled antibody L19-SIP for selective targeting of tumor vasculature. J Nucl Med. 2006;47(7): 1127–35.
128. Sauer S et al. Expression of the oncofetal ED-B-containing fibronectin isoform in hematologic tumors enables ED-B-targeted 131I-L19SIP radioimmunotherapy in Hodgkin lymphoma patients. Blood. 2009;113(10):2265–74.
129. Schliemann C et al. Complete eradication of human B-cell lymphoma xenografts using rituximab in combination with the immunocytokine L19-IL2. Blood. 2009;113(10): 2275–83.
130. Tosi DCA, Chiesa C, et al. Phase I dosimetric study of 131I-L19-SIP in solid tumors. AACR congress, Los Angeles, April 2007:Abstract 1659.
131. Bombardieri ECA, Chiesa C, et al. Phase I study with antifibronectin I-131 L19-SIP: first dosimetric and therapeutic results. SNM Meeting, Washington, June 2007:Abstract 1681.
132. Erba P, Sollini M, Boni R et al. Results of a phase I/II dose finding and efficacy study of the tumor-targeting 131-I-L19SIP human recombinant mini-antibody in patients with cancer. J Nucl Med. 2010;51 (Supplement 2): 1153
133. Brack SS, Silacci M, Birchler M, Neri D. Tumor-targeting properties of novel antibodies specific to the large isoform of tenascin-C. Clin Cancer Res. 2006;12(10):3200–8.
134. Kaczmarek J, Castellani P, Nicolo G, Spina B, Allemanni G, Zardi L. Distribution of oncofetal fibronectin isoforms in normal, hyperplastic and neoplastic human breast tissues. Int J Cancer. 1994;59(1):11–6.
135. Siri A, Carnemolla B, Saginati M, Leprini A, Casari G, Baralle F, et al. Human tenascin: primary structure, pre-mRNA splicing patterns and localization of the epitopes recognized by two monoclonal antibodies. Nucleic Acids Research. 1991;19(3):525–31.
136. Wyss MT et al. Uptake of 18F-Fluorocholine, 18F-FET, and 18F-FDG in C6 gliomas and correlation with 131I-SIP(L19), a marker of angiogenesis. J Nucl Med. 2007;48(4):608–14.

Chapter 4 Bone Imaging with SPECT-CT

Torsten Kuwert

Contents

S. Fanti et al., *Atlas of SPECT-CT*,
DOI: 10.1007/978-3-642-15726-4_4, © Springer-Verlag Berlin Heidelberg 2011

In 2004, skeletal scintigraphy was the most frequently performed nuclear medical in vivo examination in Europe and can thus also be considered the most frequently performed procedure worldwide. The quantification of bone metabolism was also among the first applications of tracers in biology. The Letter to Nature published in 1935 by George de Hevesy, which earned him the Nobel Prize in 1943, described the use of radioactive strontium to investigate bone metabolism in rats.

The ^{99m}Tc-labeled polyphosphonates that are used today were introduced into the field approximately 30 years ago; since then, the procedure has, in principle, not changed much. Scintigraphic images acquired early after intravenous injection of these tracers provide information on the perfusion and floridity of skeletal lesions. Scintigraphy performed several hours after tracer injection allows insight into bone metabolism or, more specifically, osteoblastic activity, since the polyphosphonates are adsorbed on freshly built bone tissue. Initially, bone scintigrams were planar images, acquired either as spot views or as whole-body images. Because of the sensitivity of this examination in detecting osseous lesions, skeletal scintigraphy has been widely used as a screening tool, e.g., for staging malignant disease. In the late 1980s, single-photon emission computed tomography (SPECT) became widely available. SPECT allows three-dimensional visualization of the distribution of radioactivity within the human body. This technology has considerably improved the diagnostic accuracy of bone scintigraphy by allowing a better localization of areas exhibiting pathological tracer uptake. Nevertheless, because of the limitations in spatial resolution of skeletal SPECT, still being in the range of 8–10 mm in the reconstructed images, the specificity of skeletal scintigraphy is limited. This is true particularly when compared to radiological techniques such as X-ray computerized tomography (CT) or magnetic resonance imaging (MRI).

Approximately 8 years ago, the first hybrid camera integrating a SPECT camera with a CT scanner into one gantry became commercially available. The CT component of this system was a low-dose non-spiral CT. The CT images provided by this camera were without diagnostic quality, but allowed a fairly exact localization of SPECT foci of abnormal tracer uptake and the attenuation correction of the SPECT images. Since then, technology has advanced considerably. Currently, SPECT/CT cameras with a wide array of multislice spiral CT scanners are available, and evidence of their diagnostic performance is accumulating quickly.

The SPECT examination of SPECT/CT is not performed differently from that of a stand-alone system. For skeletal CT, the intravenous injection of contrast medium is usually not necessary. With the hybrid systems featuring a multi-slice spiral CT, a CT examination of the skeleton in full diagnostic quality is, at least in principle, possible. However, since the indication for this CT examination is to elucidate unclear scintigraphic findings, low-dose CT examinations with a field of view restricted to the scintigraphic abnormalities are advocated by most authorities in the field. The mAs products reported in the literature range between 15 and 60 mAs, also depending on the indication. With this so-called SPECT-guided CT, the radiation doses delivered to the patient come down to average values between 2 and 3 mSv in most cases and thus correspond to doses caused by planar radiographs.

The advantage of SPECT/CT compared to side-by-side evaluation of data sets acquired independently from each other is the possibility for pixel-wise integration of the information from both modalities. As patient movements between the two independently performed examinations are minor, the average anatomical accuracy of alignment between both sets of images is usually better than 5 mm. This variable can also be improved by additionally applying image fusion software to the preregistered images.

Based on the CT information on tissue absorption, the SPECT images of SPECT/CT can be attenuation-corrected and a more realistic and homogeneous image of tracer distribution obtained. An important prerequisite to using this option, however, is that the alignment between CT and SPECT images is well below SPECT pixel width; otherwise, gross attenuation artifacts may lead to false interpretation of the images.

For image interpretation, both image data sets are displayed on one computer workstation. As is also the case when interpreting stand-alone SPECT images, some attention should be given to standardizing SPECT windowing. We usually use tracer uptake in the iliac crest as the reference value for evaluating tracer uptake in pathological lesions. CT images should be viewed in the bone window centered on 500 Hounsfield units (HU) with a window width of 1,500 HU. We also routinely evaluate the CT scans in the lung and soft-tissue windows, although the image quality of the low-dose CT scans may not be fully sufficient for these purposes.

One of the major indications for performing skeletal scintigraphy is staging of malignant disease, as osseous metastases frequently lead to focally increased uptake of the ^{99m}Tc-polyphosphonates. Skeletal scintigraphy has a high sensitivity to detect osseous metastases of breast and prostate cancer as well as those of primary bone tumors such as Ewing's or osteogenic sarcoma. Its sensitivity is fairly high in several other neoplasms, such as bronchial or thyroid carcinoma. Several benign lesions of the skeleton may also have increased uptake of the ^{99m}Tc-polyphosphonates, which deteriorates the specificity of scintigraphy for staging malignancies. This is in particular the case for degenerative conditions, such as those of the spine involving osteochondrosis and facet arthritis. The incidence of spinal degeneration increases sharply with age: virtually absent in the young, it may affect nearly 50% of individuals older than 60 years. Another frequent condition occurring in the elderly is vertebral fractures due to osteoporosis, which are found in nearly 25% of postmenopausal women. Further fairly frequent differential diagnoses of skeletal hot spots are osteomyelitis and benign bone tumors, such as enchondroma. Most of these conditions can be diagnosed on CT scans because of their specific morphological appearance. Therefore, SPECT/CT is very helpful in staging tumors as it reduces the frequency of indeterminate readings from roughly 30% to less than 5%. As both examinations are performed directly after another in a one-stop shop, patients are spared further examinations, and the time to definite diagnosis is considerably shortened compared to the traditional approach.

Purely lytic metastases caused by, e.g., renal carcinoma or plasmocytoma, are frequently not accompanied by increases in osteoblastic activity and can be easily missed on bone scintigrams. However, they may lead to so-called cold lesions that have reduced tracer uptake compared to normal bone. The differential diagnosis of cold lesions also includes benign lesions such as hemangioma, again presenting with typical phenomenology on CT. Therefore, also in cold lesions, SPECT/CT may increase the specificity of skeletal scintigraphy.

Skeletal pain is the leading symptom in orthopedic patients. It has a wide range of differential diagnoses, including osteoarthritis, trauma, inflammation and bone tumors. Most of these diseases exhibit increased tracer uptake. Here, as in staging, the specificity of stand-alone skeletal scintigraphy can be quite low and is much improved by SPECT/CT coregistration. It has, in fact, been shown that SPECT/CT increases diagnostic accuracy by roughly 30% in orthopedic patients when compared to stand-alone radionuclide imaging. The molecular/functional information obtained by SPECT complements structural information provided by CT. It may, in particular, help determine the floridity of lesions, such as osteoarthritis or vertebral fractures, as this information can usually not be inferred from the morphological appearance of these lesions alone.

Loosening or infection of prostheses and other metallic implants are difficult to diagnose by CT or MRI. Whereas on CT images streak artifacts may compromise image quality, MRI is practically of no value for this indication. Bone scintigraphy, therefore, is of particular interest in this clinical setting. Despite the occurrence of streak artifacts on the CT images, areas of abnormal tracer uptake may still be localized on SPECT/CT fusion images, improving the diagnostic accuracy of scintigraphy.

Suggested Reading

Bockisch A, Freudenberg LS, Schmidt D, et al. Hybrid imaging by SPECT/CT and PET/CT: proven outcomes in cancer imaging. Semin Nucl Med. 2009;39:276–89.

Even-Sapir E, Flusser G, Lerman H, et al. SPECT/multislice low-dose CT: a clinically relevant constituent in the imaging algorithm of non oncologic patients referred for bone scintigraphy. J Nucl Med. 2007;48:319–24.

Gnanasegaran G, Barwick T, Adamson K, et al. Multislice SPECT/CT in benign and malignant bone disease: when the ordinary turns into the extraordinary. Semin Nucl Med. 2009;39:431–42.

Linke R, Kuwert T, Uder M, et al. Skeletal SPECT/CT of the peripheral extremities. AJR Am J Roentgenol. 2010;194(4): W329–35.

Mohan HK, Gnanasegaran G, Vijayanathan S, et al. SPECT/CT in imaging foot and ankle pathology – the demise of other coregistration techniques. Semin Nucl Med. 2010;40: 41–51.

Römer W, Nömayr A, Uder M, et al. SPECT-guided CT for evaluating unclear foci of increased bone metabolism in cancer patients. J Nucl Med. 2006;47:1382–8.

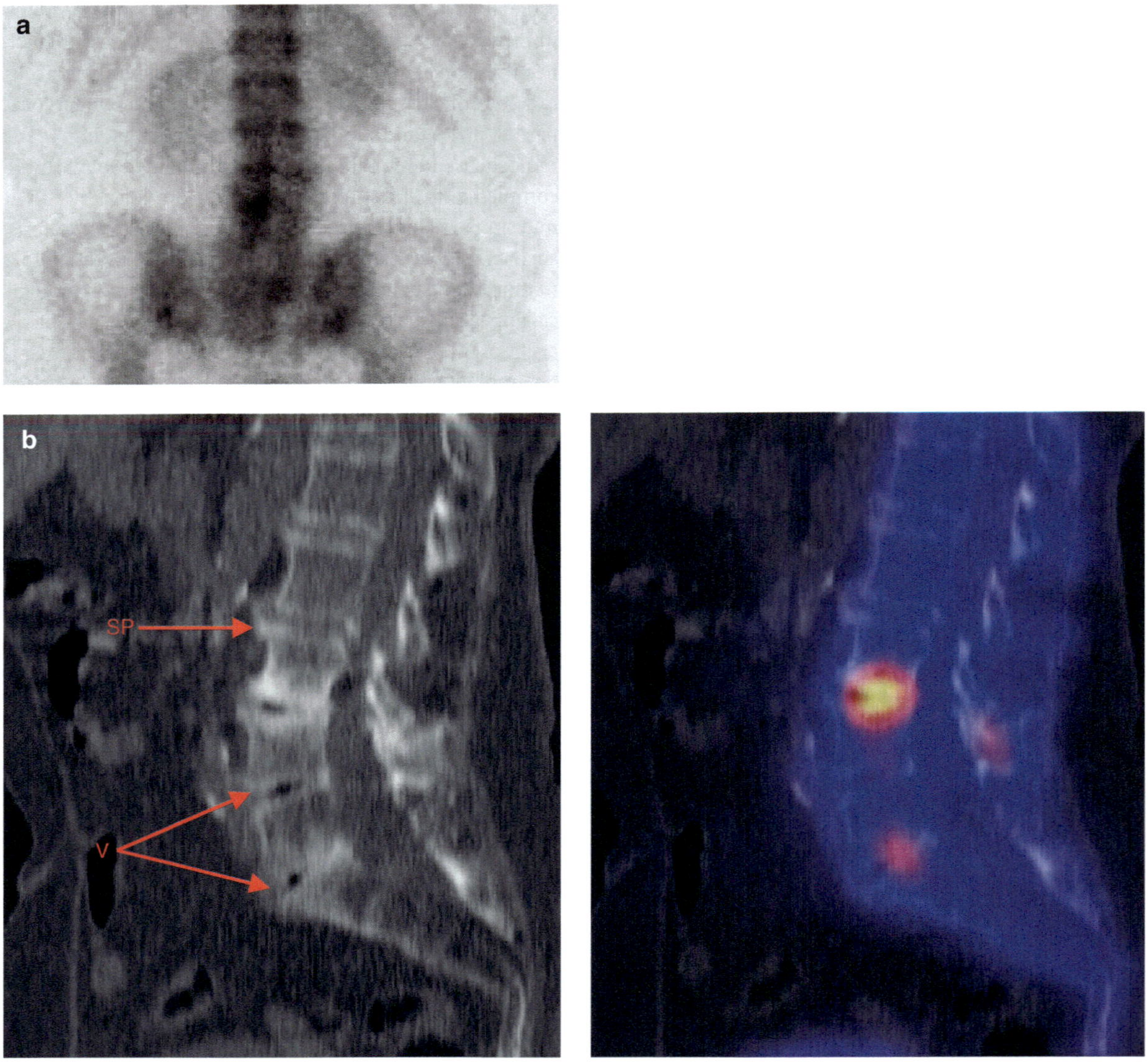

^{99m}Tc-polyphosphonate findings

Increased uptake projecting to osteochondrosis of L3/ L4 and, to lesser extent, also of L5/S1 in the skoliotic spine of a patient referred for staging breast cancer, in addition "kissing spine" L4/L5 (Baastrup's disease): (**a**) Planar; (**b**) Low-dose CT (30 mAs; *left*), SPECT/CT (*right*)

Teaching point

Note signs of spinal osteochondrosis: flattening of disk and, thus, thinning of intervertebral space, gas in disk as sign of degeneration (*V* vacuum phenomenon), subchondral sclerosis, spondylophytes (*SP* spondylosis deformans), and increased tracer uptake involving both segments.

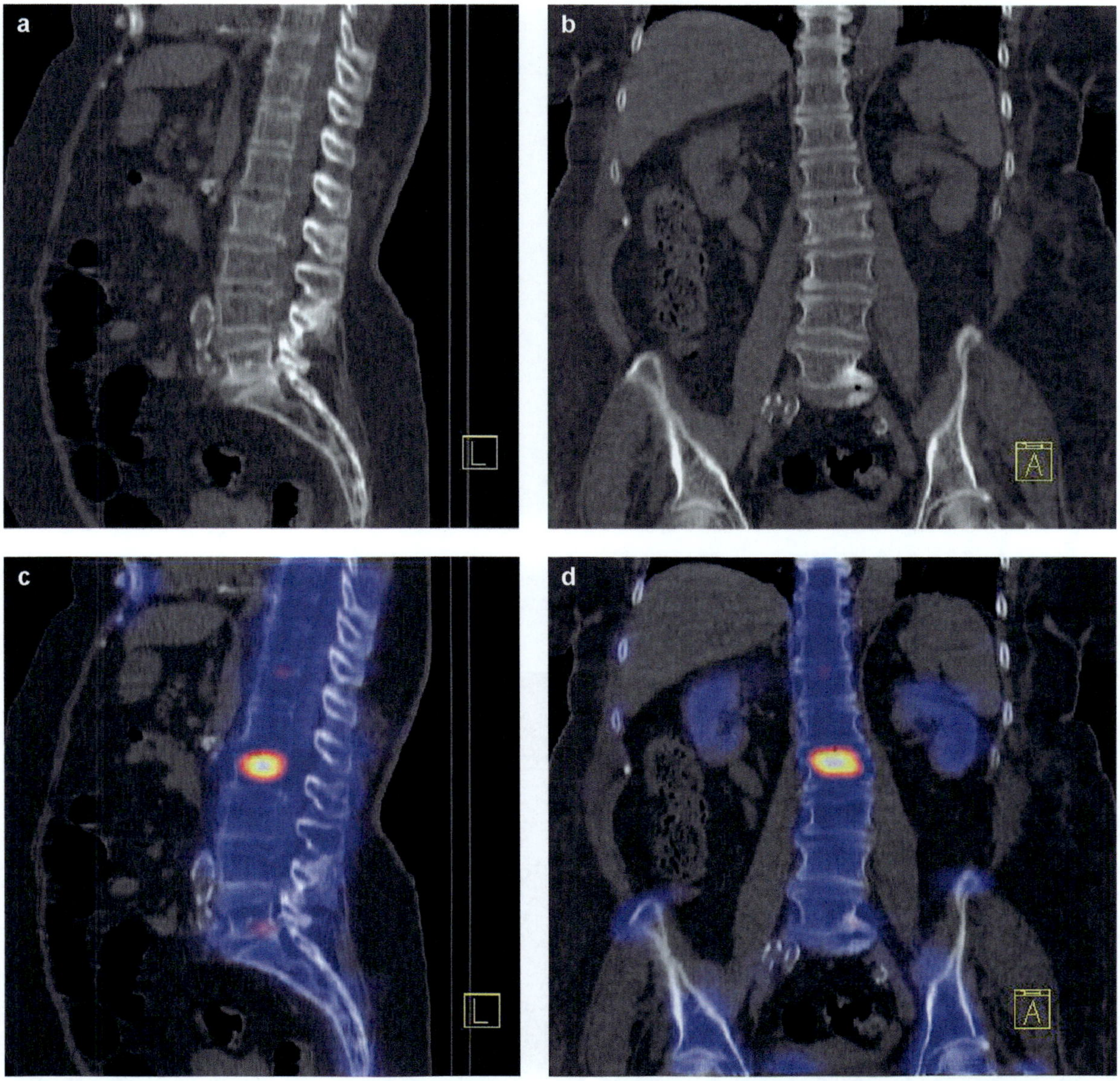

■ ^{99m}Tc-polyphosphonate findings

Increased uptake adjacent to small deck plate impression of vertebral body L2. In addition, discrete impression fracture also in T12 and slightly hypermetabolic left-sided osteochondrosis L5/S1 with osteosclerosis and spondylophytes in both vertebrae: CT (*upper row*), SPECT/CT (*lower row*); "*L*" and "*A*", view from lateral and anterior, respectively.

Teaching point

Note that in impression fractures abnormalities are usually seen only in one of the vertebral bodies adjacent to the end plate and not in both segments as in osteochondrosis. Older fractures may lack hypermetabolism.

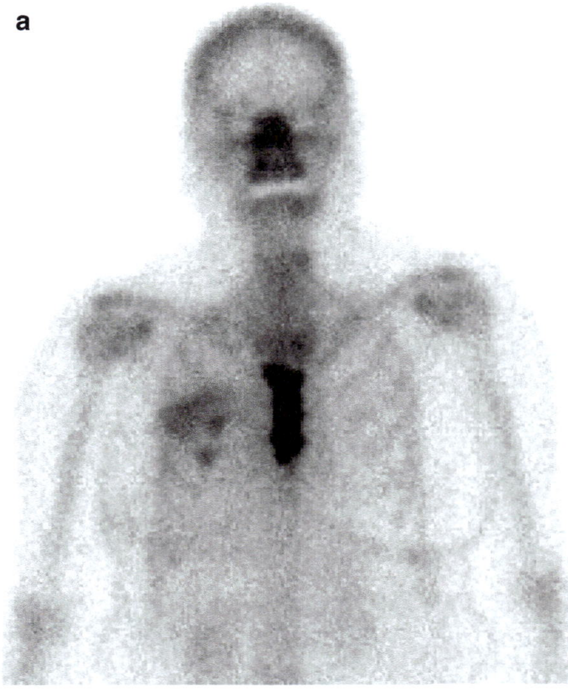
a

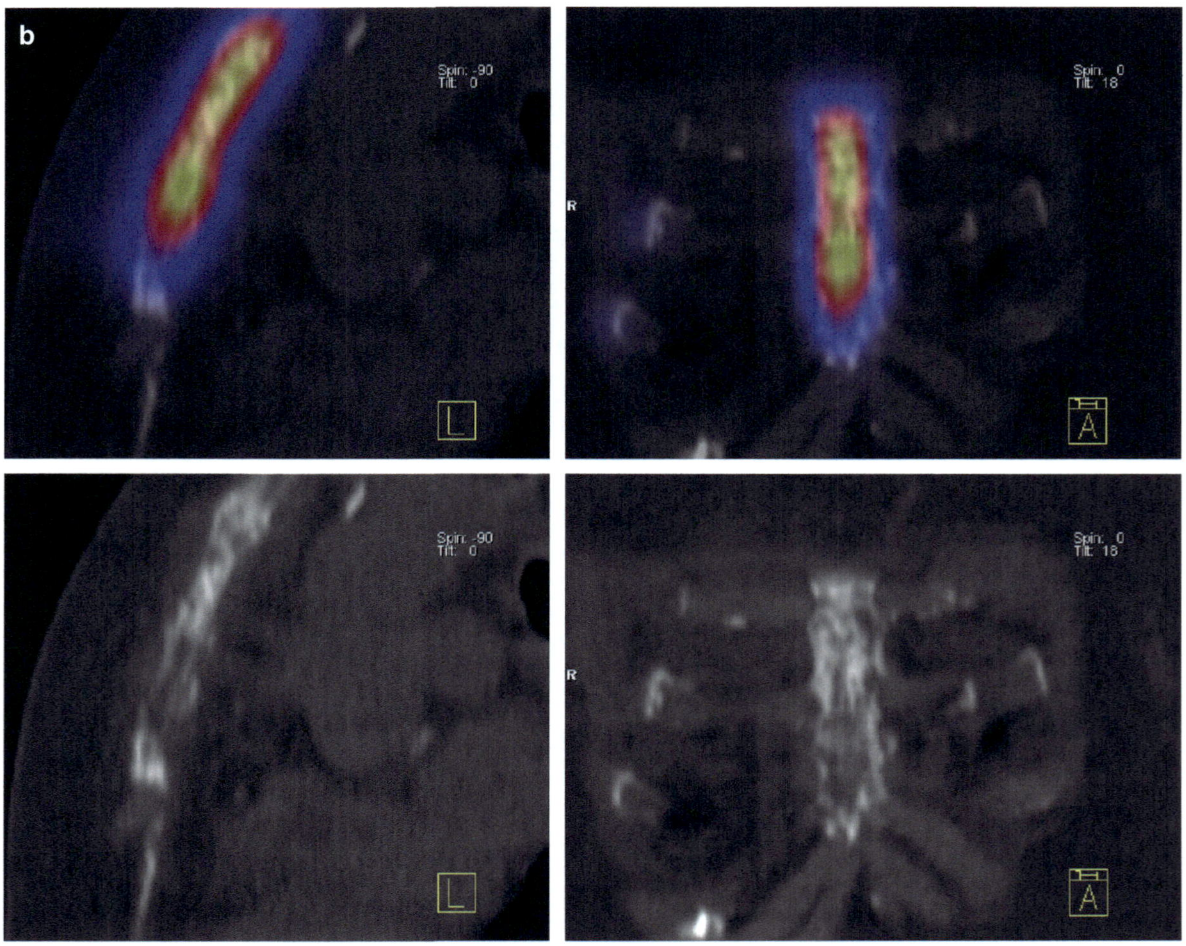
b
Spin: -90
Tilt: 0
L
Spin: 0
Tilt: 18
R
A

^{99m}Tc-polyphosphonate findings

Markedly increased uptake in the Corpus Sterni of a patient with breast cancer. CT shows predominantly lytic destruction of the bone with some reparative sclerotic changes. (**a**) Planar view from anterior; (**b**) SPECT/CT (*upper row*) and low-dose CT (30 mAs; *lower row*)

Teaching point

Osseous metastases may be osteoplastic, osteolytic, or mixed.

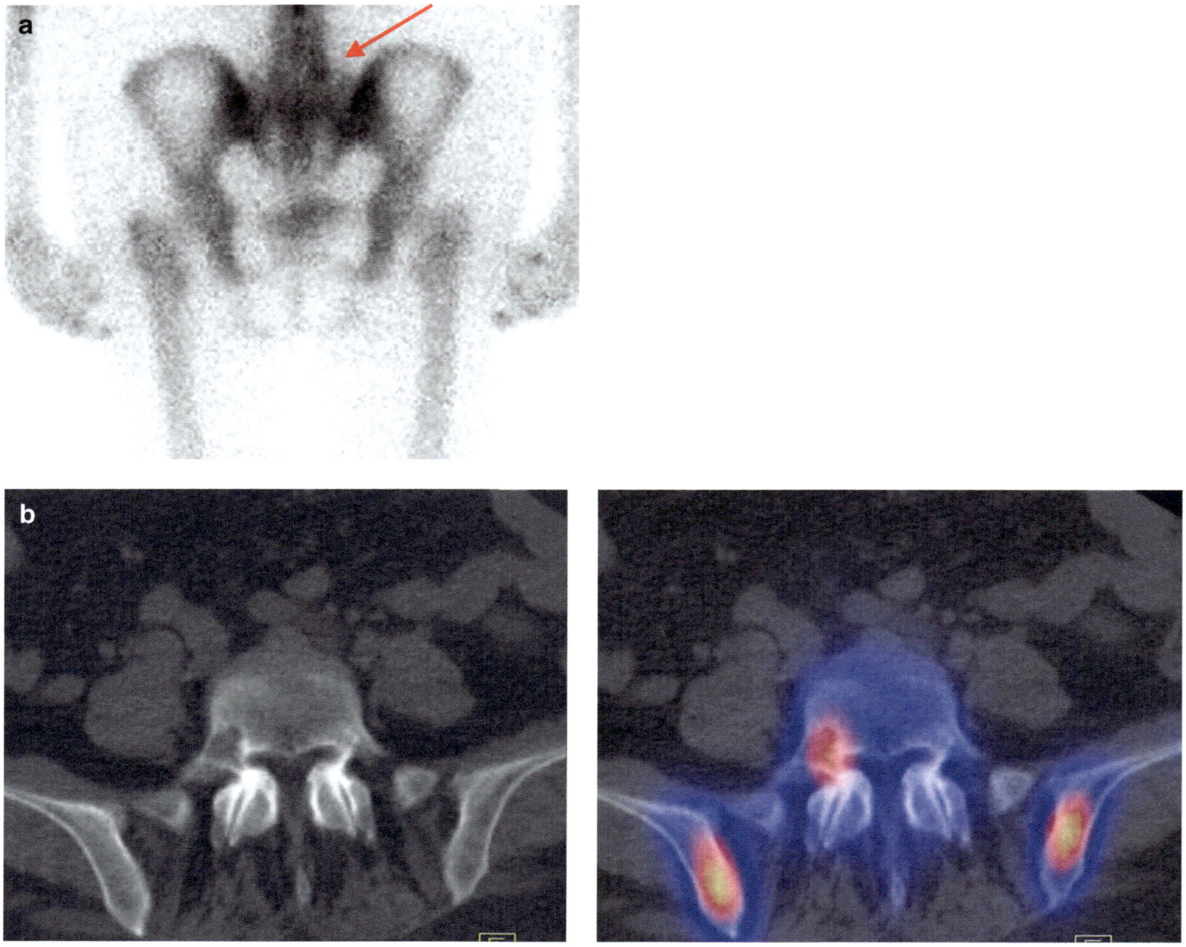

■ ^{99m}Tc-polyphosphonate findings

A focus of moderately increased uptake projecting to the lateral aspects of L5 (*arrow*) proves on SPECT/CT to be an osteolytic metastasis of breast cancer. (**a**) Planar; (**b**) CT (30 mAs; *left*) and SPECT/CT (*right*)

Teaching point

More than 90% of lesions classified as indeterminate on planar imaging can be elucidated as either benign or malignant on SPECT/CT images (cf. next case).

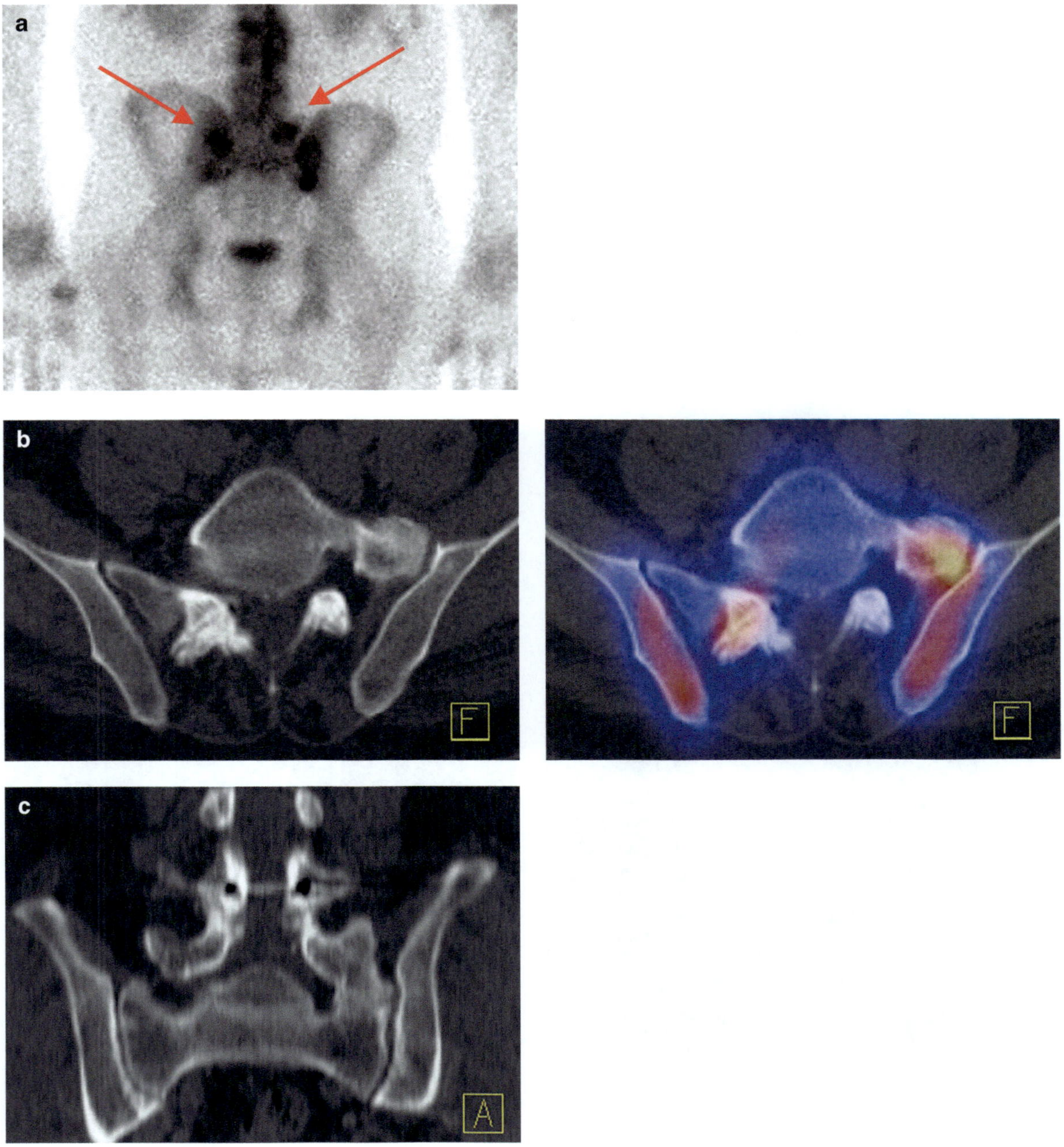

◘ ^{99m}Tc-polyphosphonate findings

Two foci of moderately increased uptake projecting to the lateral aspects of L5 and to the Os sacrum, respectively (*arrows*). The left lesion corresponds to osteoarthritis of the junction between a hemisacralized L5 and the Os sacrum, the right one to osteoarthritis of facette's joint L5/S1: (**a**) Planar; (**b**) transaxial CT (30 mAs; *left*) and SPECT/CT (*right*); (**c**) Coronal CT

Teaching point

More than 90% of lesions classified as indeterminate on planar imaging can be elucidated as either benign or malignant on SPECT/CT images (cf. previous case).

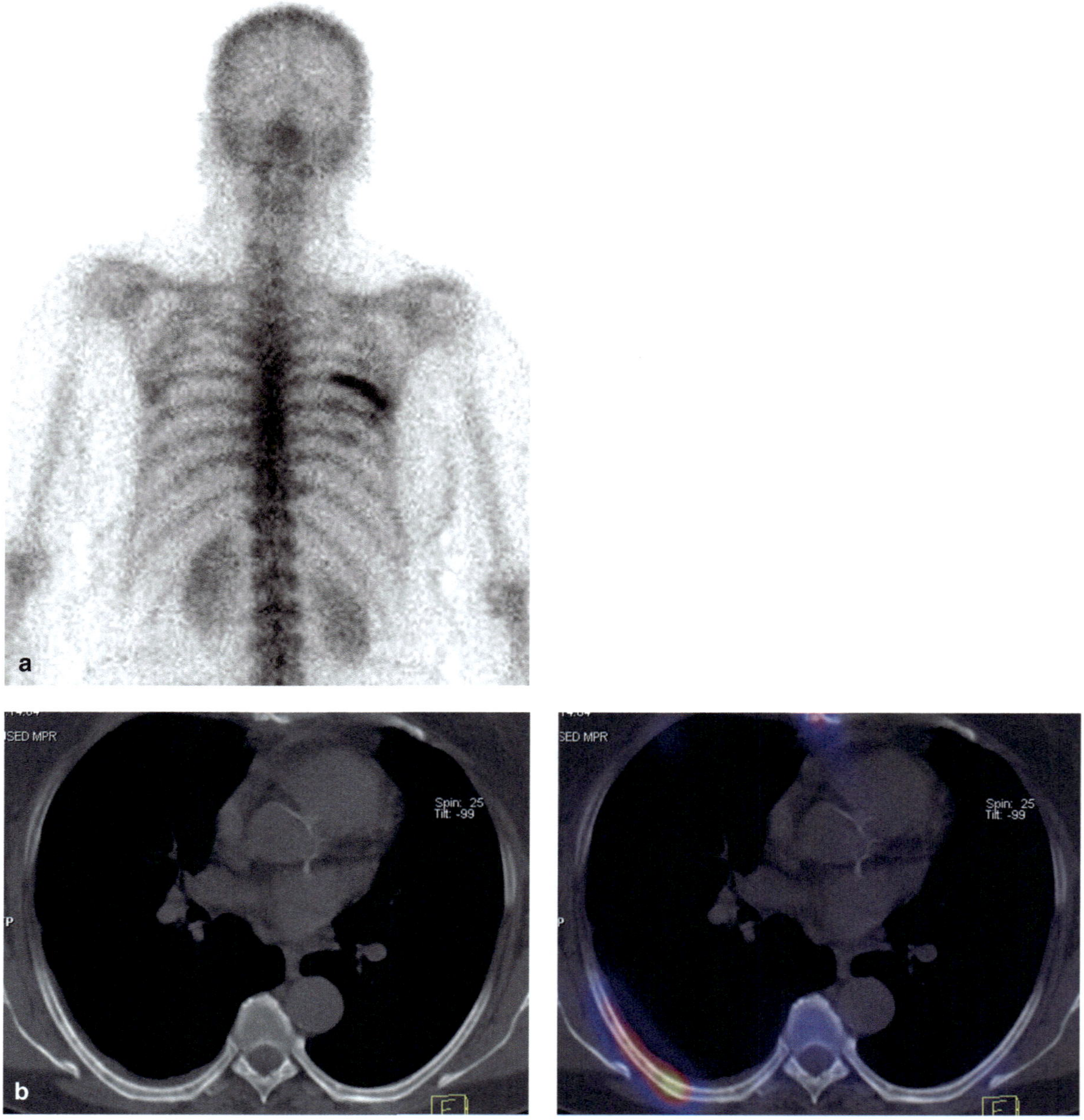

^{99m}Tc-polyphosphonate findings

Markedly increased and longitudinal uptake in right seventh rib in a patient with breast cancer. CT without easily visible lytic or sclerotic changes. (**a**) Planar; (**b**) CT (30 mAs; *left*) and SPECT/CT (*right*)

Teaching point

Some osseous metastases may be without clearcut low-dose CT abnormalities. This is the case of filiae growing in the bone marrow that have not yet grossly attacked the bone tissue. These deposits may in earlier stages also escape detection by bone scintigraphy. Filiae in the ribs or in the scapulae may, in particular, not easily be diagnosed on CT images.

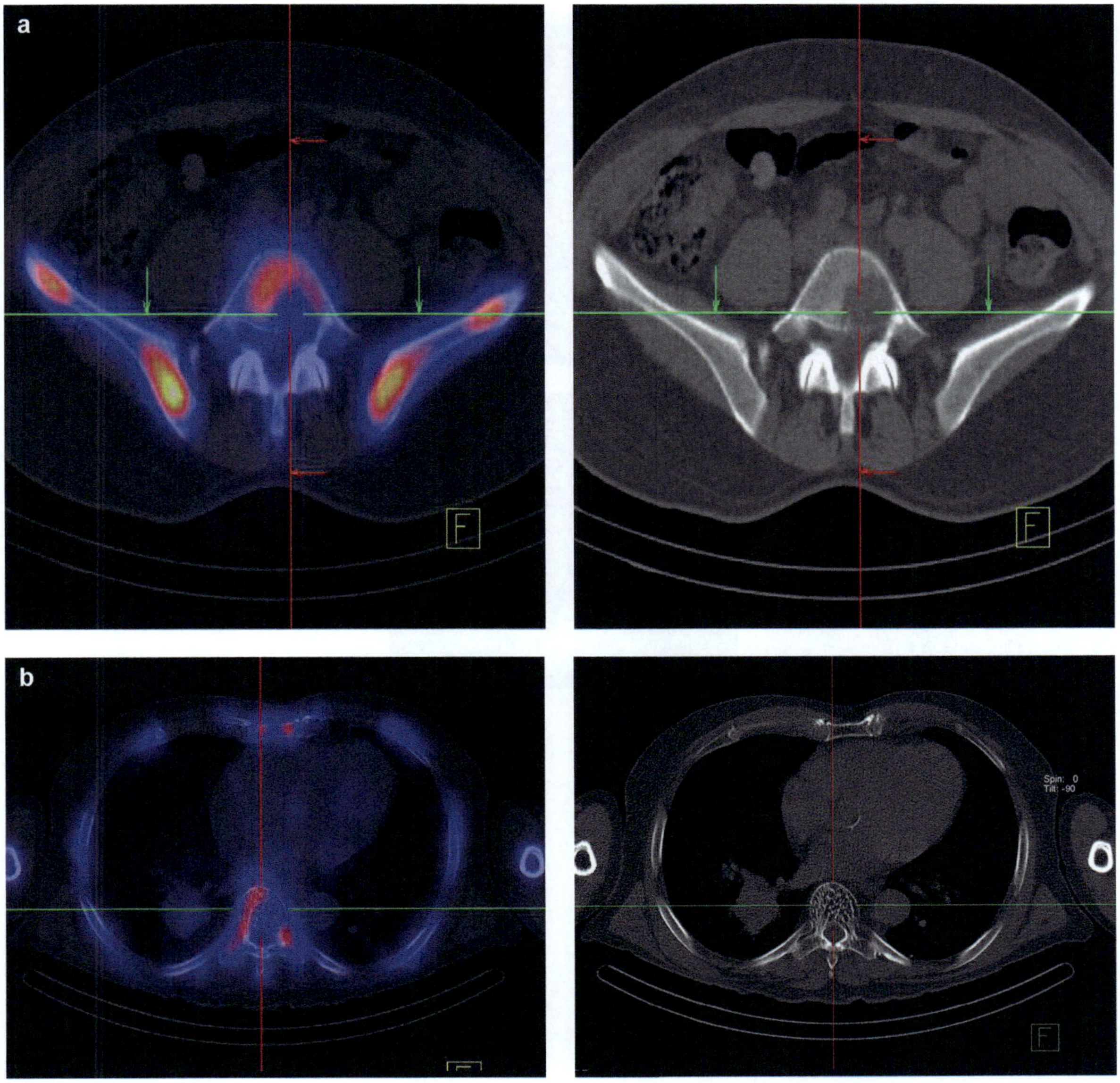

^{99m}Tc-polyphosphonate findings

(**a**) Osteolytic metastasis of renal cancer in body of L5 without tracer uptake (*left*: SPECT/CT; *right*: CT) (**b**) Cold spot due to hemangioma in thoracic vertebral body (*left*: SPECT/CT; *right*: CT). Note typical "salt and pepper" appearance of hemangioma and perihilar bronchial carcinoma

Teaching point

SPECT/CT is also helpful in the differential diagnosis of scintigraphically cold lesions.

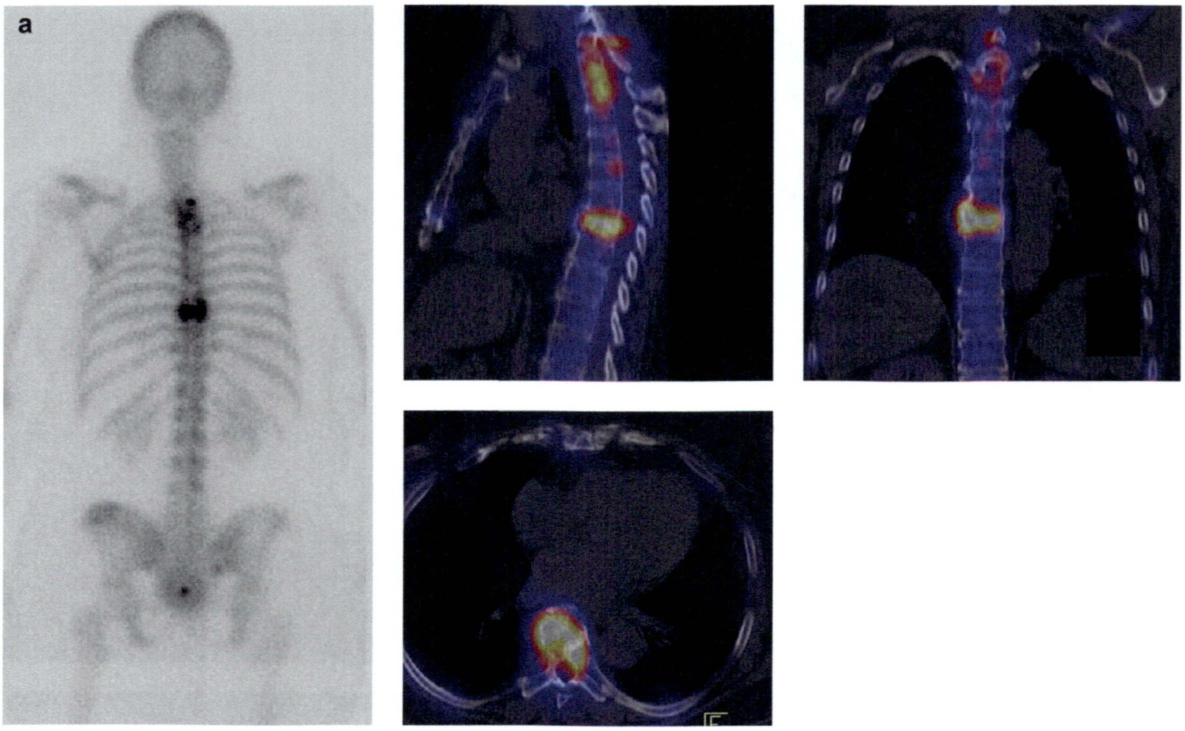

^{99m}Tc-polyphosphonate findings

Several foci of markedly increased uptake corresponding to metastases of breast cancer visible on the planar images ((**a**), left; a, right: SPECT/CT). CT (**b**) reveals that the vertebral body of T8 (arrows) is completely destroyed and has already lost in height, indicating immanent compression fracture

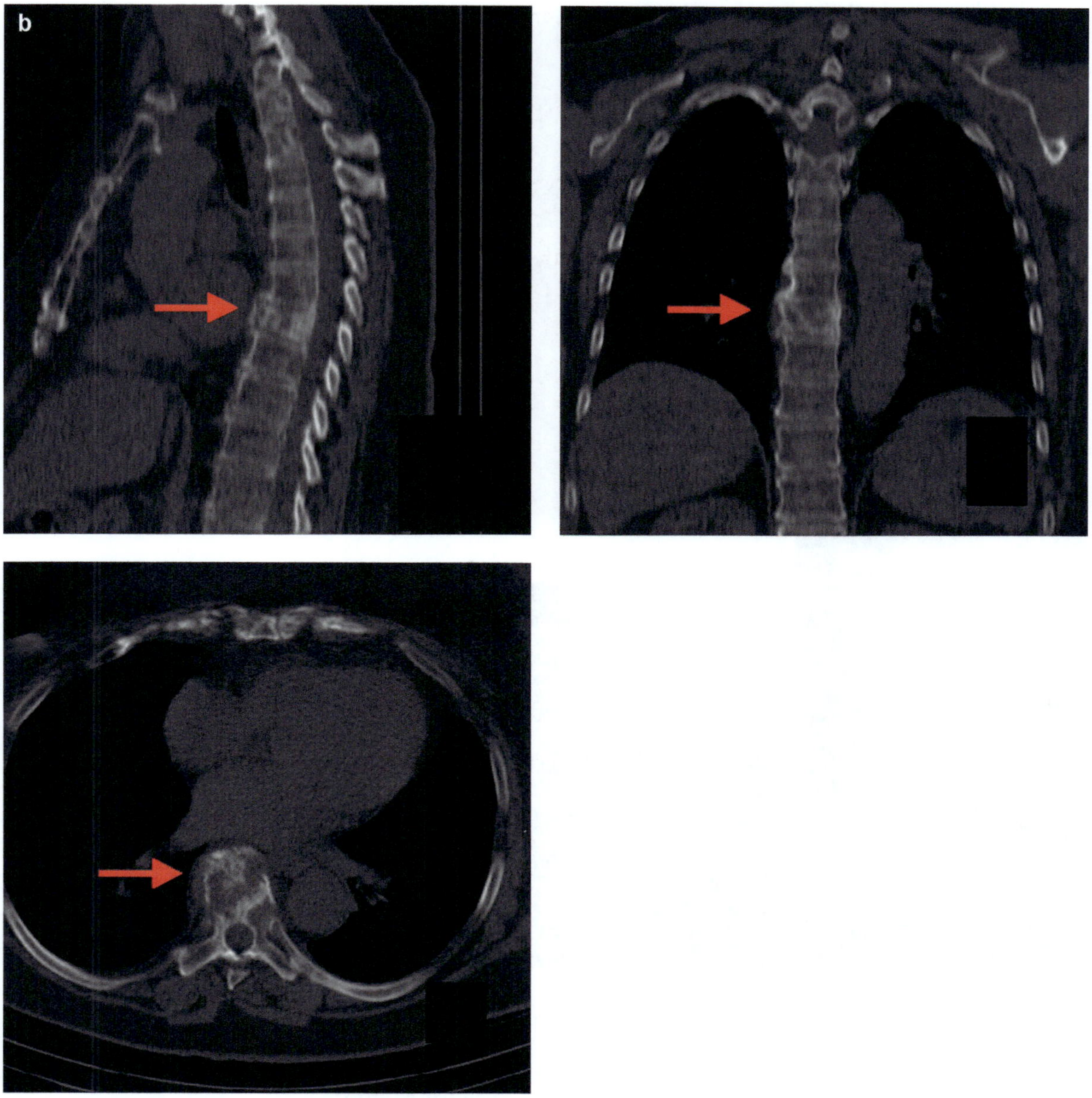

Teaching point

After detection of osseous metastases, the next question is that for stability of the bones involved. SPECT/CT allows a quick answer in a one-stop shop scenario. Metastases to the vertebrae are considered unstable when the posterior cortical rim is destroyed or when the whole body is osteolytically destroyed and a loss in height has occurred as in this case.

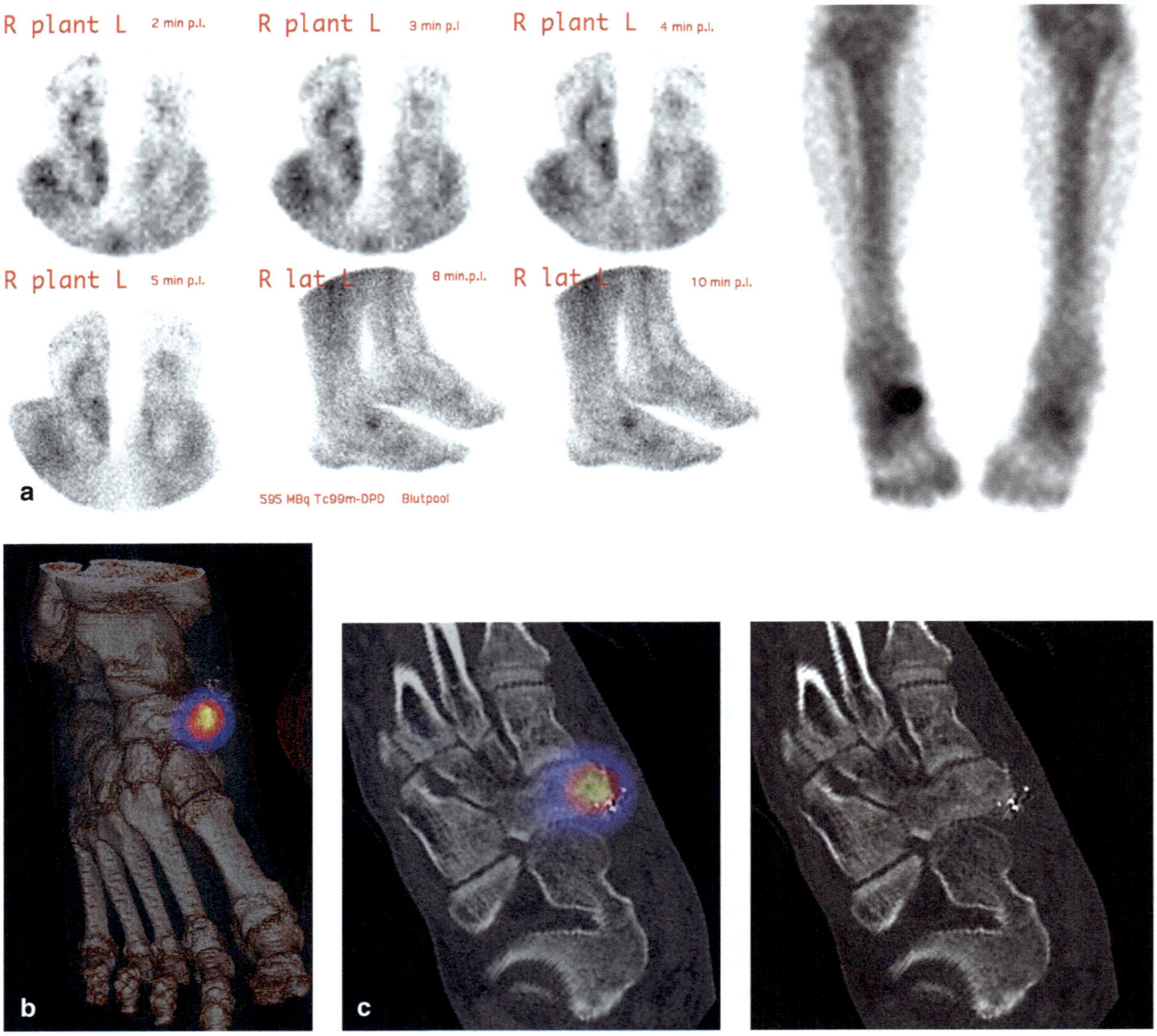

^{99m}Tc-polyphosphonate findings

Markedly increased uptake projecting to the navicular bone in all three phases on planar images (**a**) in a patient 4 months after a bullet injury to the right foot. SPECT/CT reveals that only a part of the navicular bone is hypermetabolic, thus allowing the diagnosis of osteomyelitis and the exclusion of osteonecrosis. MRI had not been helpful due to metallic artefacts left by the projectile. (**b**) Multiplanar reconstruction (MPR) of SPECT/CT fusion; (**c**) SPECT/CT on the *left*, CT on the *right*

Teaching point

The exact localization of the foci of uptake by SPECT/CT is extremely helpful in orthopedic patients, leading to a definite diagnosis in the majority of cases.

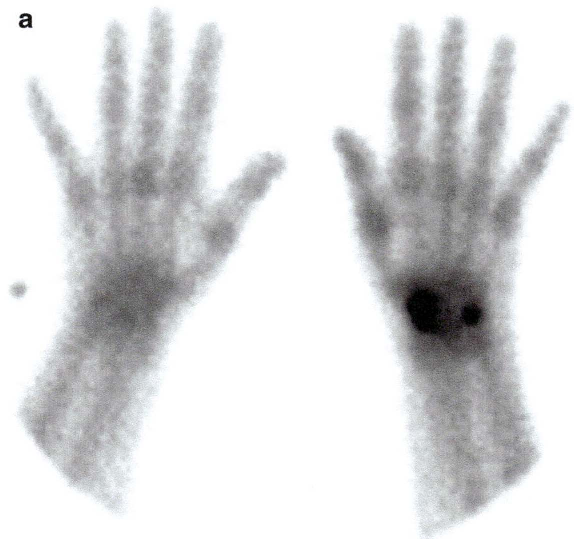

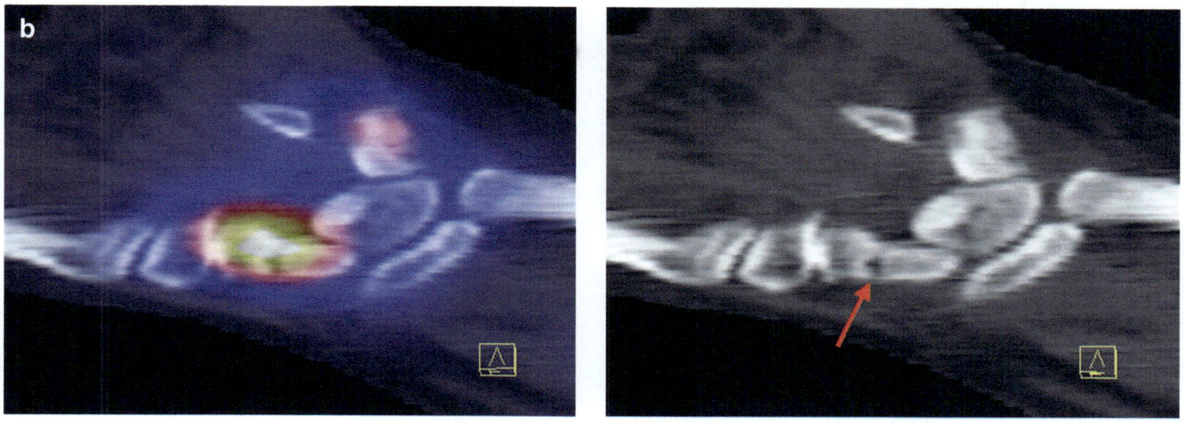

^{99m}Tc-polyphosphonate findings

Markedly increased uptake projecting to navicular and lunar bone in a patient with unremarkable planar X-rays after a fall (**a**). CT of SPECT/CT reveals a fracture line in the navicular bone (*arrow*) and a subtle irregularity also in the lunate bone. (**b**) SPECT/CT (*left*) and low-dose CT (*right*)

Teaching point

By highlighting morphological alterations indicative of fractures, the CT of SPECT/CT considerably increases the specificity of the examination. Note that the quality of low-dose CT is inferior to that of high-dose CT which may be the preferred examination in posttraumatic cases such as this one.

Chapter 5 Brain Imaging with SPECT-CT

Monica Agostini, Michela Casi,
Francesco De Lauro,
Vincenzo Mattone,
and Mirco Bartolomei

Contents

S. Fanti et al., *Atlas of SPECT-CT*,
DOI: 10.1007/978-3-642-15726-4_5,

Overexpression of somatostatin receptors has been demonstrated in various brain tumours such as meningiomas or glia-derived tumours. This evidence, following the clinical experience on neuroendocrine tumours, suggests that somatostatin analogues may also be of value for the imaging and treatment of the above-mentioned brain neoplasms.

Close to 100% of meningiomas express somatostatin receptors, especially subtype 2 (sst2), and usually do so at high density. As a result, the approach of specifically targeting receptors on meningioma cells by radiolabelled somatostatin analogues has been developed over the past 2 decades. Tracer doses of somatostatin analogues, radiolabelled with ^{111}In or ^{68}Ga via linking moieties, have been administered for diagnostic imaging, post-surgical follow-up and making the differential diagnosis against neurofibromas and neurinomas. Moreover, radiodetection of somatostatin receptors with a hand-held gamma probe has been employed to improve the surgical radicalization of somatostatin receptor-expressing meningiomas. Following these diagnostic experiences, the further obvious step was to employ radiolabelled somatostatin analogues for therapeutic purposes. Meningiomas are generally benign and, in most cases, surgery is curative. However, for high-grade histotypes or partially resected tumours, recurrence is fairly common. External beam radiation therapy is usually given in such cases, but is not always effective. Bartolomei et al. [1] have assessed peptide receptor radionuclide therapy (PRRT) using ^{90}Y-DOTATOC in a group of patients with meningioma recurring after standard treatments in all of whom somatostatin receptors were strongly expressed on cell surfaces. In particular, 29 patients with scintigraphically proven somatostatin subtype 2 receptor-positive meningiomas were enrolled: 14 had benign (grade I), 9 had atypical (grade II) and 6 had malignant (grade III) disease. Patients received intravenous injections of ^{90}Y-DOTATOC, for two to six cycles, for a cumulative dose in the range of 5–15 GBq. The treatment was well tolerated in all patients, and magnetic resonance controls, performed 3 months after treatment completion, showed disease stabilisation in 66% of cases. The authors concluded that PRRT with ^{90}Y-DOTATOC could interfere with the growth of meningiomas, supporting the adjuvant role of this treatment, to be administered soon after surgery, especially in atypical and malignant histotypes.

For many decades, glia-derived tumour cells have been studied "in vitro" to assess the presence of specific receptor panels on their surface. These investigations are aimed to develop needed alternative modalities of treatment, according to the "targeted therapy" concept. High-grade gliomas, despite the aggressive traditional modalities of treatment, present an extremely poor prognosis, with a median survival time of 6–12 and 15–27 months for glioblastoma and anaplastic astrocytoma, respectively. Low-grade gliomas show an initial better prognosis (median survival time of 5–7 years), but, because of their further genetic alterations, constantly change into high-grade forms. A few trials have focused on the presence of somatostatin receptors in glia-derived tumours. Although these studies have reported contradictory results, there is evidence that somatostatin receptors (especially subtype 2) are present in a large percentage of low-grade gliomas, and may be expressed by anaplastic astrocytomas, but are rarely detectable in undifferentiated glioblastomas. At present, the use of radiolabelled somatostatin analogues in glioma patients (both for diagnostic and therapeutic purposes) represents only an experimental approach, and no large series are reported in the literature. A pilot study performed in a group of glioma patients has proposed the use of radiolabelled somatostatin analogues with a locoregional approach [2].

Despite the expanding role of novel PET radiotracers (^{68}Ga-DOTATOC/DOTANOC), somatostatin receptor scintigraphy with ^{111}In-DTPA-Octreotide (Octreoscan®) remains the standard method to study neuroendocrine tumours and others tumours expressing somatostatin receptors. Planar and single-photon-emission computed tomography (SPECT) imaging is commonly performed in most nuclear medicine centres, but this technique often does not provide clear anatomical localisation. The availability of a modern dual-head gamma cameras equipped with an integrated X-ray transmission system (SPECT-CT) offers the opportunity to fuse the functional and morphological imaging, resulting in greatly increased diagnostic accuracy.

Herein the authors report on some SPECT-CT studies of brain lesions obtained after diagnostic and therapeutic injection of radiolabelled somatostatin analogues.

References

1. Bartolomei M, Bodei L, De Cicco C, et al. Peptide receptor radionuclide therapy with 90Y-DOTATOC in recurrent meningioma. Eur J Nucl Med Mol Imaging. 2009;36: 1407–16.
2. Schumacher T, Hofer S, Eichhorn K, et al. Local injection of the 90Y-labelled peptidic vector DOTATOC to control gliomas of WHO grades II and III: an extended pilot study. Eur J Nucl Med Mol Imaging. 2002;29:486–93.

Suggested Reading

Reardon DA, Rich JN, Friedman HS, et al. Recent advances in the treatment of malignant astrocytoma. J Clin Oncol. 2006;24:1253–65. Review.

Zalutsky MR. Current status of therapy of solid tumors: brain tumour therapy. J Nucl Med. 2005;46:151S–6. Review.

Zoller F, Eisenhut M, Haberkorn U, et al. Endoradiotherapy in cancer treatment – basic concepts and future trends. Eur J Pharmacol. 2009;625:55–62. Review.

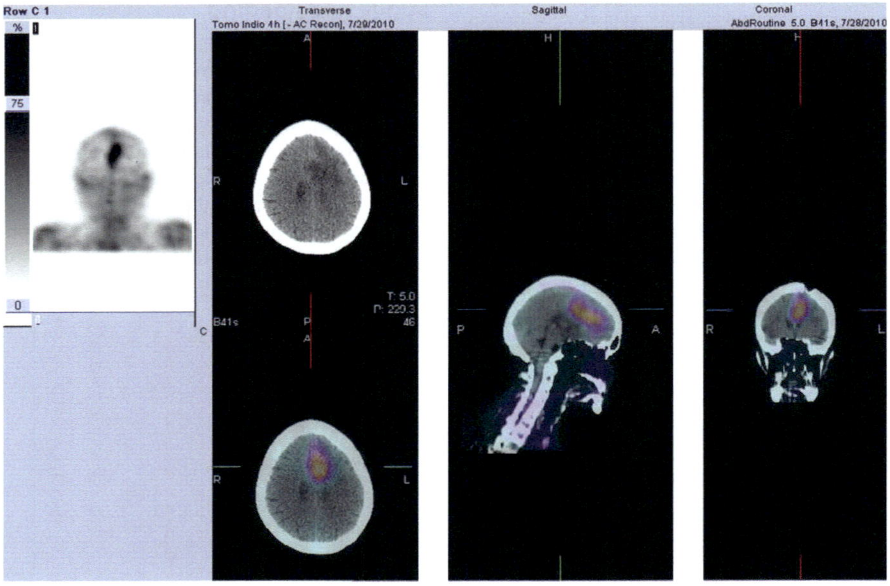

^{111}In-pentetreotide findings

3-D SPECT-CT imaging highlights an area of increased uptake of radiotracer, consistent with a recurrent anaplastic astrocytoma lesion, overexpressing subtype 2 somatostatin receptors, in the left fronto-parietal lobe.

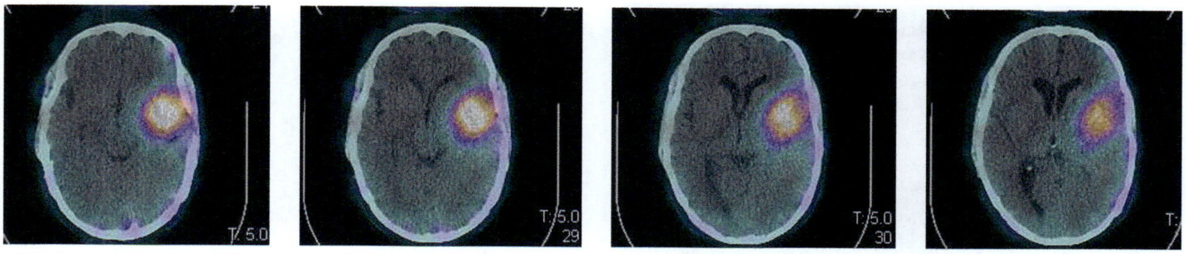

^{90}Y-DOTATOC finding

After therapeutic injection of radiolabelled somatostatin analogue (^{90}Y-DOTATOC), Bremsstrahlung-based SPECT-CT images show a high concentration of radiopharmaceuticals into a relapsing anaplastic astrocytoma of the left parietal lobe.

Teaching point

Recurrence of high-grade glioma (HGG) constantly occurs a few months after the completion of traditional therapies (surgery, radio-chemotherapy).
Scintigraphy with ^{111}In-pentetreotide has the potential to assess the presence of somatostatin receptors in HGG lesions. The tumour's high density of somatostatin receptors might allow patients bearing HGG to be enrolled for peptide receptor radionuclide therapy (PRRT).

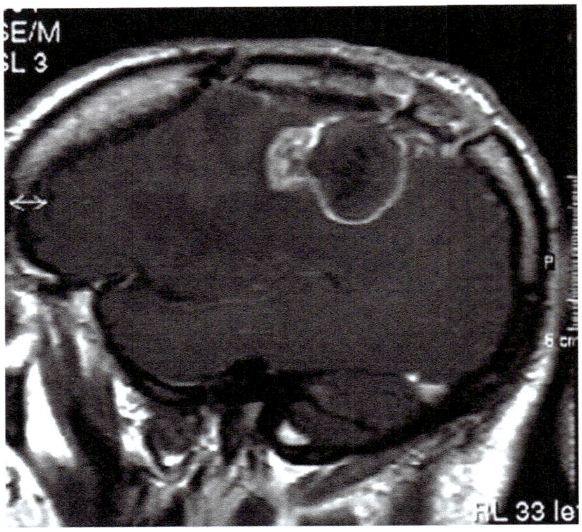

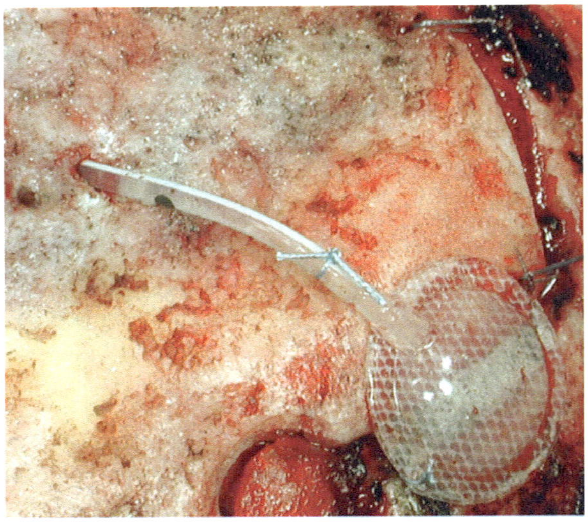

HGGs recur at or near the site of origin, and are characterised by a strong tendency to infiltrate adjacent brain tissue. Based on this evidence, locoregional therapies are fully justified.

In order to facilitate locoregional injection of drugs, a catheter into the surgical cavity, and connected with a subcutaneous reservoir, can to be implanted during surgical procedures.

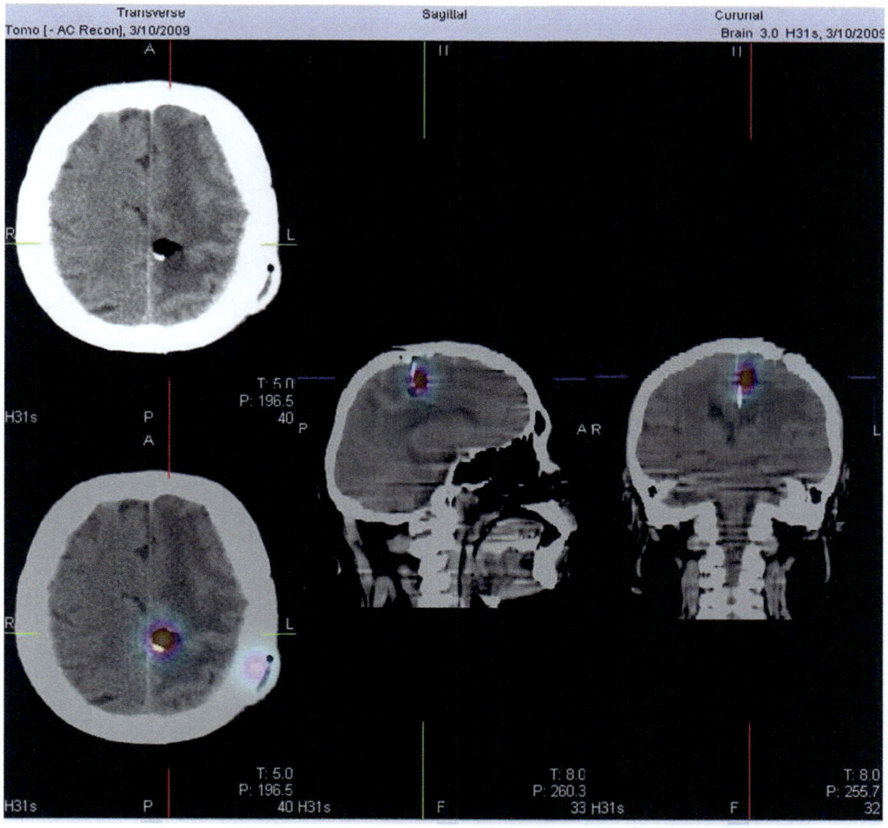

^{90}Y-DOTATOC finding

After locoregional injection of radiolabelled somatostatin analogue (^{90}Y-DOTATOC), Bremsstrahlung-based SPECT-CT images show a correct localisation of radiopharmaceuticals in the surgical cavity of the posterior-left parietal lobe.

Teaching point

Local administration of radiolabelled somatostatin analogues may circumvent the blood-brain barrier and thus potentially achieve higher intra-tumoral concentrations than are achievable following systemic administration.

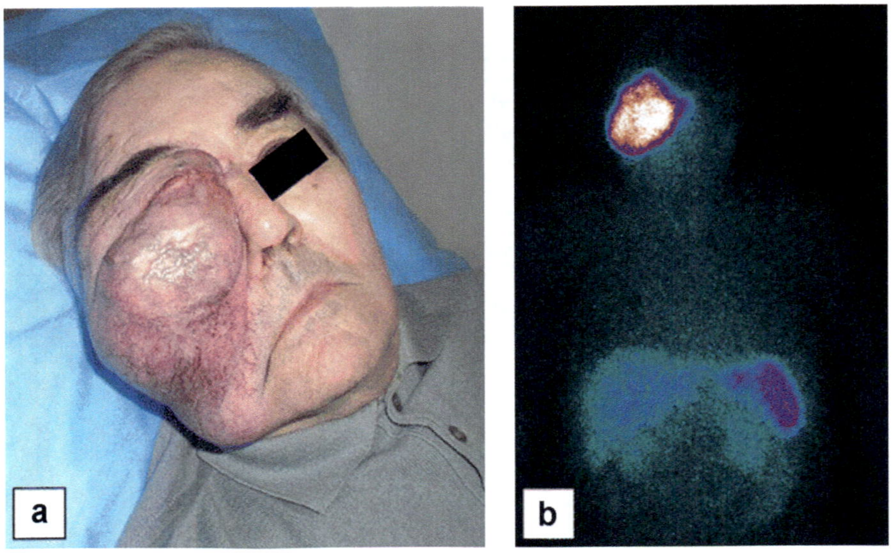

A 77-year-old man with grade I fibro-angioblastic meningioma of the right temporal lobe showing extracranial growth

^{111}In-pentetreotide finding

(**a**) The planar anterior view (**b**) after injection of ^{111}In-pentetreotide shows a focal uptake of radiotracer consistent with a large lesion overexpressing subtype 2 somatostatin receptors.

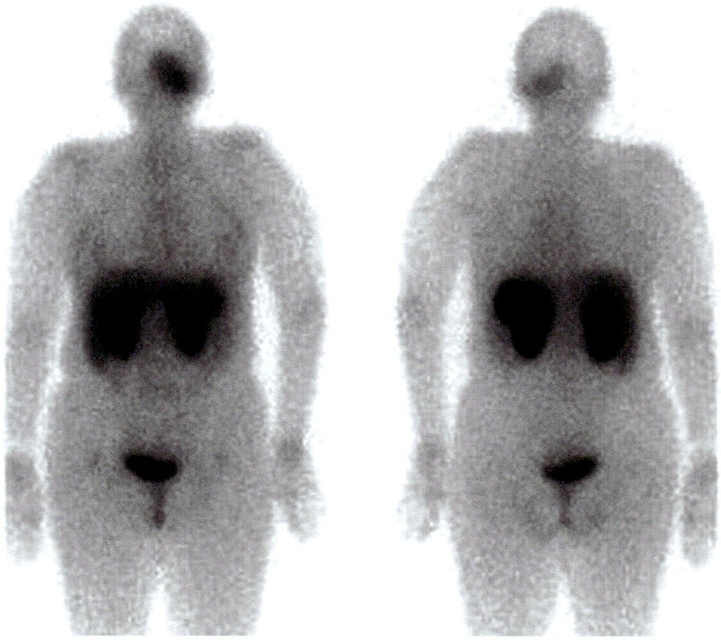

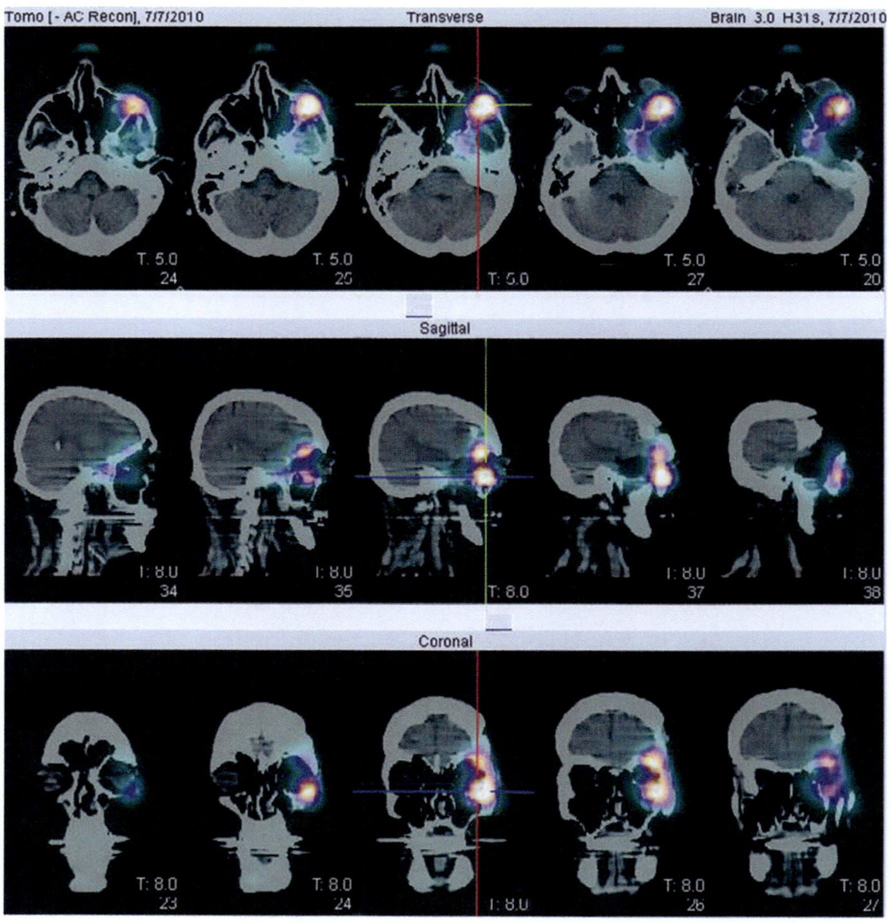
Tomo [- AC Recon], 7/7/2010
Transverse
Brain 3.0 H31s, 7/7/2010
Sagittal
Coronal

^{111}In-pentetreotide finding

Planar anterior/posterior scintigraphy and brain SPECT-CT after administration of ^{111}In-pentetreotide highlight a frontal meningioma involving the temporal bone. SPECT-TC imaging offers the possibility to better define the tumour size, shape and location, as well as infiltrating or multifocal presentation.

Teaching point

Tracer doses of somatostatin analogues, radiolabelled with ^{111}In (or ^{68}Ga) via linking moieties, are administered for diagnostic imaging, post-surgical follow-up and making the differential diagnosis against neurofibromas and neurinomas. Moreover, investigators have used radiodetection of somatostatin receptors with a hand-held gamma probe to improve the surgical radicalization of somatostatin receptor-expressing meningiomas.

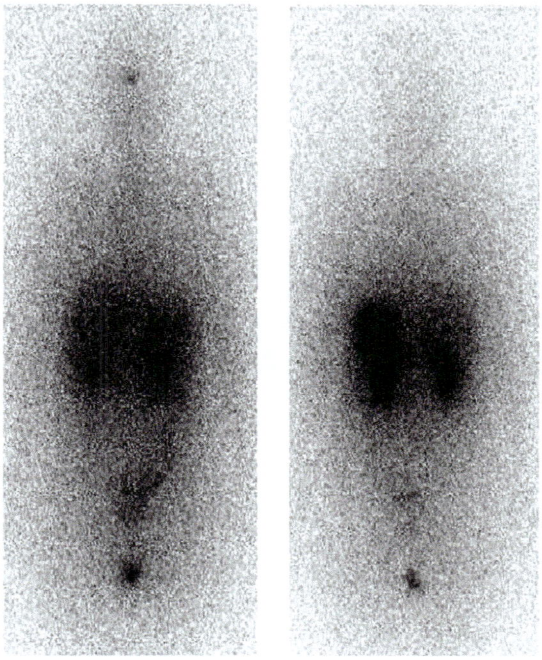

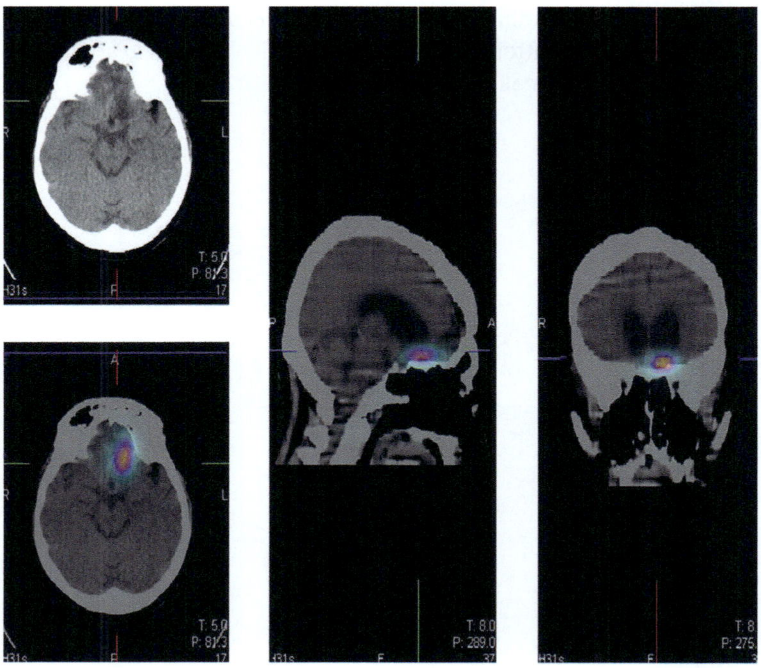

■ ^{90}Y-DOTATOC findings

Bremstrahlung-based anterior/posterior whole body and brain SPECT-CT after administration of ^{90}Y-DOTATOC show a high uptake of radiopeptide in a meningioma localised in the anterior skull fossa.

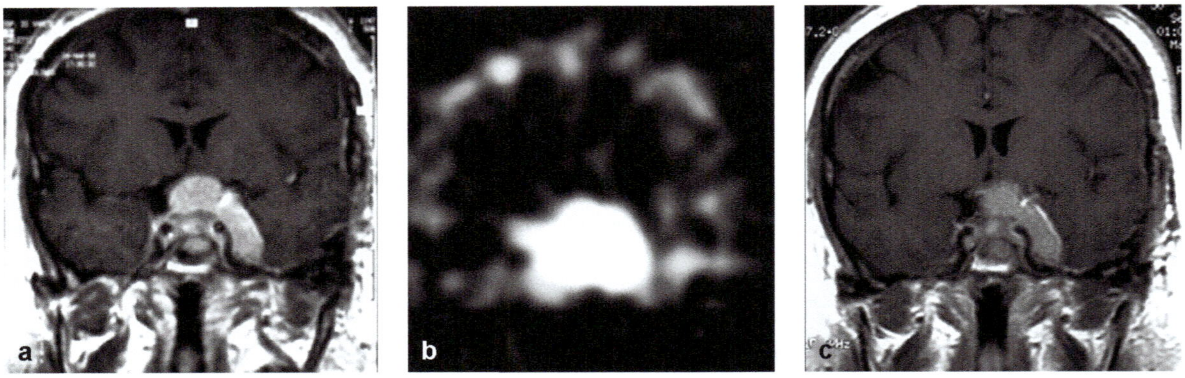

A 58-year-old woman, with skull base meningioma of the sinus cavernosus, has obtained disease stabilisation after therapy with ^{90}Y-DOTATOC. (**a**) Contrast-enhanced T1-weighted coronal MRI at baseline; (**b**) coronal view of SPECT with ^{111}In-pentetreotideat baseline; (**c**) coronal view contrast-enhanced T1-weighted MRI 12 months after treatment with ^{90}Y-DOTATOC (5 cycles, total activity administered 12.5 GBq).

Teaching point

Peptide receptor radionuclide therapy has shown the potential to interfere with the growth of meningiomas. In particular, this therapeutic option may have a role in an adjuvant setting, when it is performed soon after surgery and especially in atypical and malignant histotypes.

Chapter 6 Cardiac Imaging with SPECT-CT

Albert Flotats

Contents

S. Fanti et al., *Atlas of SPECT-CT*,
DOI: 10.1007/978-3-642-15726-4_6,

Single-photon emission tomography (SPECT) combined with computed tomography (CT) aims to provide an accurate spatial alignment between the two separate data sets into one fused image. The resultant information goes beyond that achievable with either stand-alone or side-by-side interpretation of the data sets, and beyond the information derived from attenuation correction (AC), with an equal contribution of both data sets to the image information.

Cardiac hybrid SPECT/CT imaging depicts anatomic abnormalities along with their physiologic consequences in a single setting, resulting in a decreased number of equivocal results in a patient-friendly image acquisition (only one visit to the imaging department). In addition, hybrid SPECT/CT requires fewer personnel compared with two stand-alone scanners, which may result in reduced health care costs and saves time. However, SPECT/CT has also generated controversy with regard to which patients should undergo such integrated examination for clinical effectiveness and minimization of costs and radiation dose, and whether software-based fusion of images obtained separately is a useful alternative.

SPECT myocardial perfusion imaging (MPI) and cardiac-computed tomographic angiography (CCTA) performed in one session have been proposed for dual-system scanners equipped with multidetector computed CT (MDCT). However, cardiac hybrid imaging is not used routinely because of the difficulty in predicting a priori which patients would benefit from the dual scanning. Therefore, a sequential diagnostic approach is often applied in clinical practice, with additional scans (CCTA or MPI) performed only if the results of the initial modality are equivocal. However, when CCTA is performed first, about 50% of the patients will need MPI.

Hybrid MPI and CCTA with reliable image co-registration and fusion of three-dimensional information of myocardial territories onto their subtending coronary arteries can accurately allocate the culprit lesion in multivessel coronary artery disease (CAD) (Fig. 6.1), which is particularly important because the so-called standard distribution of myocardial perfusion territories does not correspond with the real world of coronary anatomy in more than half of the cases (Fig. 6.2). Combining anatomical with perfusion data also helps to identify and correctly register possible subtle irregularities in myocardial perfusion. The reduced sensitivity of CCTA in distal coronary segments and side branches can be compensated by the MPI information. On the other hand, CCTA improves the detection of multivessel CAD, which is one of the main pitfalls of SPECT MPI. Finally, the assessment of regional myocardial perfusion and viability together with the coronary artery tree eliminates uncertainties in the relationship of perfusion defects, scar regions and diseased coronary arteries in watershed regions, which may be particularly helpful in patients with multiple perfusion abnormalities and multivessel CAD, including previous revascularization procedures.

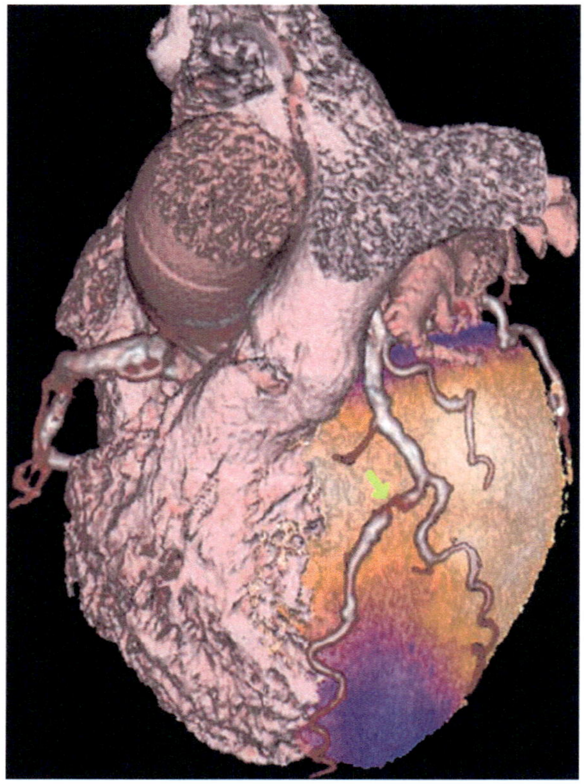

Fig. 6.1 Anterior view of stress SPECT/CT. Although massive coronary tortuosity can be observed, the culprit lesion is localized in the left anterior descending artery (*arrow*), which induces apical ischemia (*purple area*). (Courtesy of P.A. Kaufmann, Cardiac Imaging, University Hospital Zurich, Switzerland)

Teaching point

Reliable image co-registration and fusion of 3D information of myocardial territories onto their subtending coronary arteries can accurately indicate the culprit lesion.

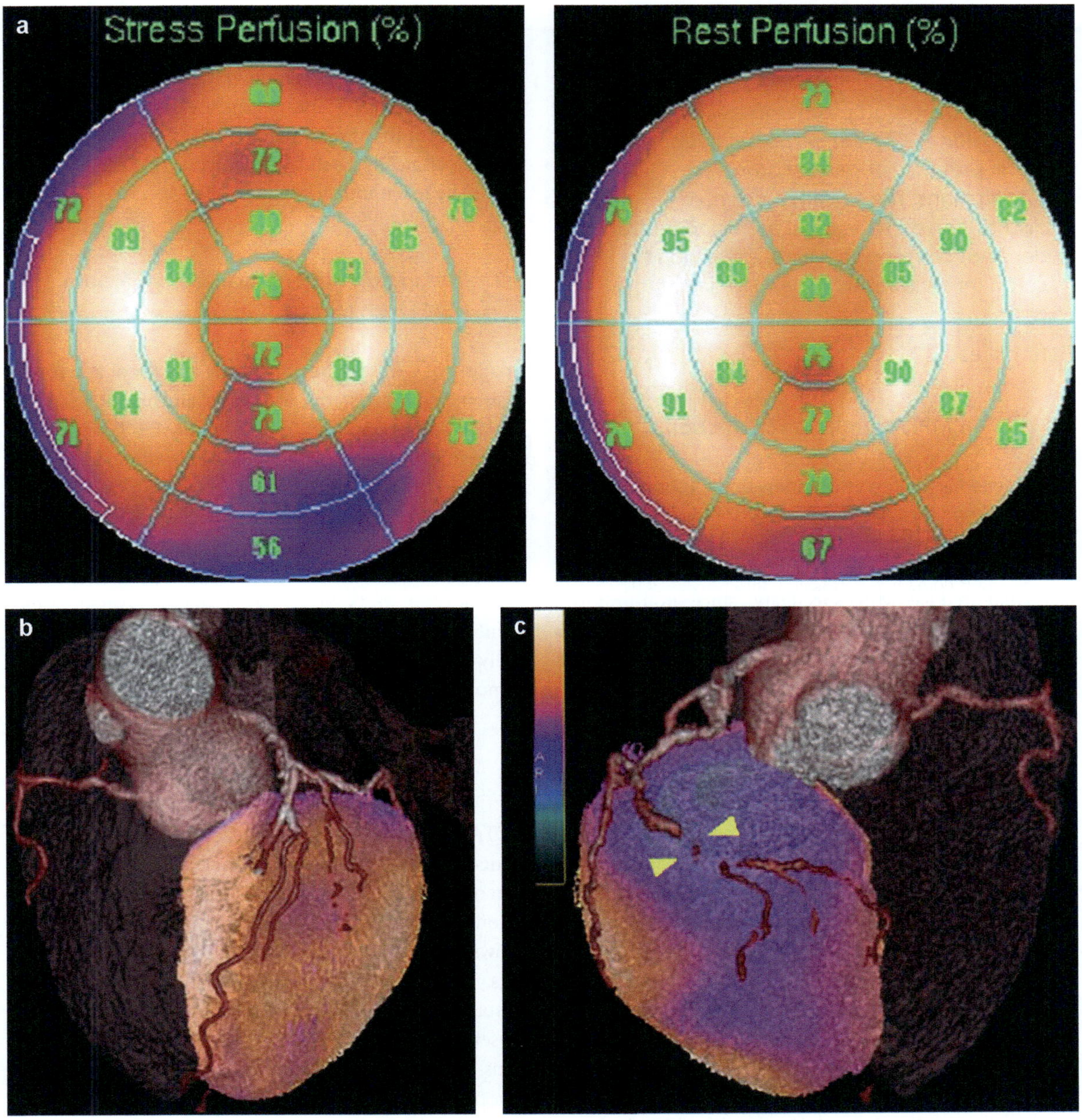

Fig. 6.2 (**a**) Adenosine/rest polar maps of ^{99m}Tc-tetrofosmin SPECT showing severe ischemia in the inferior basal wall, which suggests involvement of the right coronary artery (*RCA*). (**b**) Anterior view of the SPECT/CT with fusion of the 3D myocardial perfusion images with the volume-rendered coronary anatomy. Despite calcifications in the left anterior descending artery, there are no perfusion defects in the anterior wall. (**c**) The posterior view shows that the basal inferior ischemia is caused by a severe stenosis of the circumflex artery (*arrowheads*) and not by the RCA (courtesy of P.A. Kaufmann, Cardiac Imaging, University Hospital Zurich, Switzerland)

> **Teaching point**
>
> The specificity and positive predictive value of stand-alone CCTA are particularly suboptimal in the presence of severe coronary calcifications. The so-called standard distribution of myocardial perfusion territories does not correspond with the real world of coronary anatomy in more than half of the cases.

6.1 CT for MPI Attenuation Correction

Heterogeneous photon attenuation in the thorax is one of the most important problems of MPI, reducing the diagnostic accuracy, interpretive confidence, quantification and laboratory efficiency. On one hand, attenuation artifacts may reduce MPI specificity, since non-uniform, regional perfusion distribution can be misinterpreted as a perfusion defect. On the other hand, attenuation artifacts may also reduce MPI sensitivity when images are improperly scaled to regions suppressed by attenuation, potentially masking true perfusion defects. To overcome this problem, MPI images are corrected by determination of photon attenuation from intervening tissue in the volume of interest. Unfortunately, cardiac imaging poses a particular difficulty for AC because of respiratory and cardiac motion.

AC using the integration of CT components has represented a major step forward for SPECT MPI, improving the diagnostic accuracy and interpretive confidence (Figs. 6.3 and 6.4). It may also improve the laboratory efficiency by enabling the omission of the rest study when the stress study is normal, which may also be useful in the emergency department (i.e., single acquisition of images in the acute phase of chest pain).

Low-dose CT acquisitions are feasible for AC. However, a potential misalignment between emission and transmission data involves the risk of incomplete correction, and thus artificial perfusion defects, and requires careful quality control to avoid reconstruction artifacts (Fig. 6.5). SPECT/CT studies have shown that the frequency of misalignment is quite high and the consequences clinically significant if not corrected (Fig. 6.5). The effects of misalignment are less severe for SPECT/CT than for PET/CT, mainly because of the reduced spatial resolution of SPECT. The alignment of emission and transmission data is usually performed manually, a process that contributes to certain variability. However, automated methods for quality control are under investigation. It is relevant that even low-quality CT scans for AC can provide clinically useful extra-cardiac information that should be taken into account.

6.2 Integration of Coronary Artery Calcium (CAC) with MPI

Imaging of CAC can be a surrogate marker of atherosclerosis in hybrid systems with low- and medium-quality CT devices, as opposed to high-end MDCT suitable for the anatomic assessment of the coronary tree.

Detection of CAC has been shown to provide incremental value to MPI. Specifically, when MPI is normal, the addition of a CAC score can improve the detection of CAD, particularly severe multivessel CAD. For patients with normal stress MPI, higher major adverse cardiac event rates are associated with higher CAC scores, especially in patients with known CAD or with greater comorbidity.

6.3 Integration of CCTA with MPI

CCTA, despite having an excellent negative predictive value (NPV) to exclude CAD, is not reliable for the exclusion of myocardial ischemia. CCTA tends to overestimate coronary stenoses, and the combination with SPECT MPI allows identification of many false-positive CCTA findings. The specificity and positive predictive value (PPV) of stand-alone CCTA are particularly suboptimal in the presence of motion artifacts or severe coronary calcifications (Fig. 6.2). Non-evaluable, severely calcified vessels especially benefit from further testing because of their relatively high likelihood of obstructive disease, whereas non-evaluable vessels with motion artifacts [particularly in the right coronary artery (RCA) territory] do not usually have hemodynamic significance. Image fusion is of particular value in lesions of the distal segments, diagonal braches, RCA and left circumflex artery.

On the other hand, a normal stress SPECT MPI is a poor discriminator of patients with subclinical or "not flow-limiting" CAD. Integration of both MPI and CCTA thus have a complementary role in the evaluation of patients with suspected CAD, with improved specificity and PPV, and minor decreases in sensitivity and NPV as compared to CCTA alone.

Integration of dual imaging appears to improve both the identification of the culprit vessel (Fig. 6.1) and the diagnostic confidence for categorizing intermediate lesions and equivocal perfusion defects, and provides added diagnostic information in almost one-third of patients as compared to side-by-side analysis, thus optimizing management decisions.

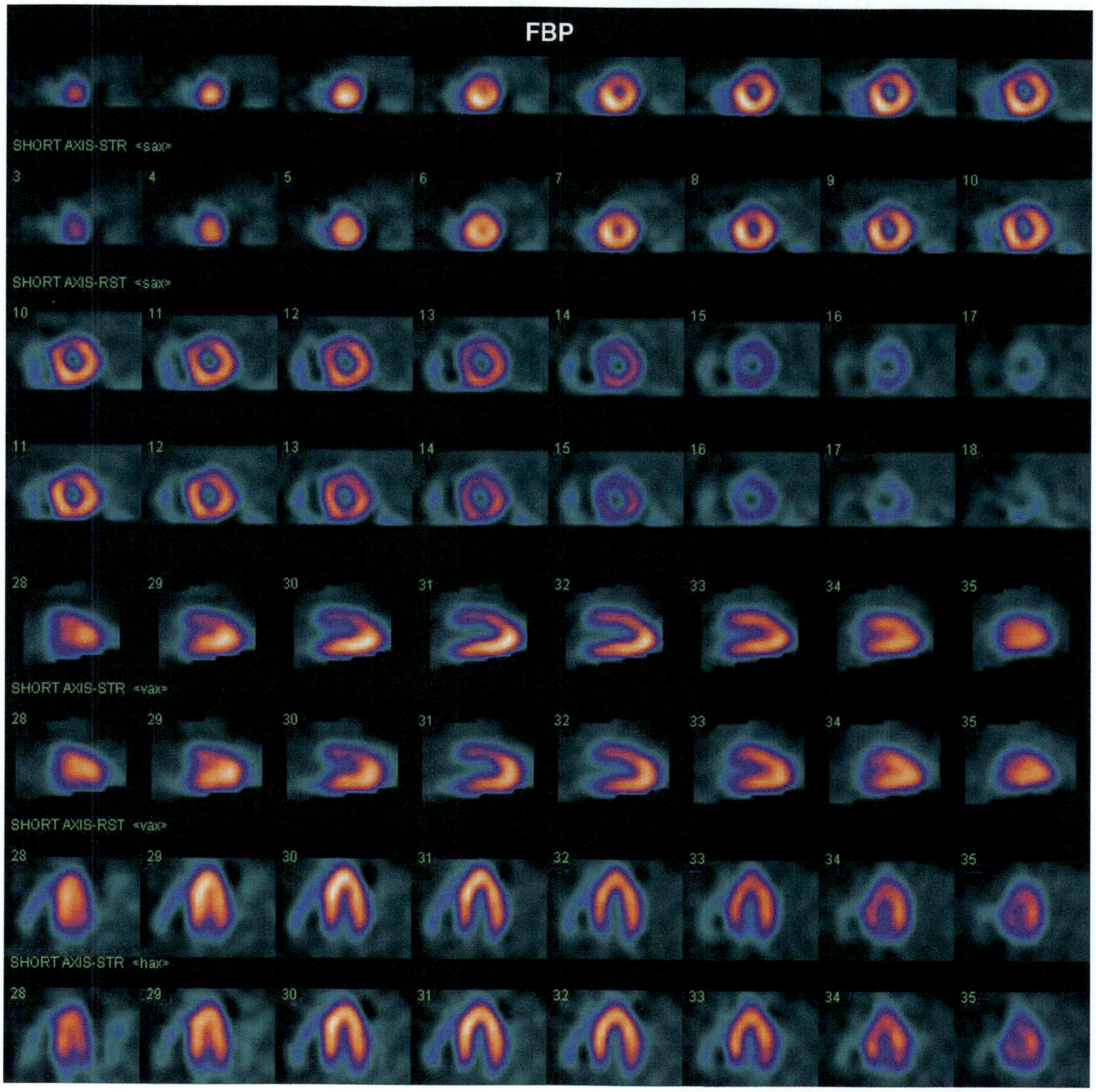

Fig. 6.3 Stress/rest slices of ^{99m}Tc-tetrofosmin SPECT of a woman with suspected coronary artery disease. *FBP* filtered back projection reconstruction without attenuation correction (*AC*). *IRACSC* iterative reconstruction with AC and scatter correction. AC was performed incorporating the CT attenuation map into a statistically based, iterative reconstruction algorithm. The mild fixed defect in the anterior wall present in the FBP images disappears in the IRACSC images, which confirms its artificial origin due to breast attenuation

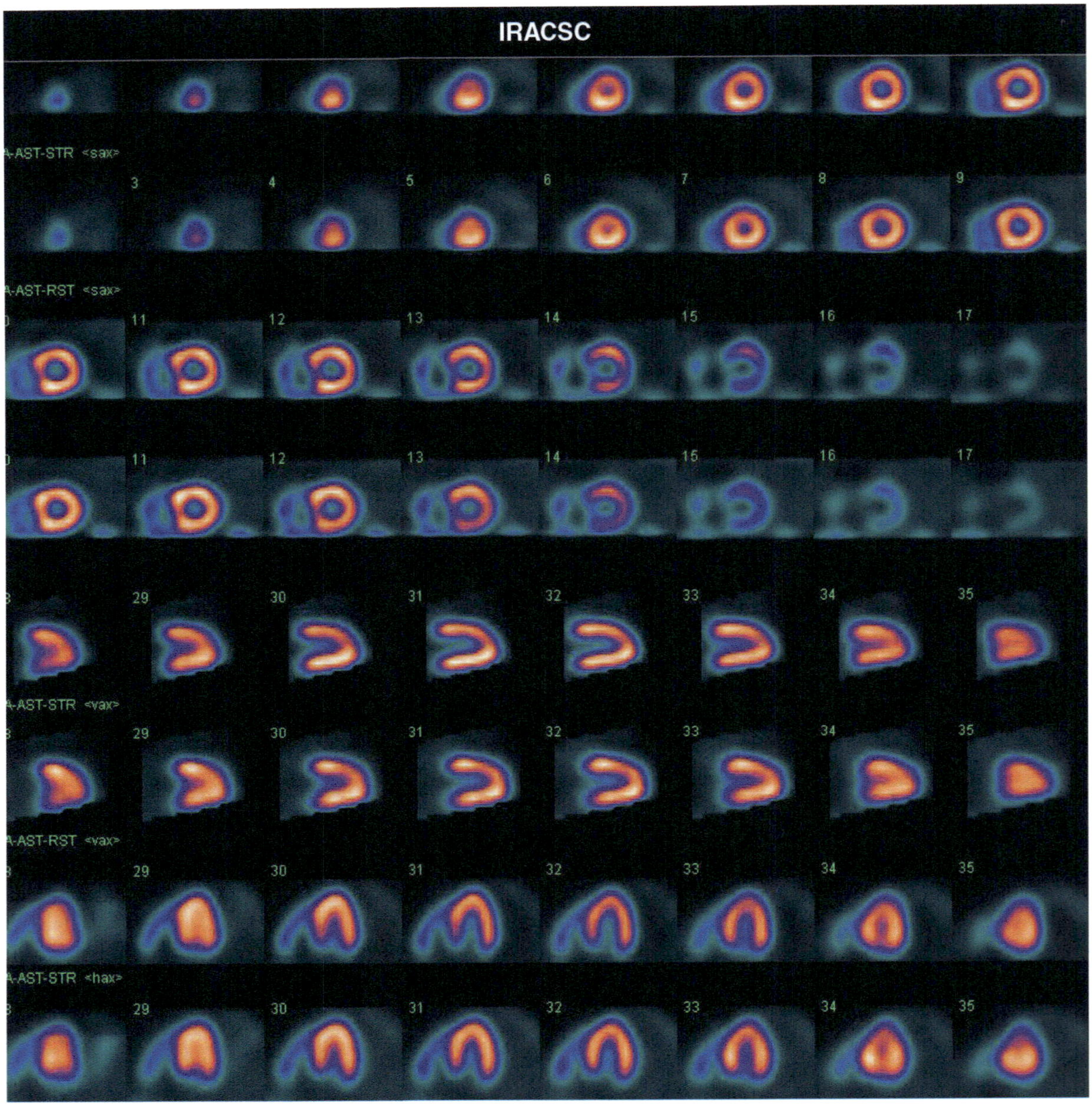

Fig. 6.3 (continued)

> **Teaching point**
>
> AC improves the diagnostic accuracy and interpretive confidence of SPECT MPI.

6.4 Radiation Exposure of Hybrid Imaging

One of the obvious concerns of hybrid imaging is related to the patient radiation dose, which can be significantly reduced considering the best practice methods. These include, for SPECT MPI, the use of ^{99m}Tc-labeled agents rather than ^{201}Tl. Furthermore, the SPECT radiation dose can be markedly reduced with the combination of new iterative reconstruction methods, and dedicated detectors and collimators optimized specifically for MPI. In addition, the omission of the rest study when the stress study is normal considerably reduces the radiation dose.

The effective patient radiation dose from cardiac CT also varies widely depending on the protocol, instrumentation and patient size. The radiation dose is minimal for a CAC scan. For CCTA, the dose tends to be higher with lower slice thickness since the radiation dosage must be increased to obtain the same signal-to-noise ratio. Implementation of modern acquisition protocols, such as prospective (step-and-shoot) ECG triggering, ECG-controlled current modulation (reduction of the tube current by 80% during systole) and body mass adapted tube voltage (reduction of the tube voltage to 100 kV in patients <90 kg of weight), allows reduction of the radiation dose from CCTA by 60–80%.

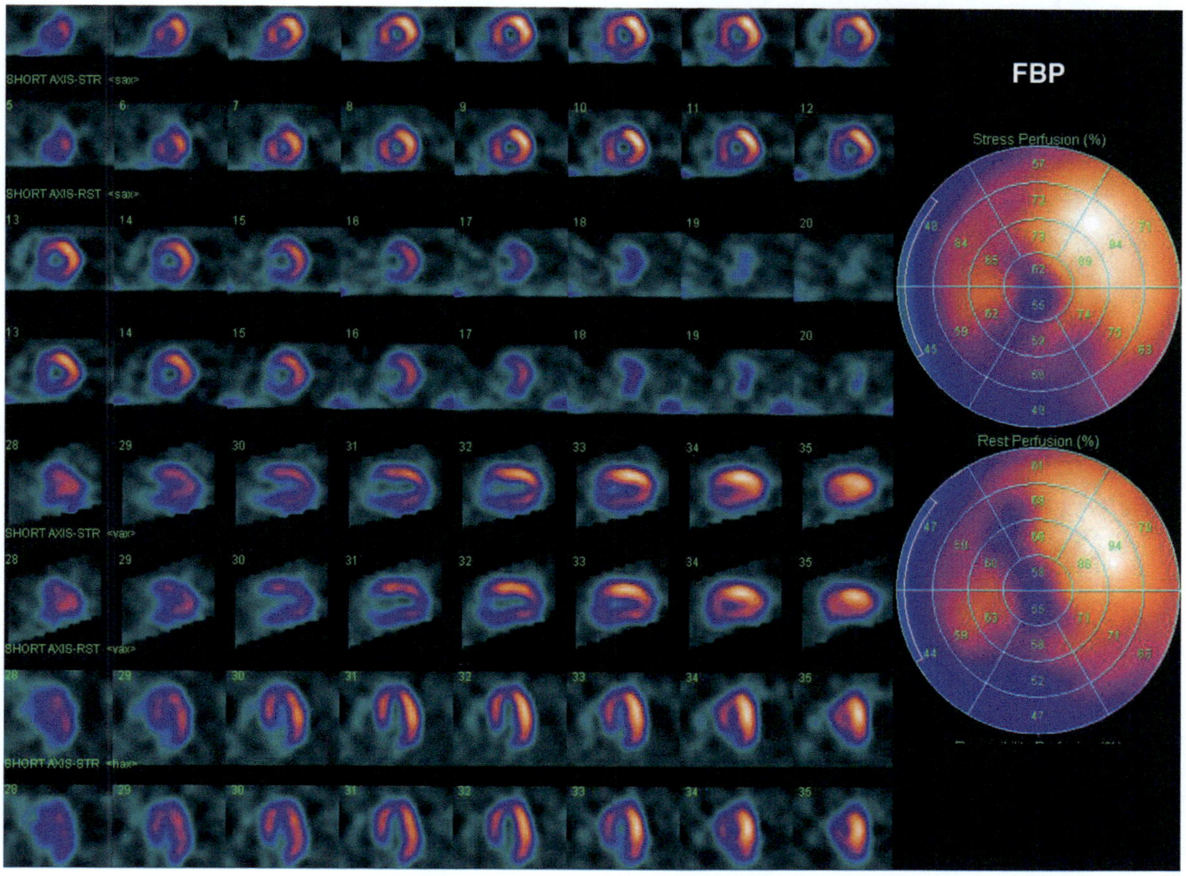

Fig. 6.4 Stress/rest slices and polar maps of ^{99m}Tc-tetrofosmin SPECT of a man with suspected coronary artery disease. *FBP* filtered back projection reconstruction without attenuation correction (*AC*). *IRACSC* iterative reconstruction with AC and scatter correction. AC was performed incorporating the CT attenuation map into a statistically based, iterative reconstruction algorithm. The mild fixed defect in the inferior wall present in the FBP images disappears in the IRACSC images, which confirms its artificial origin due to diaphragmatic attenuation

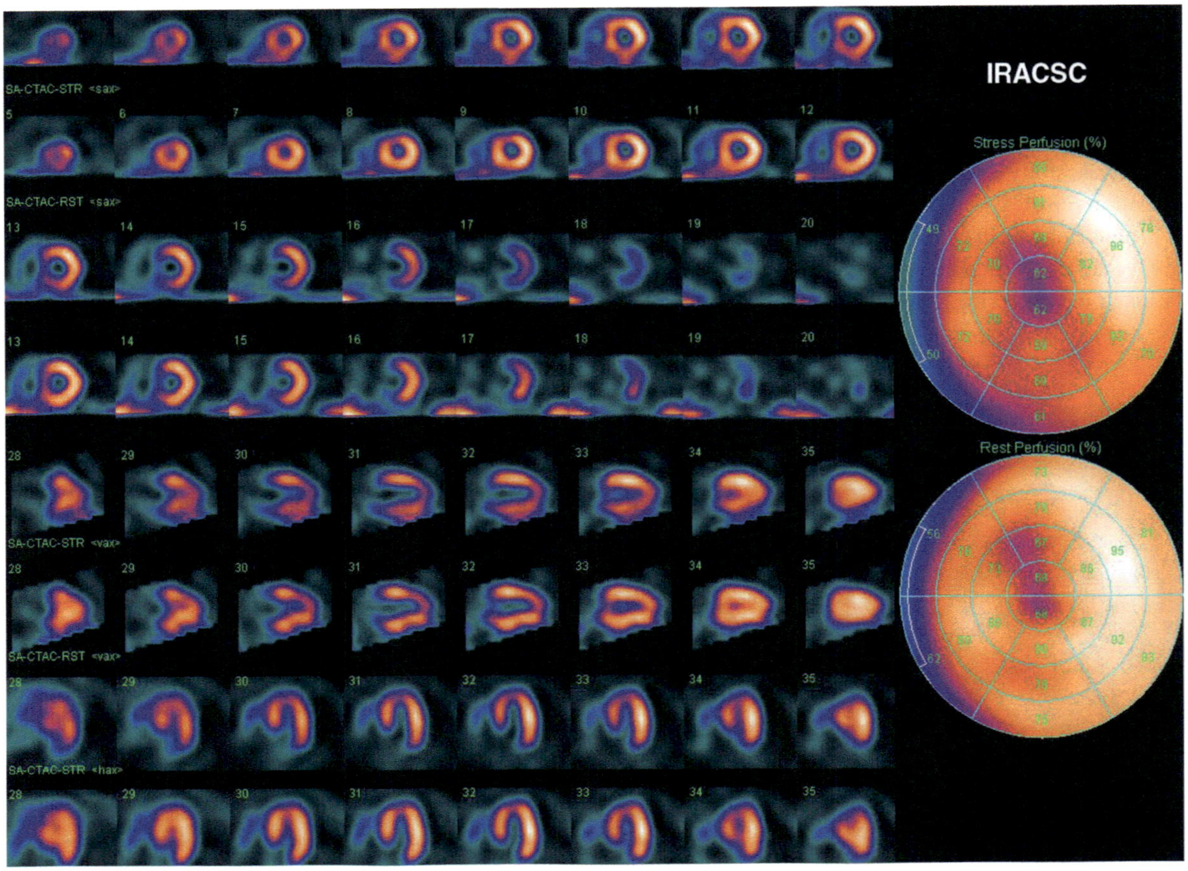

Fig. 6.4 (continued)

Fig. 6.5 Effects of different reconstruction algorithms and image co-registration in SPECT myocardial perfusion imaging. In the first column, filtered back projection (*FBP*) reconstruction without attenuation correction was used; a mild defect in the inferior wall can be seen because of diaphragmatic attenuation. In the second column, iterative reconstruction with attenuation correction and scatter correction (*IRACSC*) was used by a correct co-registration of emission and transmission data (shown in the *upper part of the column*), which results in homogeneous tracer uptake and disappearance of the former inferior defect. In the third and forth columns, mis-registration of the emission and transmission data creates artificial apical and inferolateral defects, respectively, of the IRACSC images

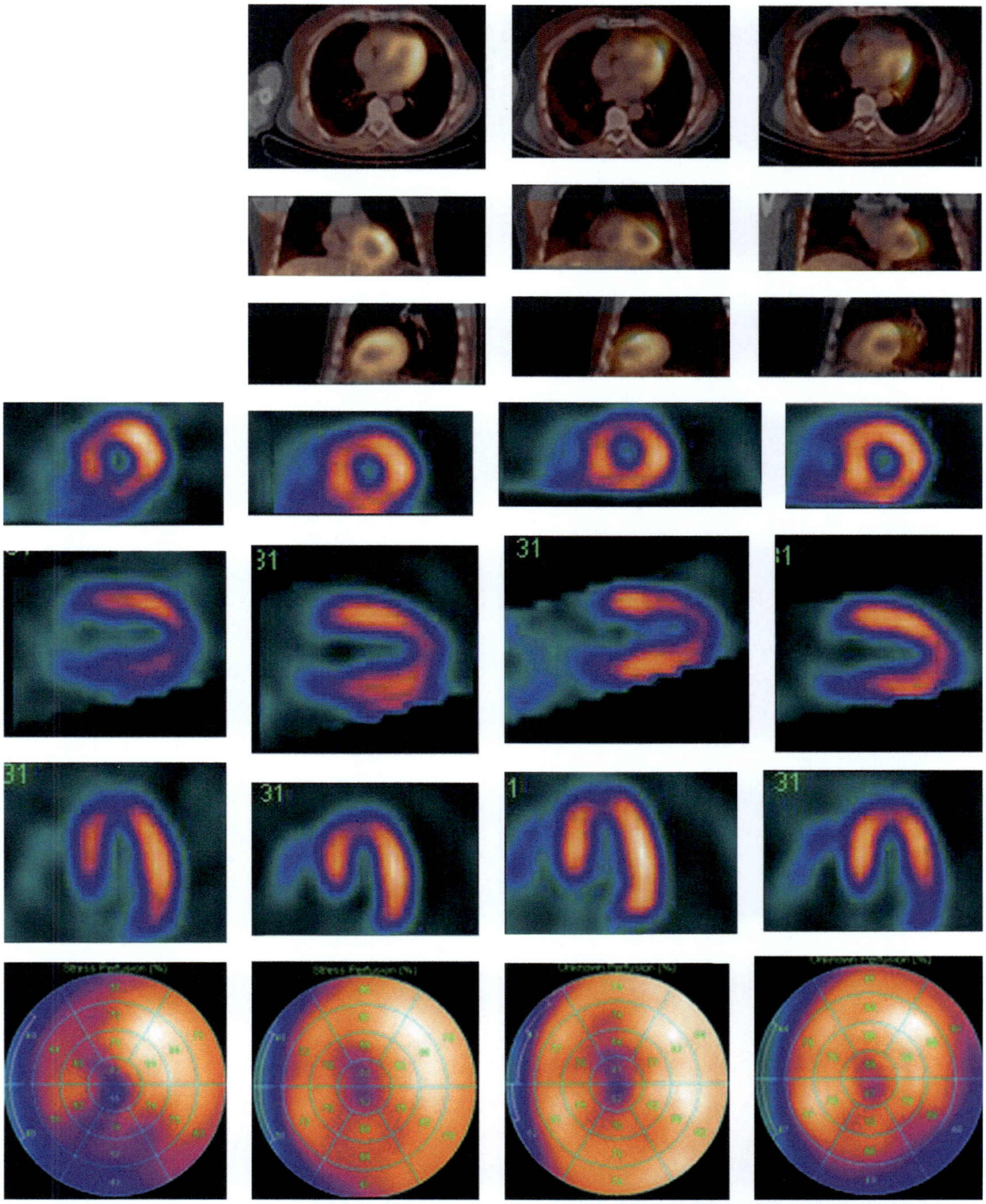

Teaching point

Misalignment between emission and transmission data can create artificial perfusion defects. Careful quality control is required to avoid reconstruction artifacts.

Chapter 7 Parathyroid Imaging with SPECT-CT

Ken Herrmann, Ivan Santi,
Andreas K. Buck,
and Ambros J. Beer

Contents

S. Fanti et al., *Atlas of SPECT-CT*,
DOI: 10.1007/978-3-642-15726-4_7, © Springer-Verlag Berlin Heidelberg 2011

Hyperparathyroidism (HPT) is a common endocrine disorder affecting approximately 1 in 500 women and 1 in 2,000 men. The clinical or chemical diagnosis is commonly seen in the 5th through 7th decades of life [1]. Primary hyperparathyroidism (pHPT) is caused by a solitary parathyroid adenoma in approximately 85% of cases, whereas the remaining cases are often secondary HPT due to glandular hyperplasia, multiple adenomas and, very rarely, also parathyroid carcinomas [2].

HPT is characterized by an increased secretion of parathyroid hormone (PTH) leading to hypercalcemia by promoting the renal tubular absorption of calcium, decreasing tubular reabsorption of phosphate, and stimulating osteoclasts and vitamin D production. The standard curative treatment approach is surgical resection, but also percutaneous ethanol injection has been reported. Therapeutic procedures are often demanding for highly accurate pre-therapeutic imaging, allowing detection and localization of abnormal parathyroid gland tissue accurately. Especially the recently developed minimally invasive surgical techniques require reliable preoperative disease localization [3, 4].

Preoperative imaging modalities comprise sonography, scintigraphy including tomographic imaging (SPECT), CT, MRI and PET. In daily clinical practice, sonography and scintigraphy have emerged as the primary means for HPT detection and localization of parathyroid adenomas [1]. Regarding preoperative sonography for the detection of solitary parathyroid adenomas, sensitivity values ranging between 72% and 89% have been reported [1, 5–8]. In a meta-analysis by Ruda et al. encompassing 54 studies performed between 1995 and 2003, the sensitivity of ultrasound for detection of primary hyperparathyroidism prior to surgery was calculated [2]. Respective sensitivity values were 79% [95% confidence interval (CI), 77–80%], 35% (95% CI, 30–40%) and 16% (95% CI, 4–28%) for detecting solitary adenoma, hyperplasia or double adenoma, respectively. Ruda et al. also investigated the value of 99mTc-sestamibi planar scintigraphy in their meta-analysis. Published sensitivities for detection of solitary adenomas, hyperplasia and double adenomas were 88% (95% CI, 87–89%), 44% (95% CI, 41–48%) and 30% (95% CI, 2–62%), respectively [2].

Introduction of subtraction techniques (administration of a second radiotracer taken up only by the thyroid gland) and SPECT of the neck using a pinhole collimator resulted in higher sensitivities by improved separation of parathyroid activity and activity of the overlying thyroid [9–11] (Fig. 7.1). Some studies reported sensitivities of ≥90% for detection of solitary adenomas by ^{99m}Tc-sestamibi SPECT [12–15]. However, also more critical reports have been published suggesting that the sensitivity of parathyroid scintigraphy without SPECT could be significantly lower than expected from the literature [16]. Gotthardt et al. conclude that apart from different trial designs (e.g., retrospective vs. prospective, varying definitions of a true positive result) and a possible bias by reevaluation of parathyroid scans by specialized physicians, the experience and routine of the reporting physician play an important role.

Recently, integrated SPECT/CT scanners have been introduced into clinical routine. With SPECT/CT, lesions visualized by functional imaging can be correlated with anatomic structures (Fig. 7.2). The addition of anatomic information increases sensitivity as well as specificity of scintigraphic findings in a widespread number of indications [17]. SPECT/CT has also been studied for presurgical imaging and precise localization of parathyroid adenomas (Figs. 7.3 and 7.4). Presurgical localization is critical especially in patients intending to have minimally invasive parathyroidectomy. Lavely et al. compared the diagnostic performance of planar imaging, SPECT, SPECT/CT, and single- and dual-phase 99mTc-MIBI parathyroid scintigraphy in 110 patients [18]. Reported sensitivities ranged from 34% for single-phase planar imaging to 73% for dual-phase studies, including an early SPECT/CT scan. Lavely et al. concluded that early SPECT/CT in combination with any delayed imaging method was significantly more accurate for parathyroid adenoma localization than any single- or dual-phase planar or SPECT study. CT coregistration was revealed to be a valuable tool for the precise delineation of parathyroid adenomas. Furthermore, it was stated that localization with dual-phase acquisition protocols was more accurate than with single-phase ^{99m}Tc-sestamibi scintigraphy for planar imaging, SPECT and SPECT/CT. Superior localization of parathyroid adenomas was also reported by Harris et al. [19]. In a series of 23 patients, SPECT/CT performed well for the detection and localization of solitary adenomas (89%), but performance for the detection of multifocal disease was limited. Less exciting conclusions were drawn in the studies by Ruf et al. [20] and Gayed et al. [21]. Ruf et al. performed low-dose CT for attenuation correction in 26 patients and reported that the sensitivity of attenuation-corrected ^{99m}Tc-MIBI SPECT/CT was only slightly higher than that of non-attenuation-corrected SPECT [20]. In the publication by Gayed et al., SPECT/CT was assumed to be only of limited additional value (8% of patients) [21]. Interestingly, in a retrospective study, Krausz et al. reported a change in therapeutic management in 39% of patients (14/36), mainly due to localization of ectopic parathyroid adenomas or accurate localization in patients with distorted neck anatomy [22]. These inconsistent results do not allow claiming a definite role of SPECT/CT in the imaging of parathyroid adenomas so far, and as previously suggested by Gotthardt and co-workers, it is still necessary to conduct well-designed prospective multi-center trials to reassess the true clinical potential of ^{99m}Tc-MIBI SPECT and ^{99m}Tc-MIBI SPECT/CT, especially in endemic goiter areas and in comparison with other imaging modalities, comprising US, MRI and potentially PET using radiolabeled amino acids (^{11}C-methionine, ^{18}F- fluoro-ethyl-thyrosine).

References

1. Johnson NA, Tublin ME, Ogilvie JB. Parathyroid imaging: technique and role in the preoperative evaluation of primary hyperparathyroidism. AJR. 2007;188(6):1706–15.
2. Ruda JM, Hollenbeak CS, Stack Jr BC. A systematic review of the diagnosis and treatment of primary hyperparathyroidism from 1995 to 2003. Otolaryngol Head Neck Surg. 2005;132(3):359–72.
3. Bergenfelz A, Lindblom P, Tibblin S, Westerdahl J. Unilateral versus bilateral neck exploration for primary hyperparathyroidism: a prospective randomized controlled trial. Ann Surg. 2002;236(5):543–51.
4. Lorenz K, Miccoli P, Monchik JM, Duren M, Dralle H. Minimally invasive video-assisted parathyroidectomy: multiinstitutional study. World J Surg. 2001;25(6):704–7.
5. Haber RS, Kim CK, Inabnet WB. Ultrasonography for preoperative localization of enlarged parathyroid glands in primary hyperparathyroidism: comparison with (99 m) technetium sestamibi scintigraphy. Clin Endocrinol (Oxf). 2002;57(2):241–9.
6. Rickes S, Sitzy J, Neye H, Ocran KW, Wermke W. High-resolution ultrasound in combination with colour-Doppler sonography for preoperative localization of parathyroid adenomas in patients with primary hyperparathyroidism. Ultraschall Med. 2003;24(2):85–9.
7. Solorzano CC, Carneiro-Pla DM, Irvin 3rd GL. Surgeon-performed ultrasonography as the initial and only localizing study in sporadic primary hyperparathyroidism. J Am Coll Surg. 2006;202(1):18–24.
8. Stephen AE, Chen KT, Milas M, Siperstein AE. The coming of age of radiation-induced hyperparathyroidism: evolving patterns of thyroid and parathyroid disease after head and neck irradiation. Surgery. 2004;136(6):1143–53.
9. Lorberboym M, Minski I, Macadziob S, Nikolov G, Schachter P. Incremental diagnostic value of preoperative 99mTc-MIBI SPECT in patients with a parathyroid adenoma. J Nucl Med. 2003;44(6):904–8.
10. Slater A, Gleeson FV. Increased sensitivity and confidence of SPECT over planar imaging in dual-phase sestamibi for parathyroid adenoma detection. Clin Nucl Med. 2005;30(1):1–3.
11. Spanu A, Falchi A, Manca A, et al. The usefulness of neck pinhole SPECT as a complementary tool to planar scintigraphy in primary and secondary hyperparathyroidism. J Nucl Med. 2004;45(1):40–8.
12. Blanco I, Carril JM, Banzo I, et al. Double-phase Tc-99m sestamibi scintigraphy in the preoperative location of lesions causing hyperparathyroidism. Clin Nucl Med. 1998;23(5):291–7.
13. Chen CC, Holder LE, Scovill WA, Tehan AM, Gann DS. Comparison of parathyroid imaging with technetium-99m-pertechnetate/sestamibi subtraction, double-phase technetium-99m-sestamibi and technetium-99m-sestamibi SPECT. J Nucl Med. 1997;38(6):834–9.
14. Pinero A, Rodriguez JM, Ortiz S, et al. Relation of biochemical, cytologic, and morphologic parameters to the result of gammagraphy with technetium 99m sestamibi in primary hyperparathyroidism. Otolaryngol Head Neck Surg. 2000;122(6):851–5.
15. Song AU, Phillips TE, Edmond CV, Moore DW, Clark SK. Success of preoperative imaging and unilateral neck exploration for primary hyperparathyroidism. Otolaryngol Head Neck Surg. 1999;121(4):393–7.
16. Gotthardt M, Lohmann B, Behr TM, et al. Clinical value of parathyroid scintigraphy with technetium-99m methoxyisobutylisonitrile: discrepancies in clinical data and a systematic metaanalysis of the literature. World J Surg. 2004;28(1):100–7.
17. Buck AK, Nekolla S, Ziegler S, et al. Spect/Ct. J Nucl Med. 2008;49(8):1305–19.
18. Lavely WC, Goetze S, Friedman KP, et al. Comparison of SPECT/CT, SPECT, and planar imaging with single- and dual-phase (99m)Tc-sestamibi parathyroid scintigraphy. J Nucl Med. 2007;48(7):1084–9.
19. Harris L, Yoo J, Driedger A, et al. Accuracy of technetium-99m SPECT-CT hybrid images in predicting the precise intraoperative anatomical location of parathyroid adenomas. Head Neck. 2008;30(4):509–17.
20. Ruf J, Seehofer D, Denecke T, et al. Impact of image fusion and attenuation correction by SPECT-CT on the scintigraphic detection of parathyroid adenomas. Nuklearmedizin. 2007;46(1):15–21.
21. Gayed IW, Kim EE, Broussard WF, et al. The value of 99mTc-sestamibi SPECT/CT over conventional SPECT in the evaluation of parathyroid adenomas or hyperplasia. J Nucl Med. 2005;46(2):248–52.
22. Krausz Y, Bettman L, Guralnik L, et al. Technetium-99m-MIBI SPECT/CT in primary hyperparathyroidism. World J Surg. 2006;30(1):76–83.

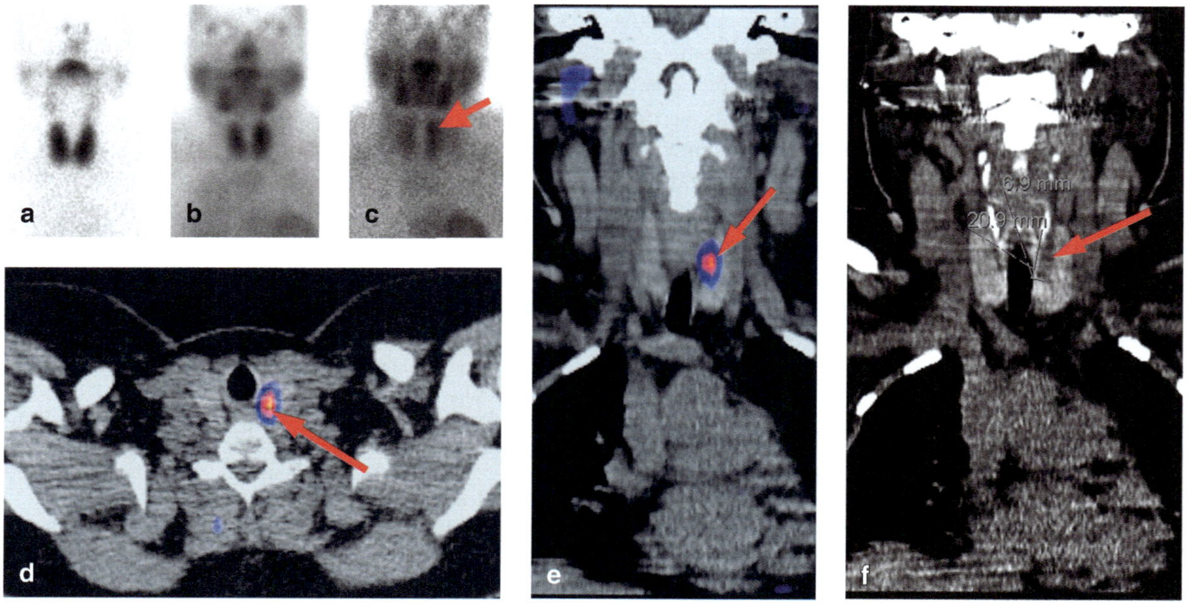

^{99m}Tc-pertechnetate and ^{99m}Tc-sestamibi findings

Dual-tracer planar scintigraphy and SPECT/CT in a patient with hyperparathyroidism. Normal findings in ^{99m}Tc planar scintigraphy (**a**). Note that in early ^{99m}Tc-sestamibi planar scintigraphy (**b**) there is a larger area of radiotracer uptake visible at the upper half of the left thyroid lobe compared to the previous image. In the late ^{99m}Tc-sestamibi planar scintigraphy (**c**) a focal but faint radiotracer uptake is present in the projection on the upper half of the left thyroid lobe, though not perfectly distinguishable. These findings however lead to the diagnosis of an upper left solitary parathyroid adenoma (*arrow*). The patient also underwent early acquisition SPECT/CT. The fused images in transaxial (**d**) and coronal (**e**) sections demonstrate the presence of the solitary parathyroid adenoma posterior to the left thyroid lobe (*arrows*), providing much more precise anatomical details than planar scintigraphy. CT alone in coronal view (**f**) shows the anatomical position of the adenoma (*arrow*) allowing exact measurements (6.9 and 20.9 mm) and precise anatomical localization for planning of surgery.

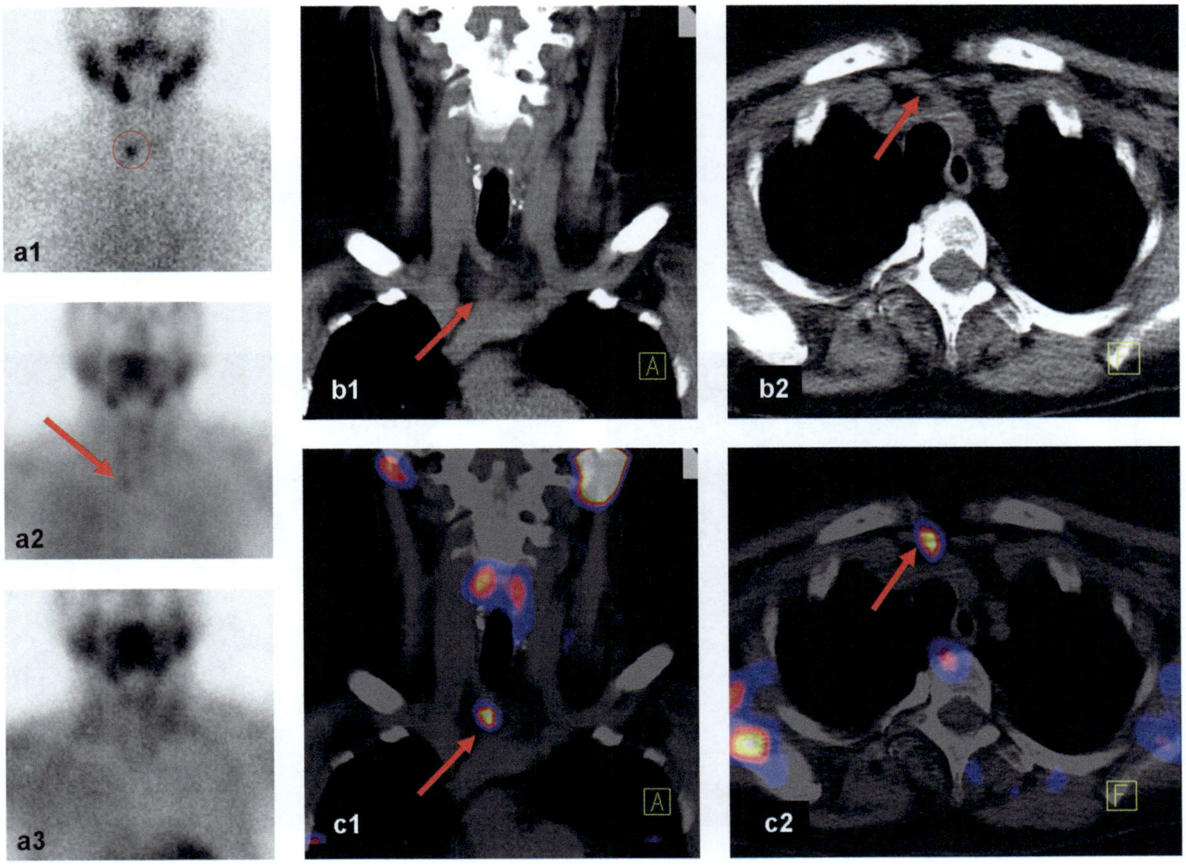

◘ ^{99m}Tc-pertechnetate and ^{99m}Tc-sestamibi findings

Patient with a diagnosis of hyperparathyroidism that underwent ^{99m}Tc-pertechnetate planar scintigraphy (**a1**) showing a thyroid nodule in the lower half of the right lobe (*circle*), not consistent with parathyroid. Subsequently early ^{99m}Tc-sestamibi planar scintigraphy (**a2**) showed a faint focal uptake located at the right paramedian upper mediastinum, which however was no longer visible at late ^{99m}Tc-sestamibi acquisition (**a3**). SPECT/CT was performed right after early planar acquisition: CT alone in coronal (**b1**) and transaxial (**b2**) sections shows the presence of a nodular structure (*arrows*) in the upper mediastinum anterior to the trachea in the right paramedial region. The respective fused images (**c1**, **c2**) demonstrate the actual correspondence between the focal radiotracer uptake and the CT finding, leading to the identification of the parathyroid adenoma (*arrows*).

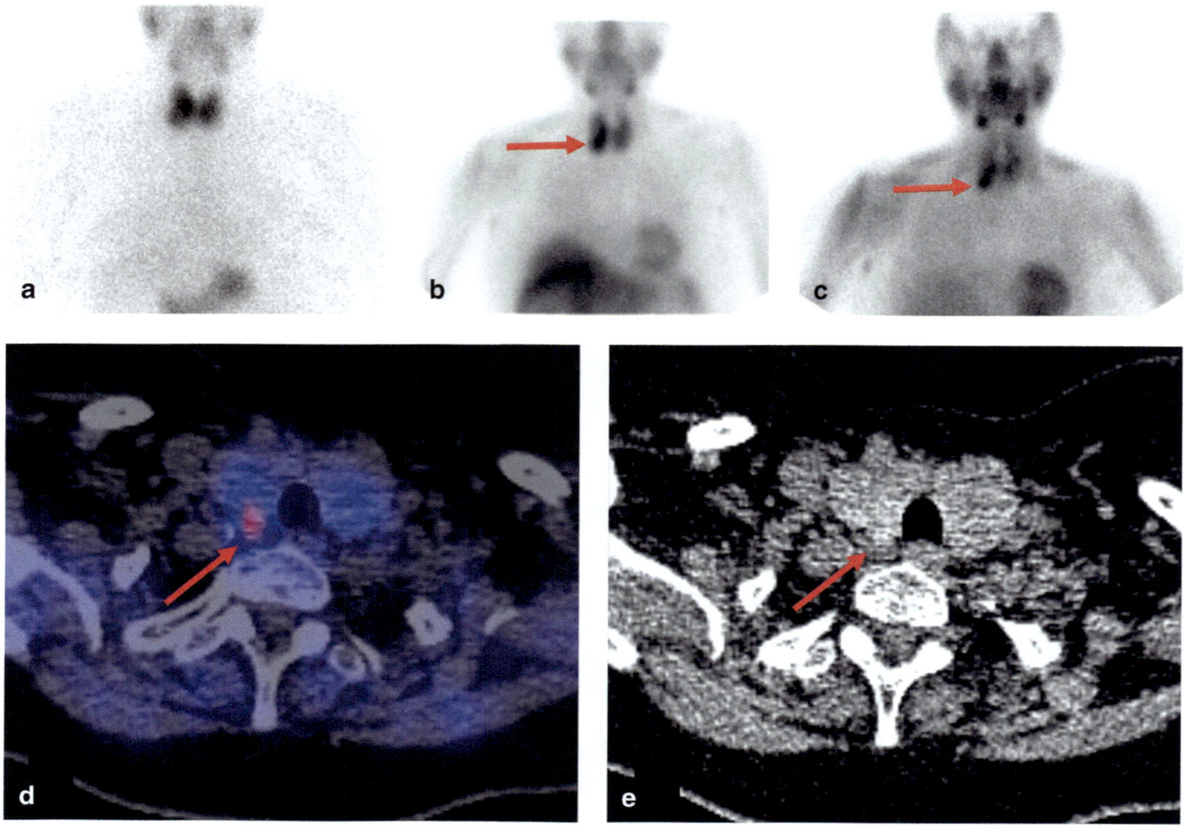

^{99m}Tc-pertechnetate and ^{99m}Tc-sestamibi findings

Patient with hyperparathyroidism studied with dual-tracer planar scintigraphy and SPECT/TC: following standard procedure thyroid planar scintigraphy (**a**) was compared to early ^{99m}Tc-sestamibi planar acquisition (**b**); the latter study showed a larger and more intense radiotracer uptake at the lower half of the right thyroid lobe (*arrow*) compared to the former. This was confirmed by the late ^{99m}Tc-sestamibi planar scintigraphy (**c**) displaying a focal uptake that however overlapped the lower pole of the right thyroid lobe (*arrow*). Thanks to the more detailed anatomical information, the SPECT/CT fused image (**d**) and CT image (**e**) demonstrated the correspondence between the tracer uptake and an enlarged parathyroid gland posterior to the right lower pole of the thyroid gland.

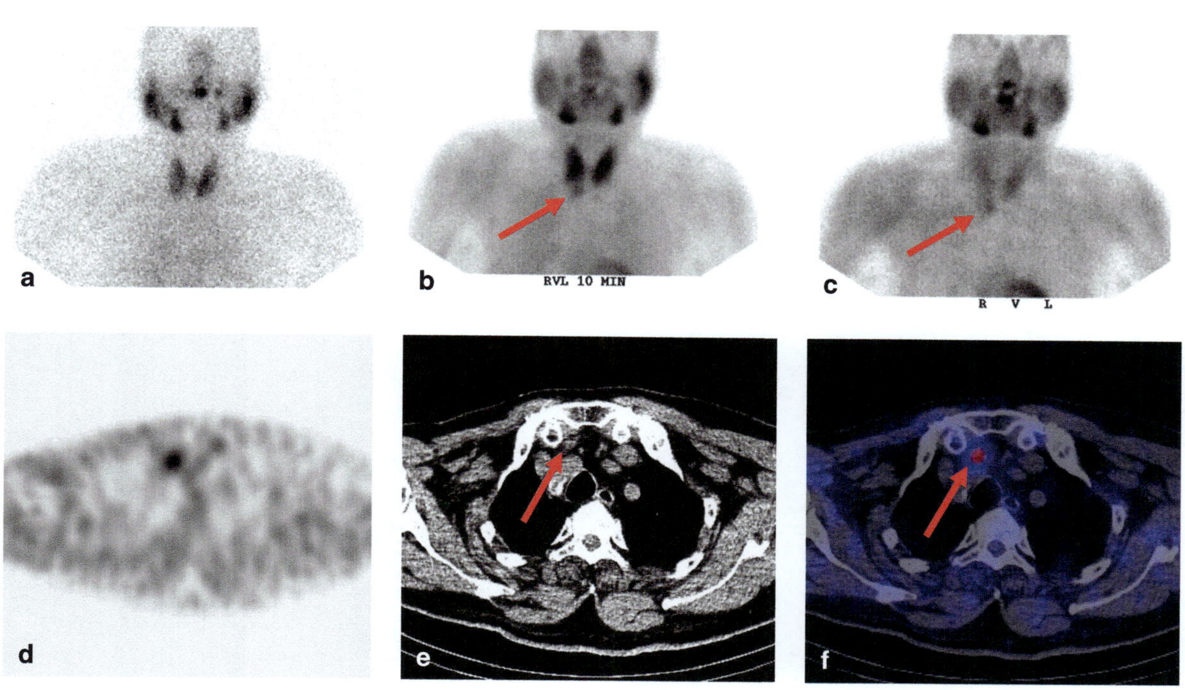

^{99m}Tc-pertechnetate and ^{99m}Tc-sestamibi findings

Patient presenting with hyperparathyroidism studied with standard dual-tracer scintigraphy: the comparison between thyroid scintigraphy (**a**) and early (**b**) and late (**c**) ^{99m}Tc-sestamibi planar acquisitions showed the presence of an area of focal MIBI uptake below the right thyroid lobe (*arrows*) not visible in the pertechnetate study, thus suggesting a parathyroid adenoma. SPECT (**d**), CT (**e**) and fused SPECT/CT (**f**) images could precisely identify a retrosternal right parathyroid adenoma (*arrows*).

Chapter 8

Sentinel Node Imaging with SPECT-CT

Cornelis A. Hoefnagel

Contents

S. Fanti et al., *Atlas of SPECT-CT*,
DOI: 10.1007/978-3-642-15726-4_8,

8.1 Introduction

The sentinel lymph node biopsy (SLNB) procedure has become an important tool in surgical oncology for staging of operable tumors at the nodal level. If the first draining node(s) is/are found to be free of tumor cells, more extensive nodal surgery, which may be associated with additional morbidity and complications, e.g., lymphoedema, can be avoided.

However, in order to base the entire treatment policy on the analysis of a single node or few nodes, it is imperative that the correct lymph node is identified as the sentinel node. Nuclear medicine plays an essential role in the preoperative mapping of sentinel nodes, which can then be selectively approached and resected, guided by an intraoperative gamma probe.

After this technique was introduced for melanoma and breast carcinoma in the early 1990s, the number of clinical indications has expanded significantly, and the sentinel lymph node biopsy is currently used in a great variety of tumor types, including penile carcinoma, vulvar carcinoma, testicular cancer, cervical carcinoma, prostatic cancer, bladder cancer, head and neck cancer, thyroid carcinoma, lung cancer, esophageal, gastric and colorectal cancers, anal carcinoma and Merkel cell tumors.

8.2 Sentinel Lymph Node Imaging and Biopsy

The sentinel node biopsy procedure in surgical oncology was introduced in early stage melanoma by Morton in 1992, although the term sentinel node had already been used by Cabanas in 1977, when he reported his approach to the management of penile carcinoma.

The procedure is based upon the concept of an orderly progression of lymph node metastases: the tumor drains directly to one or a few first lymph nodes, called sentinel node(s), from which further connections with so-called second-echelon nodes exist.

First, the lymphatic drainage pathways from the tumor are mapped, and the sentinel node(s) is/are identified by lymphoscintigraphy, so that, subsequently, these can be localized more easily during surgery, both by using an intraoperative probe and by injection of patent blue dye, and then selectively removed. Depending on the outcome of histological examination (including hematoxyline-eosine and immunohistochemical staining), subsequently radical lymphadenectomy will follow in case of metastases or may be refrained from, when the sentinel node(s) is/are normal. This procedure represents a sensitive staging method.

Literature shows that the combined use of lymphoscintigraphy, intraoperative probe and blue dye is the most reliable approach, with a detection rate varying from 93% to 100%, versus 66–82% for blue dye only and 84–93% for using the probe without lymphoscintigraphy. The number of false-negative results is inversely related.

In order to make this procedure as successful and reliable as possible, the lymphoscintigraphic studies must meet the highest quality criteria, which can be achieved by using the right radiopharmaceutical (generally Technetium-99m-labeled microcolloids with a diameter ranging from 5 to 75 nm are preferred), meticulous tracer administration (depending on the indication), the use of a modern gamma camera, performing imaging at several time intervals both in the anterior and lateral projection (and for breast carcinoma in prone position), defining the body contour by means of transmission scanning using a ^{57}Co-flood source, and identifying and localizing the sentinel node(s) with the aid of a marker source or pen, marking its site on the skin with non-erasable ink in the position in which the patient will be operated.

The major success determining factors for the sentinel node biopsy procedure are: the administered dose, colloid size, number of colloid particles (concentration), route of administration, protocol and quality of the lymphoscintigram. As there is a distinct learning curve for nuclear medicine physicians, technologists and surgeons, experience is an equally important factor, as is teamwork between nuclear medicine, surgery and pathology departments. The yield of this procedure may be significantly enhanced by introducing new tools and three-dimensional orientation.

8.3 New Tools

For some of the more recent indications for sentinel lymph node biopsy, the procedure as described above will not suffice. To locate and access sentinel nodes in more difficult locations, new technologies have been developed. For instance, to dissect an intraabdominal sentinel node, laparoscopic probes have become available. But for this approach, it makes no sense to mark the location of the sentinel node on the abdominal skin; the surgeon requires more accurate anatomical localization of the sentinel node, which can be provided by adding SPECT/CT to the scintigraphic node mapping.

An additional improvement is the use of a portable mini gamma camera in the surgical theater. This portable camera can be positioned above the patient undergoing surgery and can be set to display both the Technetium-99m signal from the sentinel node and the signal from an Iodine-125 seed on the tip of the laparoscopic probe. This way the laparoscopic probe can be guided to the sentinel node, and the effective resection of this node can be monitored real-time.

More recently, also the use of 3D mini gamma cameras has been investigated and software for 3D display of SPECT/CT images utilized.

8.4 Why SPECT/CT?

For some of the more traditional indications (melanoma, breast cancer, penile and vulvar carcinoma) planar lymphoscintigraphy, both in anterior/posterior and lateral projections and at several time intervals after administration of ^{99m}Tc-nanocolloid, often suffices to locate the sentinel node and mark its position on the skin.

However, for tumors or lymphatics located in anatomically more challenging regions, e.g., the head and neck, abdominal and pelvic areas, more advanced technologies, such as SPECT/CT and intraoperative mini gamma camera are required to provide surgeons with more detailed information about the location of the sentinel node(s).

In prostate cancer, for instance, the tumor generally drains to pelvic lymph nodes, but drainage outside the area of the extended pelvic lymphadenectomy (e.g., to the aortic-iliac junction, paraaortic lymph nodes, abdominal wall) may also be observed. It is relevant to know the exact location in relation to other structures (in particular, to the large vessels), in order to be able to locate and identify the sentinel node successfully and to remove it safely during operation.

In this respect, SPECT/CT has significant value to localize the sentinel node(s) preoperatively and guide the surgeon during surgery. Evaluating the role of SPECT/CT in a series of patients with prostatic carcinoma [1], SPECT/CT was found to reveal additional sentinel nodes in 63% of the patients, and sentinel nodes located outside the area of extended pelvic lymphadenectomy were detected in 35% of the patients. In 56% of the cases, these were only detected by SPECT/CT. In other words, without the addition of SPECT/CT, sentinel nodes would be missed in 20% of all patients, even with the performance of extended pelvic lymphadectomy.

In case of positive sentinel nodes, postoperative radiotherapy may be indicated, and also here the SPECT/CT images can serve as guidance to determine the correct radiotherapy target volume.

Another complex area for sentinel node detection and localization is the head and neck region. Again, SPECT/CT will detect more sentinel nodes than planar lymphoscintigraphy and provides better anatomical localization.

Also in selected patients with melanoma or breast carcinoma, there is additional value of SPECT/CT. For melanoma, this may be particularly true for head and neck and truncal locations of the primary tumor. In breast carcinoma, SPECT/CT may be very helpful to detect and localize non-axillary sentinel nodes, e.g., internal mammary, intramammary, interpectoral and subpectoral nodes, and to exclude false-positive findings due no non-nodal tracer accumulation (e.g., intralymphatic or contamination). Moreover, in case of nonvisualization of a sentinel node on the planar lymphoscintigram, SPECT/CT may still reveal and localize the sentinel node, especially when it is not so active and/or deeply located.

Nevertheless, sequential images of planar lymphoscintigraphy will remain important to identify lymph nodes appearing early as sentinel nodes. However the anatomical localization of these sentinel nodes is better achieved by SPECT/CT. It may provide new insight into the lymphatic spread of tumors, such as cervical, prostatic and testicular cancer, bladder and renal cell carcinoma.

8.5 Three-Dimensional Imaging

Taking the SPECT/CT study one step further, it is possible to display the SPECT/CT fusion images in a two-dimensional way (transaxial, coronal and/or sagittal sections) or in a three-dimensional way. For the latter, SPECT/CT fusion images are stacked and displayed in a volume-rendered way. The software allows choosing from a variety of parameters, by which the sentinel node(s) can be displayed within its surrounding environment, highlighting anatomical structures, such as bone, muscle and/or skin. Although the 3D volume-rendered images (either displayed in a static, rotational or tilted mode) contain essentially the same information as the 2D tomographic fusion images, the 3D volume-rendered display provides the surgeon with a three-dimensional roadmap, which is attractive and more easily interpretable. Improved anatomical information to the surgeon may influence the surgical approach with the aim of preserving important and fragile normal anatomical structures.

Evaluating the use of combined 2D SPECT/CT and 3D volume-rendered images in 30 consecutive patients, the anatomical localization of the sentinel node was improved in 77% and the surgical approach was altered in 50% of the patients.

It is concluded that SPECT/CT is more sensitive and accurate than planar lymphoscintigraphy in locating the sentinel node(s), in particular in tumors of the head and neck, abdomen and pelvis, as well as in the localization of non-axillary sentinel nodes in breast carcinoma.

By several cases presented in this chapter, the complementary role of SPECT/CT in sentinel node lymphoscintigraphy in a variety of tumor types will be demonstrated, showing how the SPECT/CT fusion image and 3D volume rendering can highlight the exact location of the sentinel node, which would often be difficult to mark on the skin, in relation to essential anatomical structures relevant to the surgeon.

Reference

1. Vermeeren L, Valdés Olmos RA, Meinhardt W, Bex A, van der Poel HG, Vogel WV, Sivro F, Hoefnagel CA, Horenblas S. Value of SPECT/CT for detection and anatomic localization of sentinel lymph nodes before laparoscopic sentinel node lymphadenectomy in prostate cancer. J Nucl Med. 2009;50:865–870.

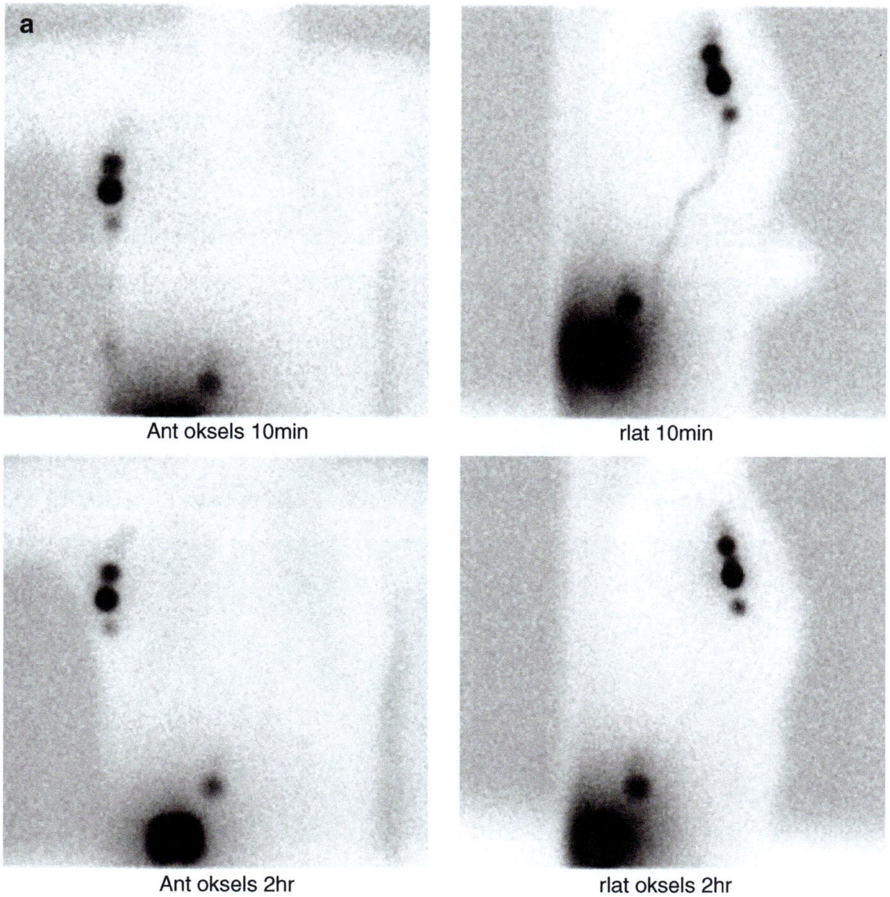
a
Ant oksels 10min
rlat 10min
Ant oksels 2hr
rlat oksels 2hr

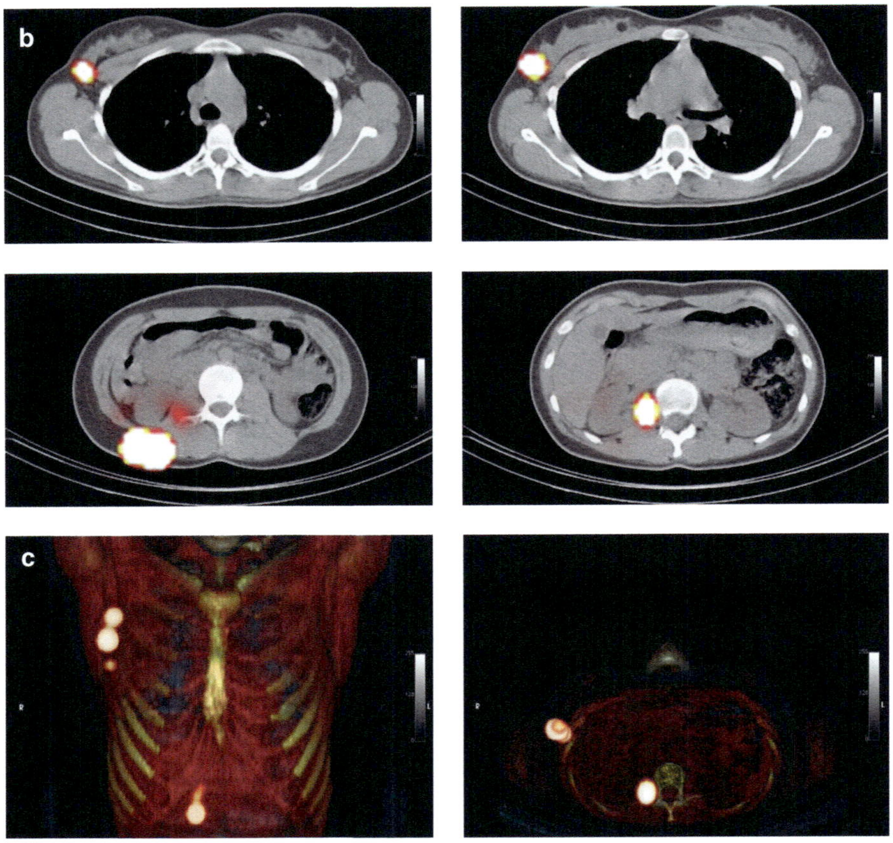

Sentinel lymph node mapping in an 18-year-old female patient with a cutaneous melanoma in the right lumbar region

Sentinel node scintigraphy findings

Planar scintigraphy (**a**) shows lymphatic drainage to the right axilla, but also reveals a lymph node close to the injection site: subcutaneous sentinel node, interval node? SPECT/CT (**b**) and 3D volume rendering (**c**) localize this node more deeply in the right paravertebral region, which alters the surgical approach.

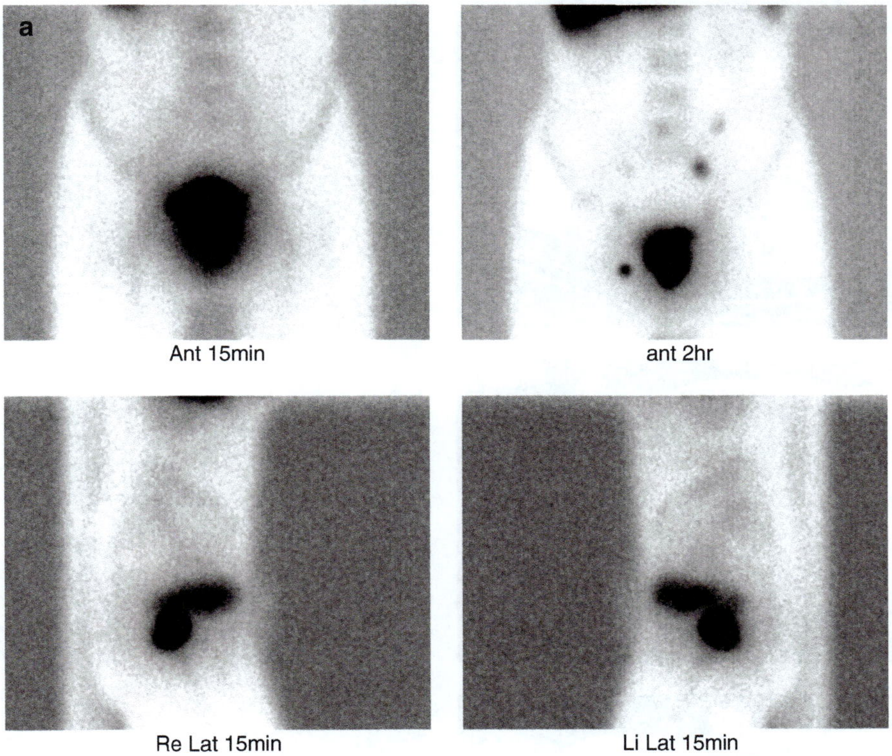

A 67-year-old male with a recurrent prostatic carcinoma

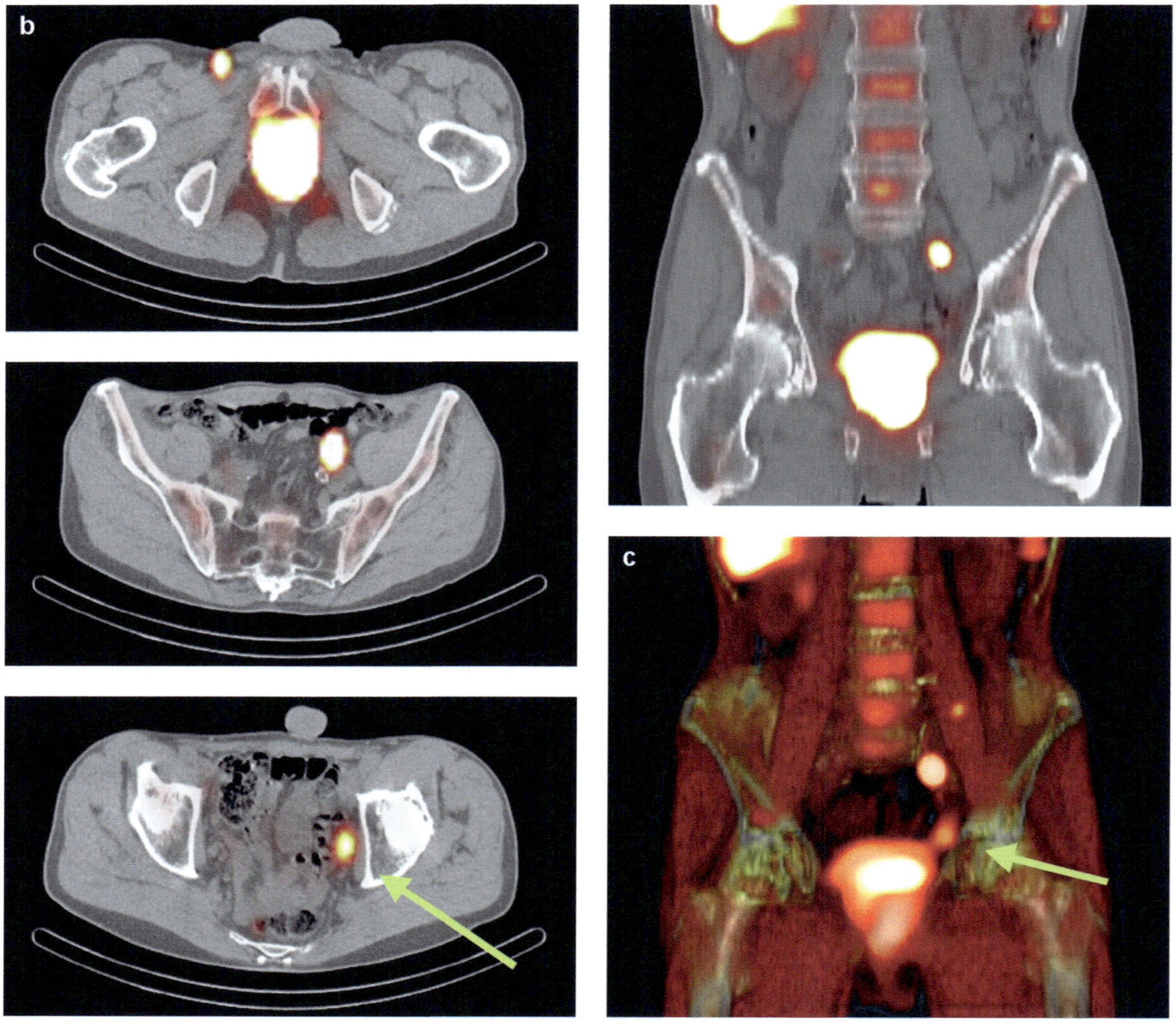

Sentinel node scintigraphy findings

After ultrasound-guided transrectal administration into both prostatic lobes, planar lymphoscintigraphy (**a**) shows unilateral drainage to a quite cranially located left parailiac sentinel node, as well as deviation of lymphatic drainage on the right towards the right groin, probably due to previous brachytherapy with 125I-seeds. SPECT/CT (**b**) and 3D volume rendering (**c**) localize this sentinel node and reveal an additional sentinel node below it (*arrow*). The sentinel nodes were successfully removed by laparoscopic probe, guided by an intraoperative mini gamma camera.

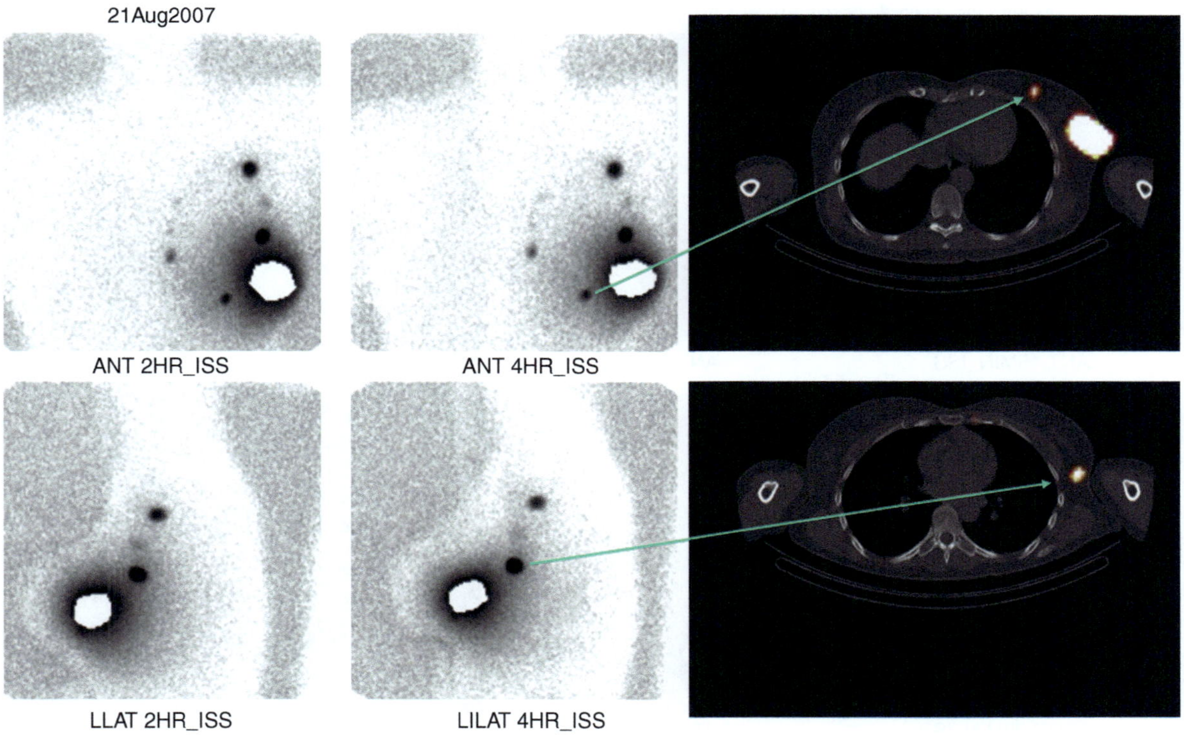

Female patient, 43 years old, with left-sided breast carcinoma

Sentinel node scintigraphy findings

Planar lymphoscintigraphy shows sentinel nodes in the left axilla, as well as an additional sentinel node medial to the injection site: subcutaneous, intramammary or intercostal node? SPECT/CT confirms that it is an intramammary sentinel node.

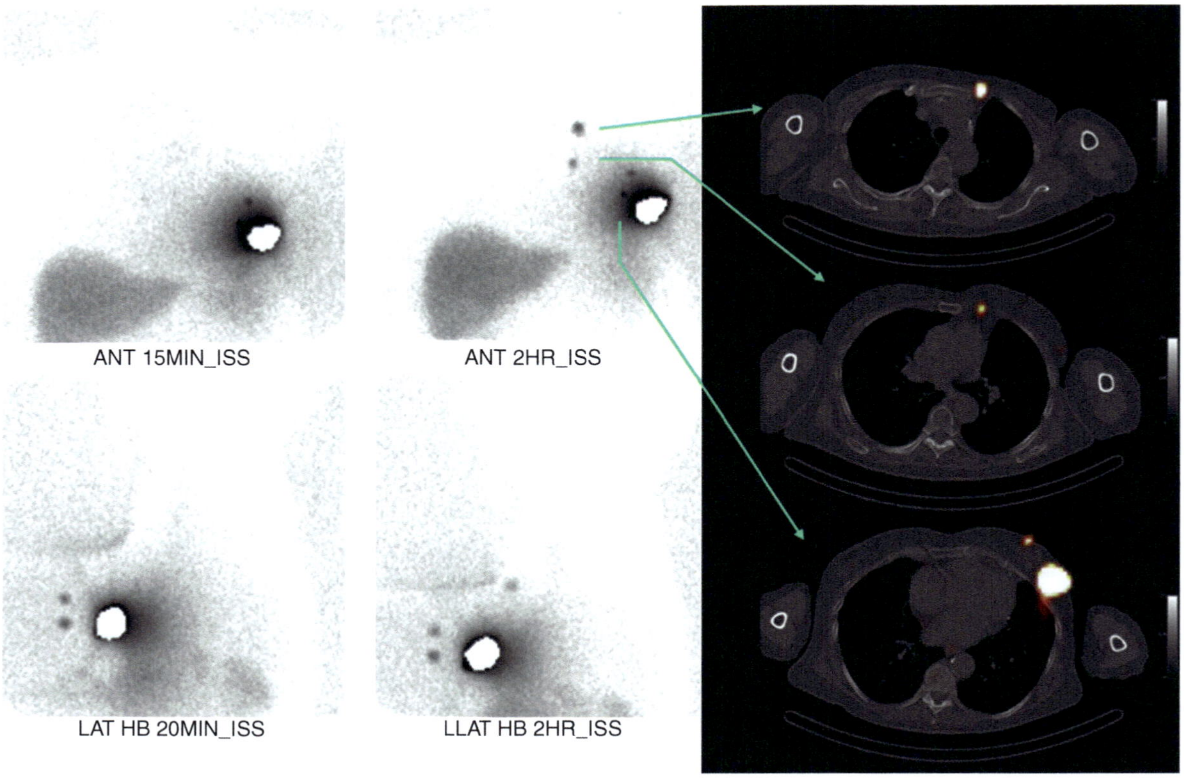

Female patient, 33 years old, with leftsided breast carcinoma

Sentinel node scintigraphy findings

Planar lymphoscintigraphy shows sentinel nodes in the left internal mammary chain, no axillary nodes, and two nodes close to the injection site: intramammary nodes? SPECT/CT confirms that the hot spots are caused by contamination on the skin.

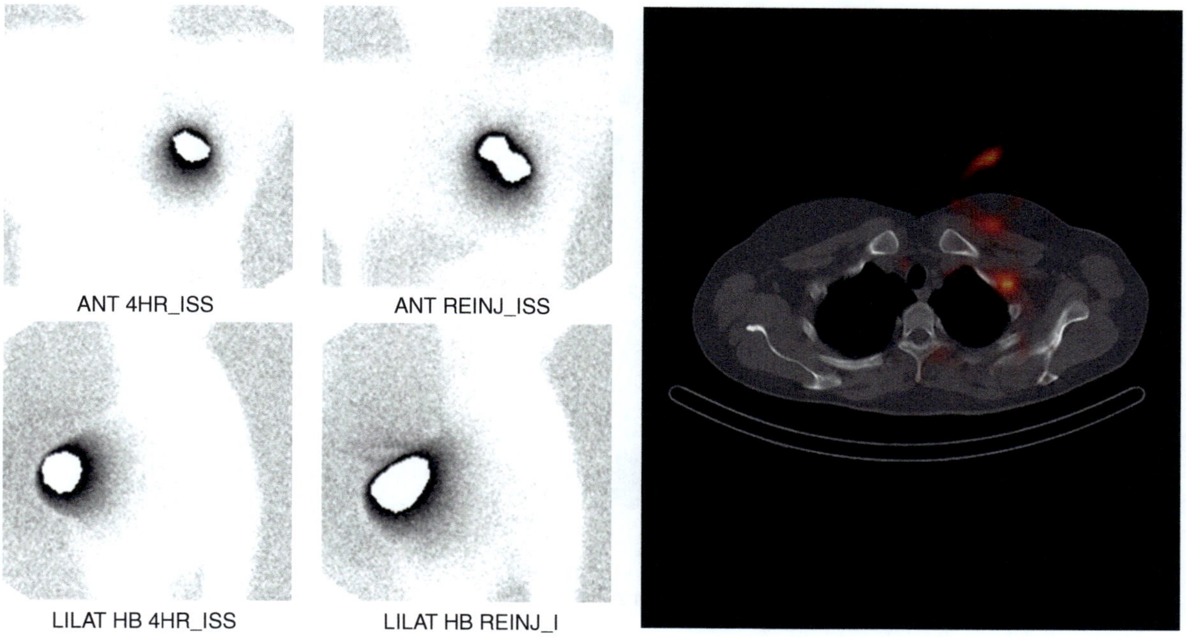

Female patient, 49 years old, with a small tumor in the upper medial quadrant of the left breast

Sentinel node scintigraphy findings

Despite reinjection, planar scintigraphy does not visualize any nodes. SPECT/CT reveals a sentinel node, located deeply in the left axilla against the thoracic wall.

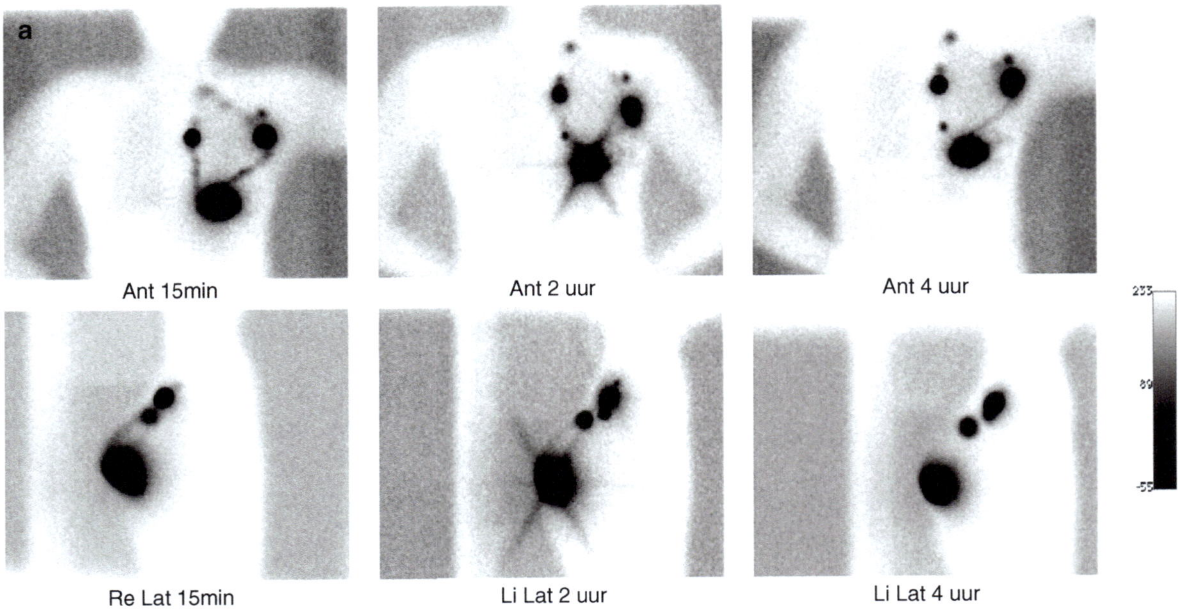

Female patient, 35 years old, with breast carcinoma in the left lower medial quadrant

Sentinel node scintigraphy findings

Early planar lymphoscintigraphy (**a**) shows drainage to the internal mammary chain and to the left axilla with clear afferent lymphatic vessels. The late images reveal an additional sentinel node between the tumor and the internal mammary sentinel node. SPECT/CT (**b**) shows that this is also an internal mammary sentinel node and, together with 3D volume rendering (**c**), provides better localization to the surgeon.

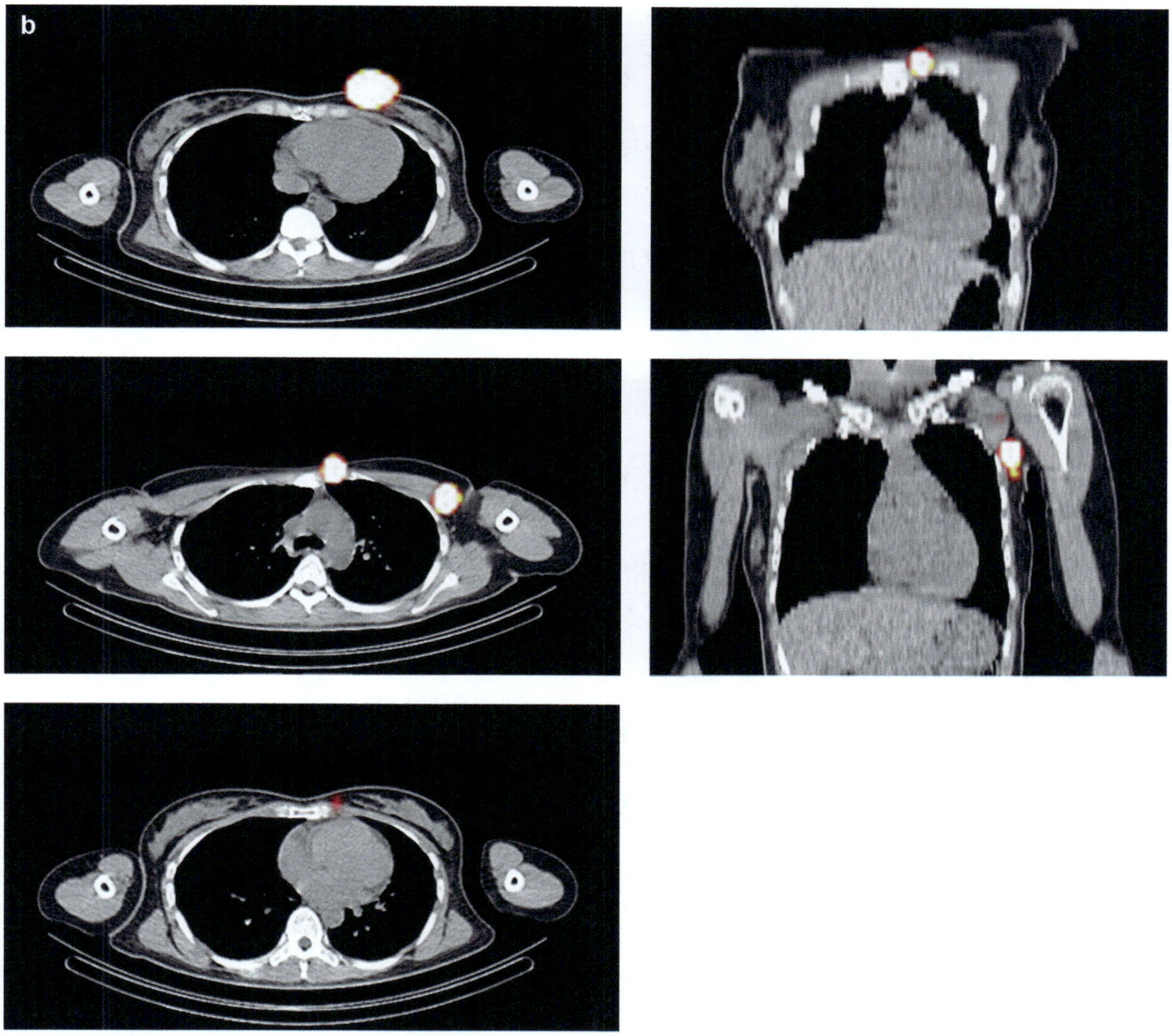
b

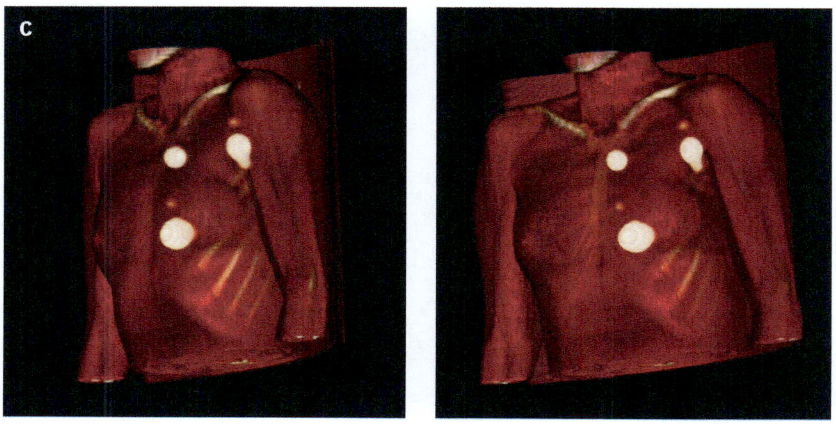
c

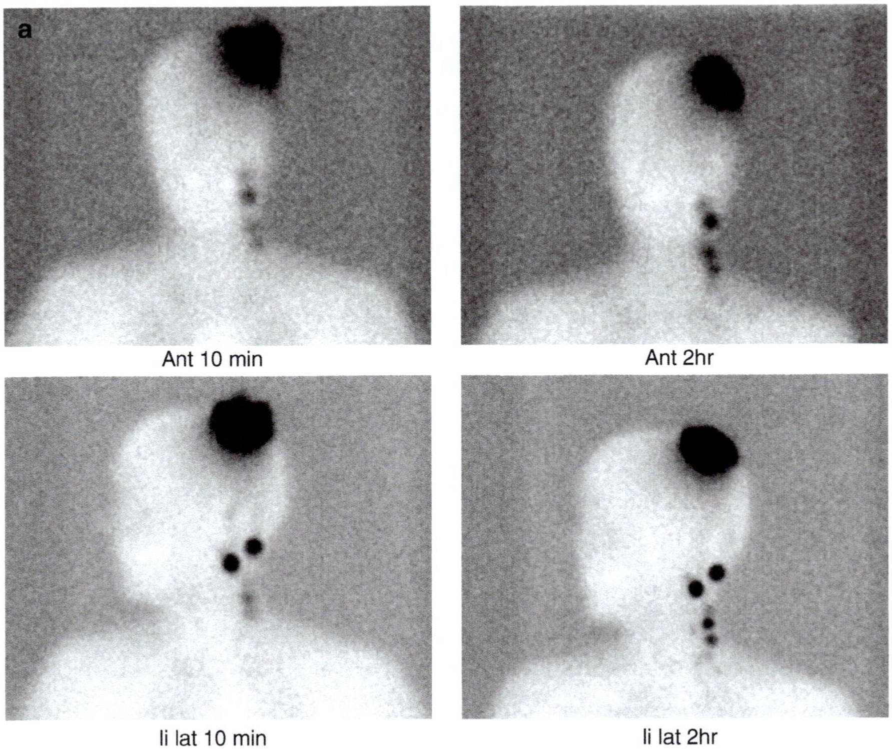
a
Ant 10 min
Ant 2hr
li lat 10 min
li lat 2hr

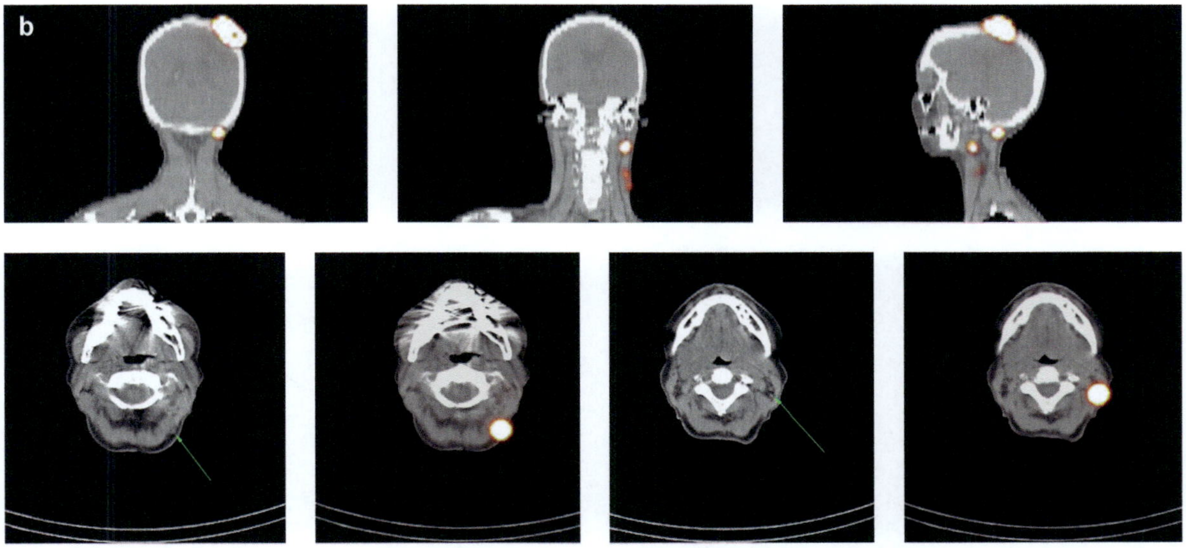

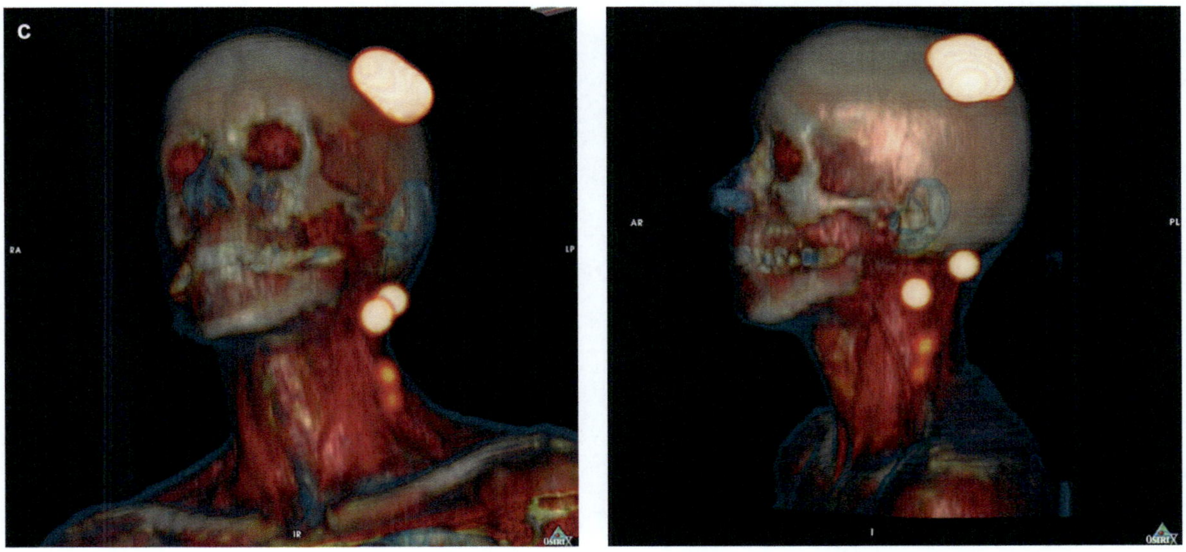

Male, 55 years old, with a tumor of the hairy skin of his head

Sentinel node scintigraphy findings

Planar lymphoscintigraphy (**a**) shows lymphatic drainage to two sentinel nodes high in the left posterior neck and two second-echelon nodes below them in the left posterior triangle, localized better by SPECT/CT (**b**) and 3D volume rendering (**c**).

Chapter 9 Infection Imaging Using SPECT-CT

Onelio Geatti,
Andor W.J.M. Glaudemans,
Fernando Di Gregorio,
Elena Lazzeri, and Alberto Signore

Contents

S. Fanti et al., *Atlas of SPECT-CT*,
DOI: 10.1007/978-3-642-15726-4_9, © Springer-Verlag Berlin Heidelberg 2011

9.1 White Blood Cell SPECT-CT

Onelio Geatti, Andor W.J.M. Glaudemans,
Fernando Di Gregorio, and Alberto Signore (✉)

The clinical use of radiolabelled white blood cells (WBC) is of invaluable importance for the diagnosis and follow-up of many diseases and for research purposes. In the field of inflammation and infection imaging, radiolabelled white blood cell scintigraphy (WBC-S) is the gold standard technique for infection detection [1–4]. The body of evidence accumulated so far about the use of WBC-S all over the world makes this technique the method of choice, and it will be the standard technique for many years to come. Over the past 30 years, there has been phenomenal growth in the use of this technique to satisfy clinical demands.

In the mid 1970s, ^{111}In-oxine was introduced as a non-selective labelling for WBC-S. This complex is a nonspecific agent, as it is neutral and lipid-soluble, which enables it to penetrate through the bilayer cell membrane. Within the cell, indium becomes firmly attached to cytoplasmic components, such as lactoferrin. After injection, about 60% of the radioactivity is immediately taken up by the liver, spleen, bone marrow and other tissues. There is only a very short transient hold-up in the bowel. The remainder shows exponential clearance from the circulation with a half-life between 5 and 10 h, resulting in a final uptake of 20% in the liver, 25% in the spleen, 30% in the bone marrow and 25% in other organs. Clearance of activity from the liver and spleen is very slow, resulting in a very low excretion of activity in both the urine and faeces. The advantages of ^{111}In-oxine-labelled WBCs are the high labelling efficiency (LE), the low efflux of activity from the labelled WBCs, and – if a bone marrow scan is required at 24 h – that they do not interfere with imaging, because different energy windows can be used. ^{111}In-labelled WBCs are preferentially indicated for imaging abdominal infections and inflammatory bowel diseases because of the low intestinal excretion. Disadvantages however are the low quality of the planar and SPECT images, the need to order ^{111}In in advance, and the high radiation exposure of labelled cells, critical organs (spleen) and the whole body [5].

Although ^{111}In-oxine-labelled WBCs have been successfully used in the field of infection/inflammation, over the years the labelling agent has been largely replaced by ^{99m}Tc-HMPAO because of the favourable physical characteristics, availability, costs and lower radiation burden. ^{99m}Tc-HMPAO kit preparations have been commercially available since 1988. This lypophilic complex can freely cross the cell membrane of WBCs and is subsequently trapped inside the cell by two mechanisms: (1) conversion into a hydrophilic complex by reducing agents, such as glutathione, and (2) binding to nondiffusible proteins and cell organelles. After reinjection in the patients, some release of ^{99m}Tc-HMPAO from the WBCs is observed, resulting in accumulation of radioactivity in the gastrointestinal and urinary tracts [6]. Normal physiological uptake is seen in the spleen, liver, bone marrow, lungs (in early images) and, as mentioned above, the bowel, kidneys and bladder.

The common clinical indications for WBC-S (both ^{99m}Tc-HMPAO and ^{111}In-oxine, the latter being preferable for the detection of inflammatory sites in the abdomen) include osteomyelitis of the appendicular skeleton, infected joint and vascular prosthesis, inflammatory bowel disease, intra-abdominal infections, diabetic foot, fever of unknown origin, postoperative abscesses, lung infections, endocarditis, neurological infections, and infected central venous catheters or other devices [5, 6].

Regardless of which tracer is used, uptake of labelled WBCs depends on intact chemotaxis, the number and types of cells labelled, and the cellular component of a particular inflammatory response. Labelling of WBCs does not affect their chemotactic response. A total white blood cell count of at least 2,000/μl is needed to obtain satisfactory images. In most clinical settings, a mixed leukocyte population is labelled. Hence, the majority of cells labelled are neutrophils, and therefore the procedure is most useful for identifying neutrophil-mediated inflammatory processes, such as bacterial infections. The procedure is less useful for those diseases in which the predominant cellular response is not neutrophilic, i.e., opportunistic infections, tuberculosis and sarcoidosis.

The whole labelling procedure has some major disadvantages. It is laborious and time-consuming, relatively expensive, and exposes the patient and the operator to several potential risks. Waterproof gloves should be worn throughout the procedure, and special caution should be taken when handling needles. Strict aseptic conditions are required, with only sterile reagents and disposable plastic ware used. This implies that the whole procedure should be performed by trained personnel under strict regulations in a class A laminar flow cabinet in a class B or class C environment [7]. Recently, guidelines from the EANM for the whole labelling procedure (both with ^{99m}Tc-HMPAO and ^{111}In-oxine) became available to guide the labelling of WBCs in accordance with currently effective European Union regulations [5, 6]. The whole procedure and precautions can be read there.

To overcome the disadvantages of the labelling procedure, a sterile single-use closed disposable device was developed (Leukokit®; GIpharma, Italy) and recently became available; it is easier to use compared to the standard techniques and will make WBC labelling available for more clinical centres and patients [8]. This is a licensed medical device distributed worldwide that may allow simplification of the required infrastructure, although to date there is no defined legislation for the use of this type of product in a different way from that of open systems. The kit includes a sterile GMP-produced vial of anticoagulant agent (ACD-A), a vial of 10% HES and a vial of PBS for cell washing and resuspension, thus avoiding possible causes of contamination of the labelled product [5, 6].

At the time of sampling, patients should preferably be fasting. A careful history must be obtained from the referring physician to ensure that the correct procedure will be applied, e.g. the use of ^{111}In-oxine- or ^{99m}Tc-HMPAO-labelled WBCs, and the type and time of acquisition. The blood results of the patient have to be checked to determine if infection parameters in the blood are elevated and enough white blood cells are available for labelling. The possible interaction of high levels of cholesterol and glucose in the blood has to be taken into account. Further on, the possible interference of some drugs and antibiotics has to be checked [9].

For the image acquisition a large-field-of-view camera with a low-energy high-resolution collimator for ^{99m}Tc-HMPAO and medium-energy high-resolution collimator for ^{111}In-oxine is usually preferred. The recommended injection dose is 10–18.5 MBq ^{111}In-oxine-labelled WBCs and 370–740 MBq ^{99m}Tc-HMPAO-labelled WBCs. Planar whole body images should include anterior and posterior views of the head, chest, abdomen and pelvis, and when clinically indicated also the extremities. In some cases (e.g. vascular grafts) oblique views may help to differentiate between uptake in the graft itself and surrounding tissue. Images are performed 30 min–1 h after injection (diffuse and intense lung uptake should be seen to check if the labelling was satisfactory), 3–4 h after injection (early image) and 20–24 h after injection (delayed image). Early and delayed images should be acquired in time mode and corrected for the radioisotope half-life. SPECT imaging of the suspected area is recommended, and for some indications (e.g. endocarditis) even obligatory. Usually 20–30 s per step is used for early images and 40–50 s per step for delayed images.

Accurate interpretation of WBC-S requires knowledge of the normal and abnormal variants of WBC localisations. The diagnosis of an infection is made by comparing early and delayed images. Visually images are classified as negative when no uptake is seen at all or when a decrease in uptake is seen from the early to delayed image, and classified positive when the uptake increases with time. Quantitative evaluation may also be performed. A region of interest (ROI) is drawn over the suspected region (target ROI) and over the same region contralateral or in presumed normal reference tissue, e.g. the iliac bone (background ROI). The target-to-background (T/B) ratio can be calculated in early and in delayed images. When the T/B ratio increases with time, the scan is considered positive for an infection; when it decreases, it is classified negative.

The recent development of the SPECT-CT camera also is a major push forward in the imaging of inflammation/infection. Using a combined system, one can now sequentially acquire both anatomic and functional information that is accurately fused in a single examination. For imaging infection, early reports indicate that SPECT-CT increases specificity and may significantly affect disease management. Fusion of the WBC images with the CT images may be helpful for a more accurate localisation of the WBC uptake, particularly for differentiating soft tissue uptake from bone uptake, e.g. in the diabetic foot. Another important feature is the ability to correct the nuclear emission images for attenuation and scatter to obtain more accurate image data. The benefits of using CT for attenuation correction as opposed to a radionuclide transmission source include less noise, faster acquisition, no influence on CT data by the SPECT radionuclide, and no need to replace decayed transmission sources [10]. In case of prosthesis, both attenuated and non-attenuated images must be carefully analysed in order to avoid false positives.

Radionuclide imaging procedures are routinely performed as part of the diagnostic workup in musculoskeletal infections. Bone scintigraphy is sensitive with accuracy in unviolated bone. In the setting of underlying osseous abnormalities, however, the specificity of the test decreases [11]. Currently, WBC-S is the radionuclide procedure of choice for diagnosing osteomyelitis, often performed in conjunction with bone marrow imaging to maximise accuracy. The overall accuracy of combined WBC/bone marrow scintigraphy is approximately 90% [12]. WBC-S is especially useful in the evaluation of prosthetic joint infections, neuropathic joint infections and infections of the diabetic foot. In suspected joint replacement infections, the accuracy ranges from 88% to 98%. Although inflammation may be present in both the infected and aseptically loosened device, neutrophils are usually absent in aseptic loosening. This critical difference between infection and aseptic loosening accounts for the high sensitivity and specificity of WBC-S for diagnosing prosthetic joint infection.

Recent publications confirm also the incremental value of SPECT/CT-labelled WBC imaging. WBC-S with and without SPECT/CT was performed in 26 patients with suspicion of musculoskeletal infections. SPECT/CT significantly changed the interpretation of the study in ten patients, excluded osteomyelitis in seven and provided a more precise delineation of the extent of infection in three [13]. In contrast to other sites in the skeleton, WBC-S is of limited value for detecting spinal osteomyelitis or spondylodiscitis. Although increased uptake is virtually diagnostic of the disease, 50% or more of all cases present as areas of decreased, or absent, activity. However photopenia is not specific for vertebral osteomyelitis; it can also be associated with tumours, infarction and previously treat osteomyelitis [11].

High sensitivity and specificity values were also reported for WBC-S with ^{99m}Tc-HMPAO for the assessment of activity in inflammatory bowel diseases (Crohn's disease and colitis ulcerosa) [14]. Some discussion has been raised about the best imaging time. The overall tendency is a high sensitivity and specificity if imaging is performed within 3 h. Moreover, scanning after 1 and 3 h may be helpful as the pathological accumulation in actively inflamed segments becomes more pronounced. On the other hand, false-positive findings may occur after 3 h because of excretion of ^{99m}Tc-HMPAO into the bowel. WBC labelled with ^{111}In-oxine has also been used for inflammatory bowel diseases and has been shown suitable for the assessment of presence and location of active inflammation. In children, WBC-S is a useful tool in the diagnosis and therapeutic strategy of CD, and provides information on the presence, intensity and extent of the disease, particularly in the terminal ileum [14]. Very few studies investigated the role of SPECT in inflammatory bowel diseases. One study compared SPECT images after 2 h with planar images after 30 min and 2 h. Both planar and SPECT images were comparable in terms of detecting the presence of an active inflammation, but SPECT images showed a higher uptake and provided more detailed visualisation of lesions. SPECT may better discriminate between intestinal and bone marrow uptake, and thus is useful for assessing lesions within the pelvis, including perianal disease [15]. Compared with spiral CT, both WBC-S and CT are valuable non-invasive diagnostic methods in cases involving severe, active CD. WBC-S seems better for the detection of segmental inflammatory activity, whereas CT displayed excellent suitability for the recognition of complications such as abscesses, stenosis and fistula. Using the combined SPECT-CT camera may provide better sensitivity and specificity, but no reports can be found in the literature yet.

Fever of unknown origin (FUO) is an illness of at least 3-week duration with several episodes of fever exceeding 38.3°C and no diagnosis after an appropriate evaluation. Underlying causes are numerous and include infections, malignancies, granulomatous diseases and collagen vascular diseases. Both ^{111}In- or ^{99m}Tc-labelled WBC have been successfully used in patients with FUO. A study already performed in the early 1990s with ^{111}In-labelled WBCs in 68 patients with FUO demonstrated an accuracy of 76% and was helpful in reaching a final diagnosis in 28% of these patients [16]. Other studies found a somewhat lower overall accuracy. In the recent years, ^{18}F-FDG-PET is increasingly considered the best radionuclide imaging method for FUO; however, a study from Kjaer et al. in 19 FUO patients showed that ^{111}In-labelled WBC-S was 71% sensitive and 92% specific, which was significantly higher than ^{18}F-FDG-PET (50% and 46% sensitivity and specificity, respectively). The authors concluded that ^{111}In-WBC-S has a superior diagnostic performance compared to ^{18}F-FDG-PET for the diagnosis of a localised infectious/inflammatory or neoplastic cause of FUO [17].

WBC-S plays also an important role in various vascular diseases. Several studies demonstrated the use of WBC-S for the detection of myocardial abscesses in infective endocarditis patients. In a recent study, 78 patients with suspected endocarditis or infection of cardiac devices were evaluated with ^{99m}Tc-labelled WBC SPECT/CT, and this study concluded that the SPECT/CT allows an accurate diagnosis of cardiac and additional unsuspected extra-cardiac infection sites. WBC-S also demonstrated high sensitivity (ranging from 82% to 100%) and specificity (ranging from 75% to 100%) for the diagnosis of vascular graft infection [10].

The recent availability of radiolabelled anti-granulocyte antibodies (Scintimun®, CIS bio, France) allows fast and accurate detection of infection. Particularly for peripheral osteomyelitis, the diagnostic accuracy is comparable to that of WBCs, and all acquisition and interpretation criteria mentioned above can also be applied, including the use of SPECT/CT techniques.

In the examples of WBC-S, the normal body distribution and the qualitative and quantitative evaluation will be explained. This will be followed by some examples of a positive WBC-S. The advantages of the use of SPECT and SPECT-CT will be demonstrated with some examples.

References

1. Annovazzi A, Bagni B, Burroni L, D'Alessandria C, Signore A. Nuclear medicine imaging of inflammatory/infective disorders of the abdomen. Nucl Med Commun. 2005;26: 657–64.
2. Prandini N, Lazzeri E, Rossi B, Erba P, Parisella MG, Signore A. Nuclear medicine imaging of bone infections. Nucl Med Commun. 2006;27:633–44.
3. Cascini GL, De Palma D, Matteucci F, Biggi A, Rambaldi PF, Signore A, Mansi L. Fever of unknown origin, infection of subcutaneous devices, brain abscesses and endocarditis. Nucl Med Commun. 2006;27:213–22.
4. Capriotti G, Chianelli M, Signore A. Nuclear medicine imaging of diabetic foot infection: results of meta-analysis. Nucl Med Commun. 2006;27:757–64.
5. Roca M, De Vries EFJ, Jamar F, Israel O, Signore A. Guidelines for the labelling of leucocytes with ^{111}In-oxine. Eur J Nucl Med Mol Imaging. 2010;37:835–41.
6. De Vries EFJ, Roca M, Jamar F, Israel O, Signore A. Guidelines for the labelling of leucocytes with ^{99m}Tc-HMPAO. Eur J Nucl Med Mol Imaging. 2010;37:842–48.
7. Roca M, Martin-Comin J, Becker W, Bernardo-Filho M, Gutfilen B, Moisan A, Peters M, Prats E, Rodrigues M, Sampson C, Signore A, Sinzinger H, Thakur M. A consensus protocol for white blood cells labelling with technetium-99m hexamethylpropylene amine oxime. Eur J Nucl Med. 1998;25:797–99.
8. Signore A, Glaudemans AWJM, Lazzeri E, Prandini N, Viglietti AL, Devicienti A, De Vries EFJ, Dierckx RAJO. Development and testing of a new disposable sterile device for labelling white blood cells. Submitted
9. IAEA Guidelines Radiolabelled autologous cells.
10. Signore A, Mather SJ, Paiggio G, Malviya G, Dierckx RA. Molecular imaging of inflammation/infection: nuclear medicine and optical imaging agents and methods. Chem Rev. 2010;110:3112–45.
11. Palestro CJ, Love C, Bhargava KK. Labeled leukocyte imaging: current status and future directions. Q J Nucl Med Mol Imaging. 2009;53:105–23.
12. Palestro CJ, Love C, Tronco GG, Tomas MB, Rini JN. Combined labeled leukocyte and technetium-99m sulfur colloid marrow imaging for diagnosing musculoskeletal infection: principles, technique, interpretation, indications and limitations. RadioGraphics. 2006;26:859–70.
13. Filippi L, Schillaci O. Tc-99m HMPAO-labeled leukocyte scintigraphy for bone and joint infections. J Nucl Med. 2006;47:1908–13.
14. Glaudemans AWJM, Maccioni F, Mansi L, Dierckx RAJO, Signore A. Imaging of cell trafficking in Crohn's disease. J Cell Phys. 2010;223:562–71.
15. Biancone L, Schillaci O, Capoccetti F, Bozzi RM, Fina D, Petruzziello C, Geremia A, Simonetti F, Pallone F. Technetium-99m-HMPAO labeled leukocyte single photon emission computerized tomography (SPECT) for assessing Crohn's disease extent and intestinal infiltration. Am J Gastroenterol. 2005;100:344–54.
16. Syrjälä M, Valtonen V, Liwendahl K, Myllylä G. Diagnostic significance of Indium-111 granulocyte scintigraphy in febrile patients. J Nucl Med. 1987 ;28(2): 155–60.
17. Kjaer A, Lebech AM, Eigtved A, Hojgaard L. Fever of unknown origin: prospective comparison of diagnostic value of 18F-FDG PET and ^{111}In-granulocyte scintigraphy. Eur J Nucl Med Mol Imaging. 2004;31(5):622–6.

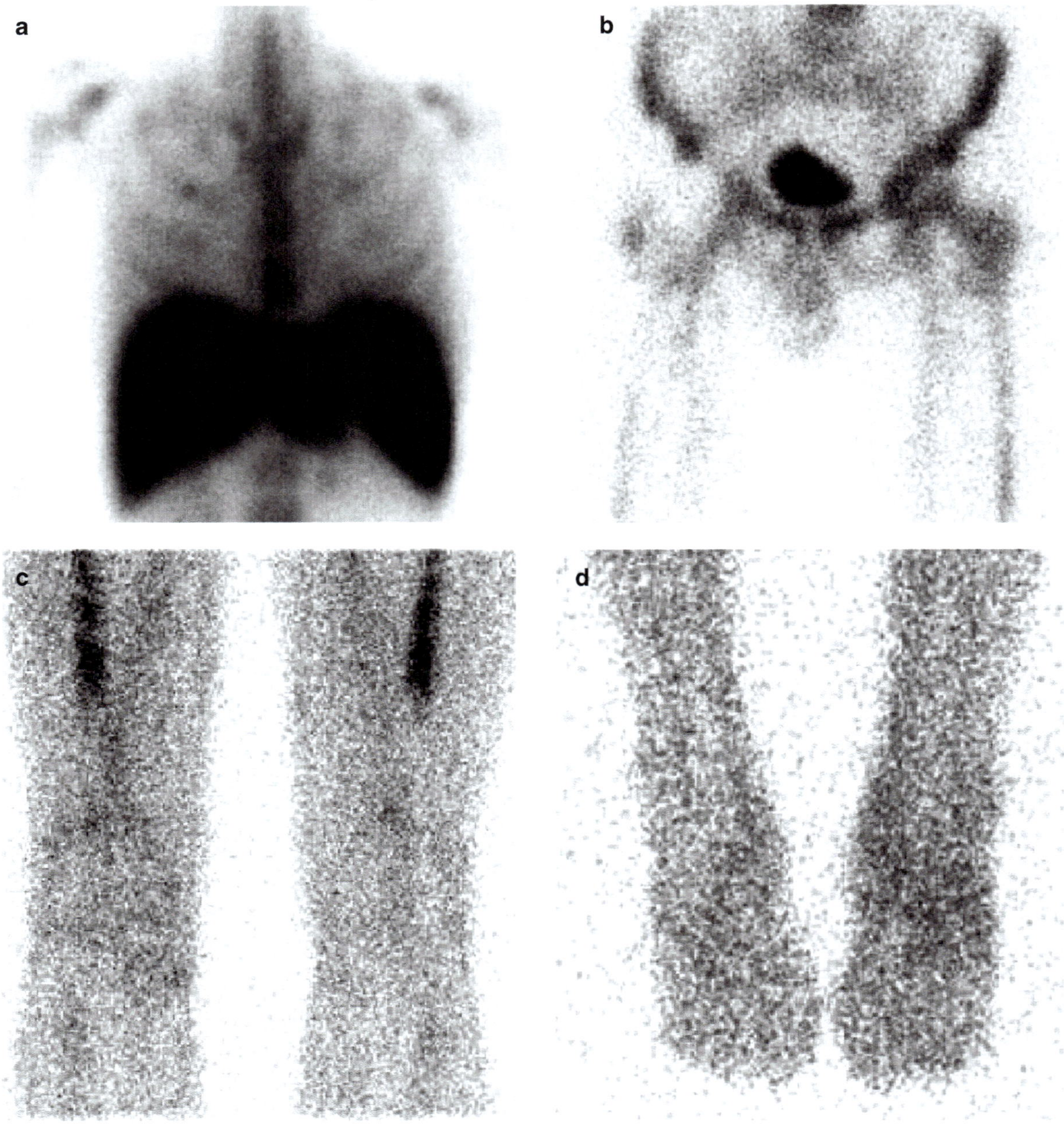

^{99m}Tc-HMPAO-WBC scintigraphy

Physiological biodistribution of ^{99m}Tc-HMPAO-WBC in (**a**) thorax, (**b**) pelvis and hip region, (**c**) knees, and (**d**) ankles and feet. All anterior early views (after 3 h), different patients.

Teaching point

Note the normal increased uptake in the liver and spleen (spleen must always be more than the liver) (**a**), in the bone marrow (**a**–**c**), in the bladder (**b**) and in the large vessels in early images (**b**)

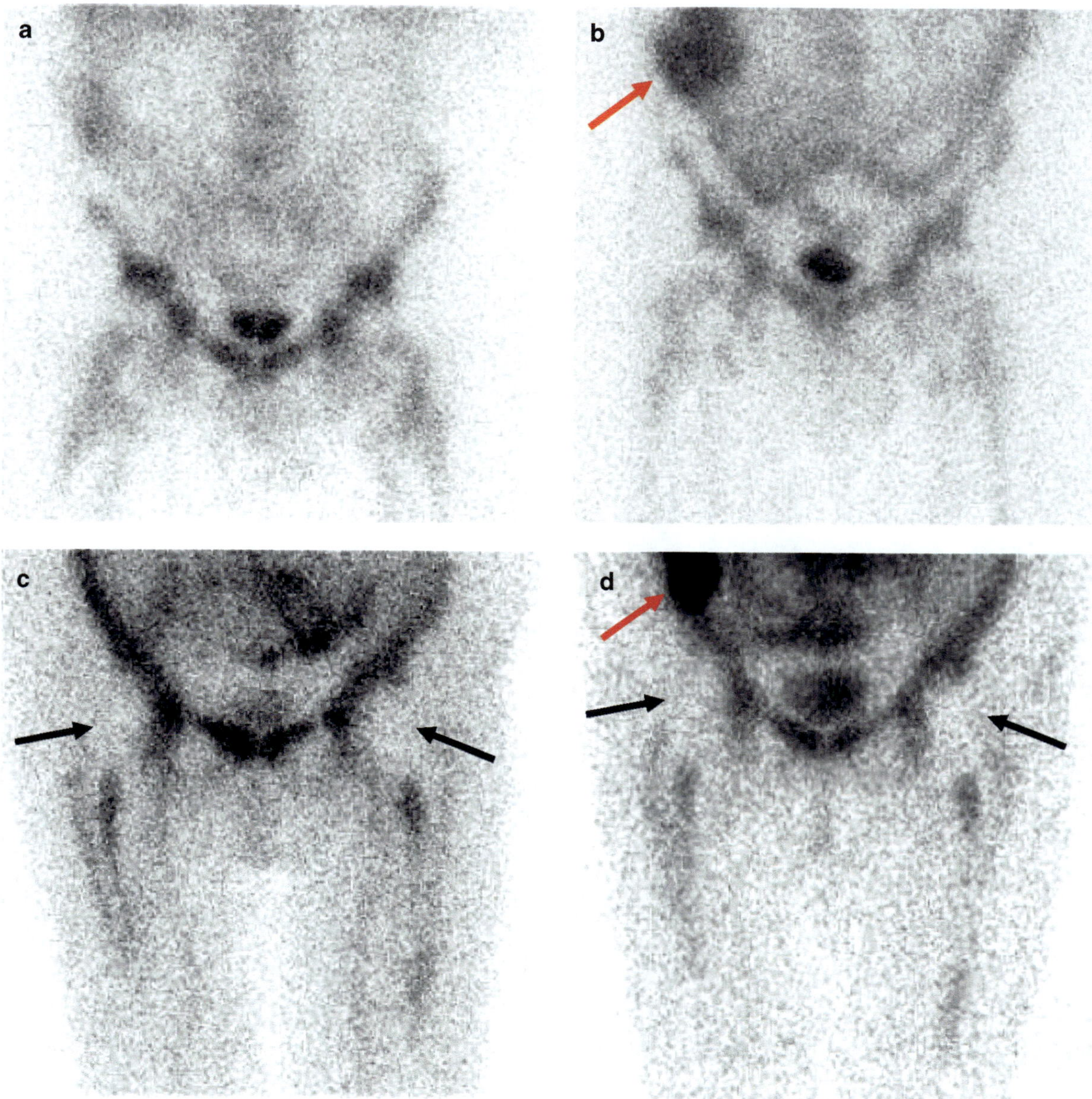

^{99m}Tc-HMPAO-WBC scintigraphy

Physiological biodistribution of ^{99m}Tc-HMPAO-WBC in (**a**) early (3 h) and (**b**) late (24 h) anterior images of the pelvic region of the same patient, (**c**) early (3 h) and (**d**) late (24 h) anterior image of patient with two hip prostheses. All images acquired in time-mode corrected for Tc decay.

Teaching point

1. Note the normal uptake in the bone marrow and the bladder on all images
2. Note that there is no increased uptake on the late images compared to the early images, meaning that there is no infection
3. Note the cold areas in **c** and d (*black arrows*) in the region of the prostheses
4. Note the increased uptake in the bowel in **b** and **d** (*red arrows*) because of physiological bowel uptake

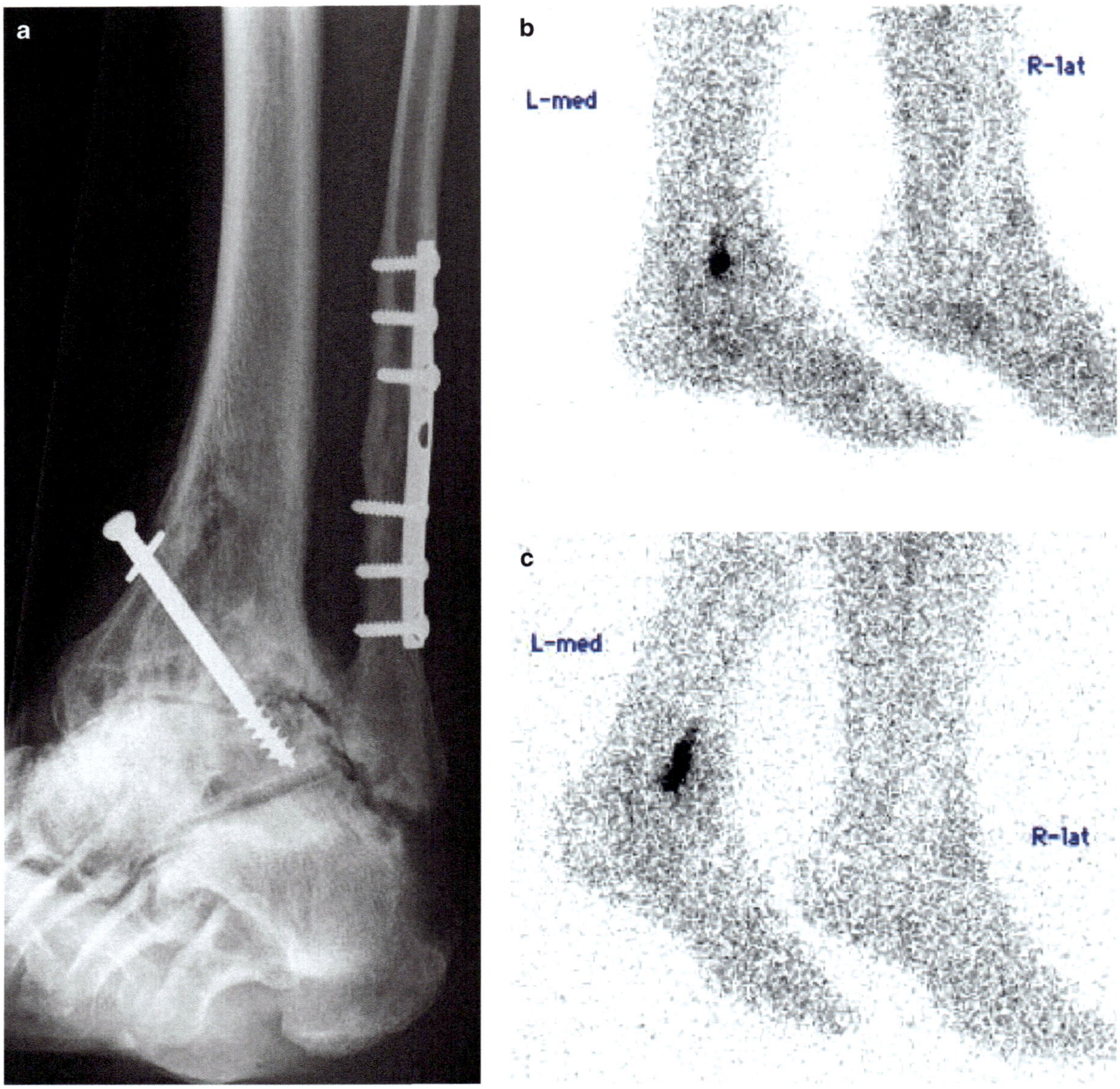

Patient with a non-healing fracture of the upper jump joint after a sports trauma and after a surgical arthrodesis with osteosynthesis

^{99m}Tc-HMPAO-WBC-scintigraphy findings

(**a**) X-ray of the left ankle joint, (**b**) early image after 3 h and (**c**) late image after 24 h. Decay-corrected acquisitions show abnormal focal uptake on the medial site of the left ankle. There is an increased uptake on the late images compared to the early image, meaning that there is an infection, possibly in the region of the distal part of the screw in the upper jump joint. The exact anatomical localisation cannot be determined based on this image only. Here you see the need for SPECT-CT images.

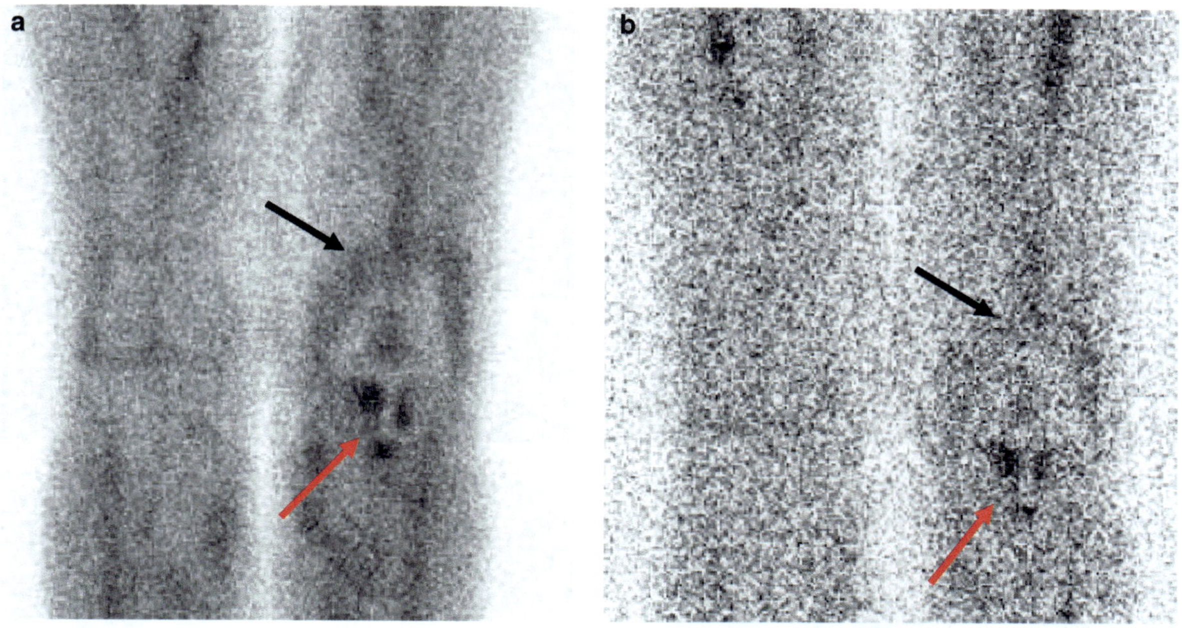

Patient 2 years after surgery for a knee prosthesis on the left side who still had pain complaints

^{99m}Tc-HMPAO-WBC-scintigraphy findings

(**a**) Early anterior image (after 3 h) and (**b**) late anterior image (after 24 h) of the knee region. Decay-corrected acquisitions. Decay-corrected acquisitions show abnormal high uptake around the femoral part of the knee prosthesis (*black arrow*) that decreases with time (sterile inflammation). Increased uptake in three small areas around the tip of the tibial part of the knee prosthesis (*red arrow*) was also detected. The ratio (area of uptake/background uptake on the other side) of these three spots increases in time, making it suspicious for an infection of the tibial part of the knee prosthesis on the left side.

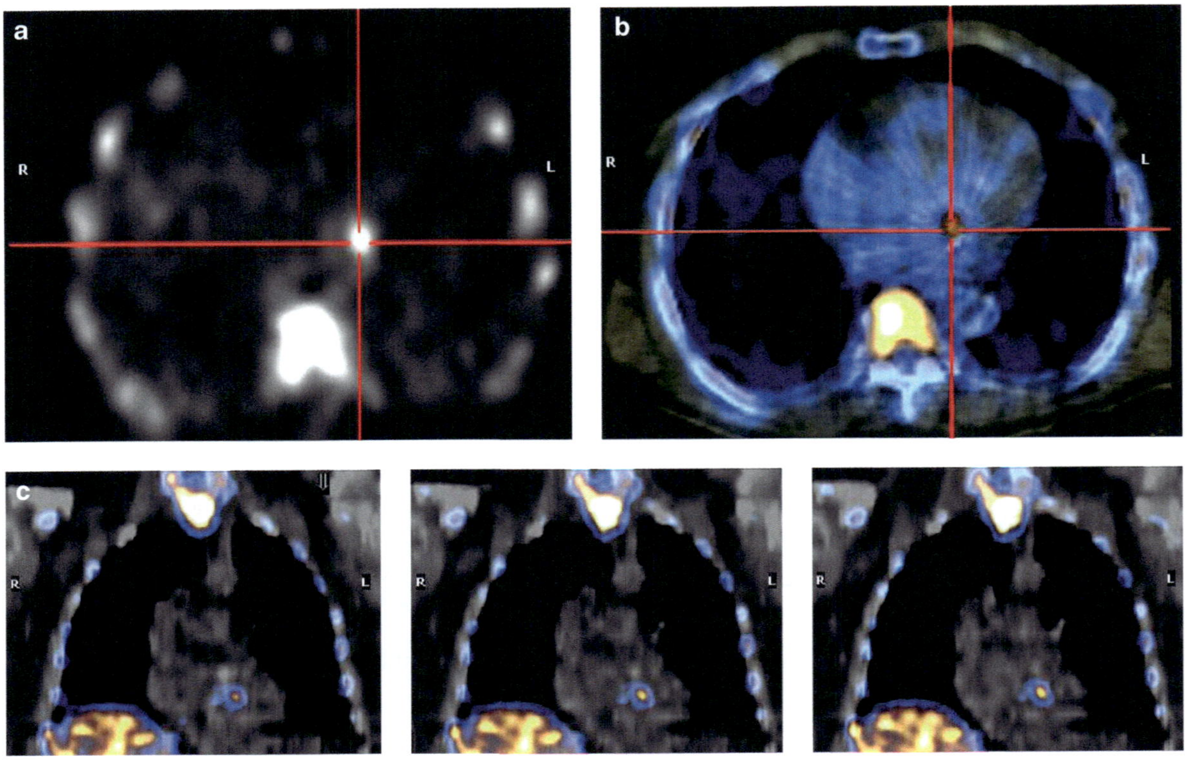

Patient with a suspected endocarditis

^{99m}Tc-HMPAO-WBC scintigraphy findings

(**a**) Late transaxial SPECT slice, (**b**) fused transaxial SPECT-CT slice and (**c**) three sequential coronal fused SPECT-CT slices show normal uptake in the bone marrow and in the liver. An increased uptake in the heart region (between the red lines) was detected, which was fused with the CT located around the mitral valve, suspicious for an endocarditis.

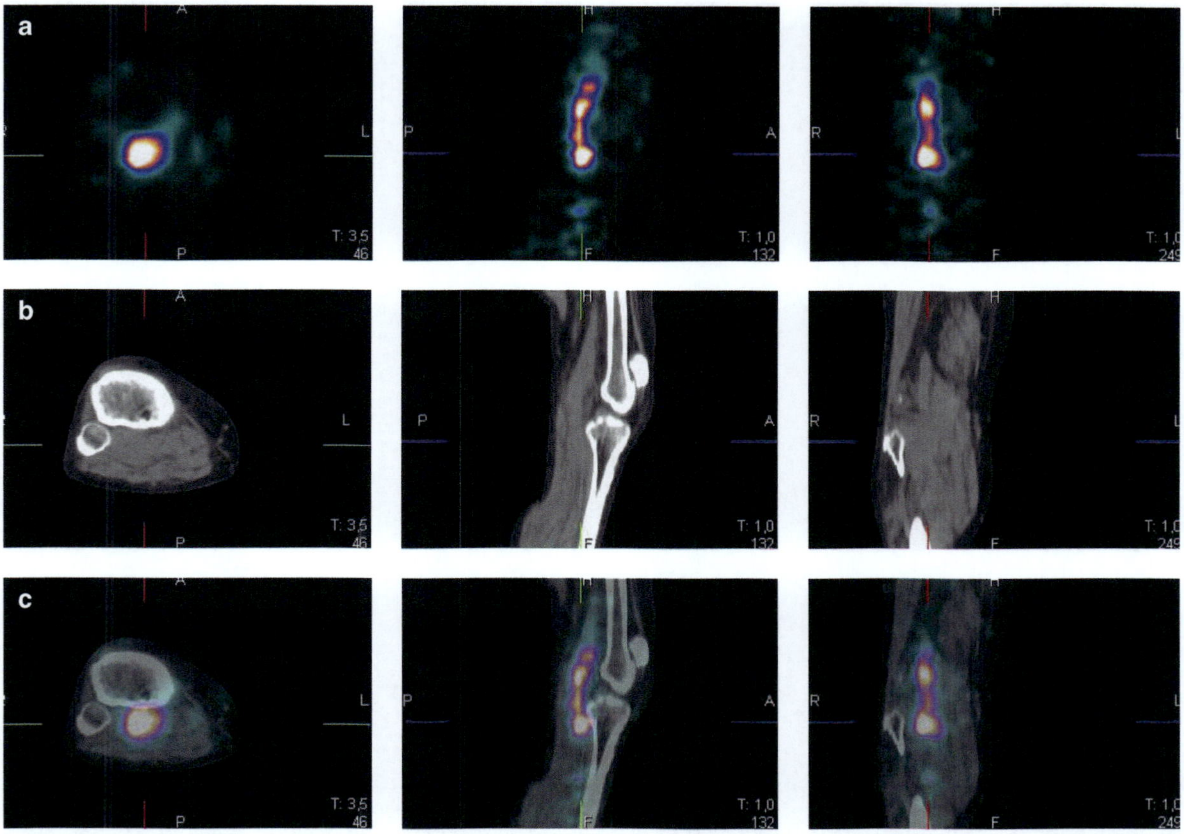

Patient with pain complaints and right lower leg claudicatio intermittens without fever and serum parameters of infection. Echo Doppler showed a thrombosis of the A. poplitea

^{99m}Tc-HMPAO-WBC scintigraphy findings

(**a**) SPECT transaxial, coronal and sagittal slice, (**b**) CT slices and (**c**) fusion images show abnormal uptake located behind the osseus structures in the knee region. CT fused images correctly located the uptake in the right popliteal artery, consistent with infected thrombus. The diagnosis was further confirmed as after antibiotic treatment the patient felt well, and echo Doppler showed normal popliteal artery flow.

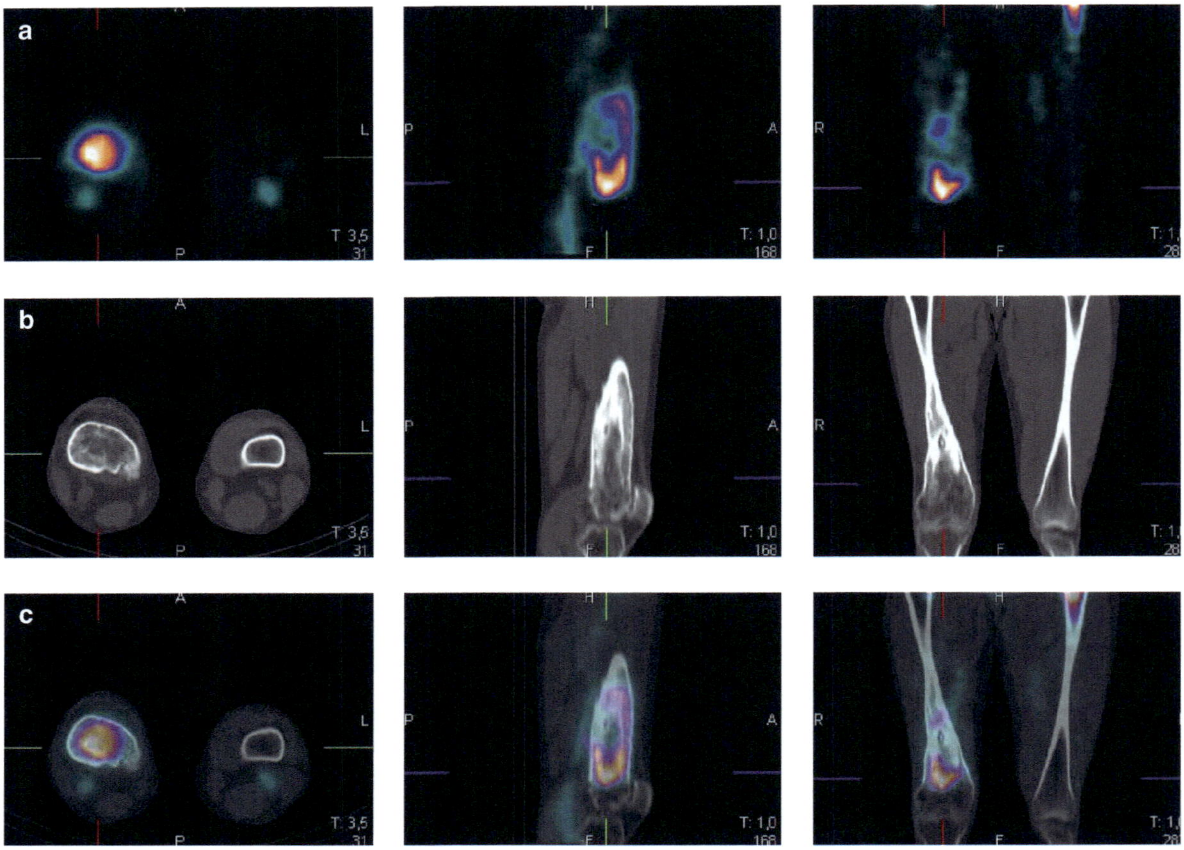

Patient suspected to have an osteomyelitis of the right lower leg

^{99m}Tc-HMPAO-WBC scintigraphy findings

(**a**) SPECT (transaxial, coronal and sagittal view), (**b**) CT slices and (**c**) fusion images show abnormal intense uptake located in the distal part of the right femur indicating an osteomyelitis. CT images clearly demonstrated structural alteration in the affected bone.

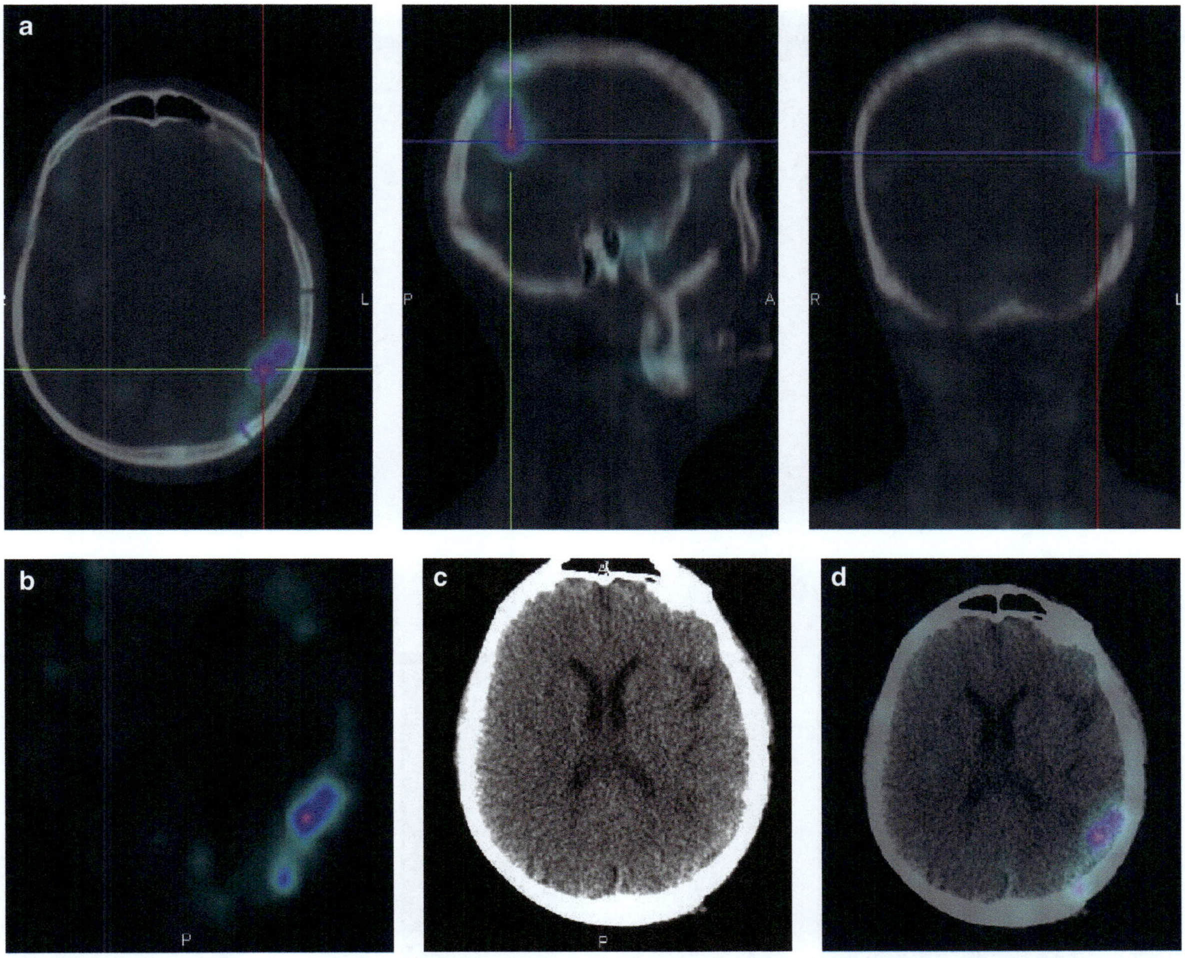

Patient suspected to have an intra-cerebral abscess

^{99m}Tc-HMPAO-WBC scintigraphy findings

(**a**) SPECT-CT fusion images with CT in bone setting, transaxial, sagittal and coronal view, (**b**) SPECT transaxial slice, (**c**) CT transaxial slice and (**d**) fused image show high uptake located in the the left occipital lobe, consistent with an intracerebral abscess. No abnormal uptake was demonstrated by SPECT-CT repeated after 3 months of antibiotic therapy.

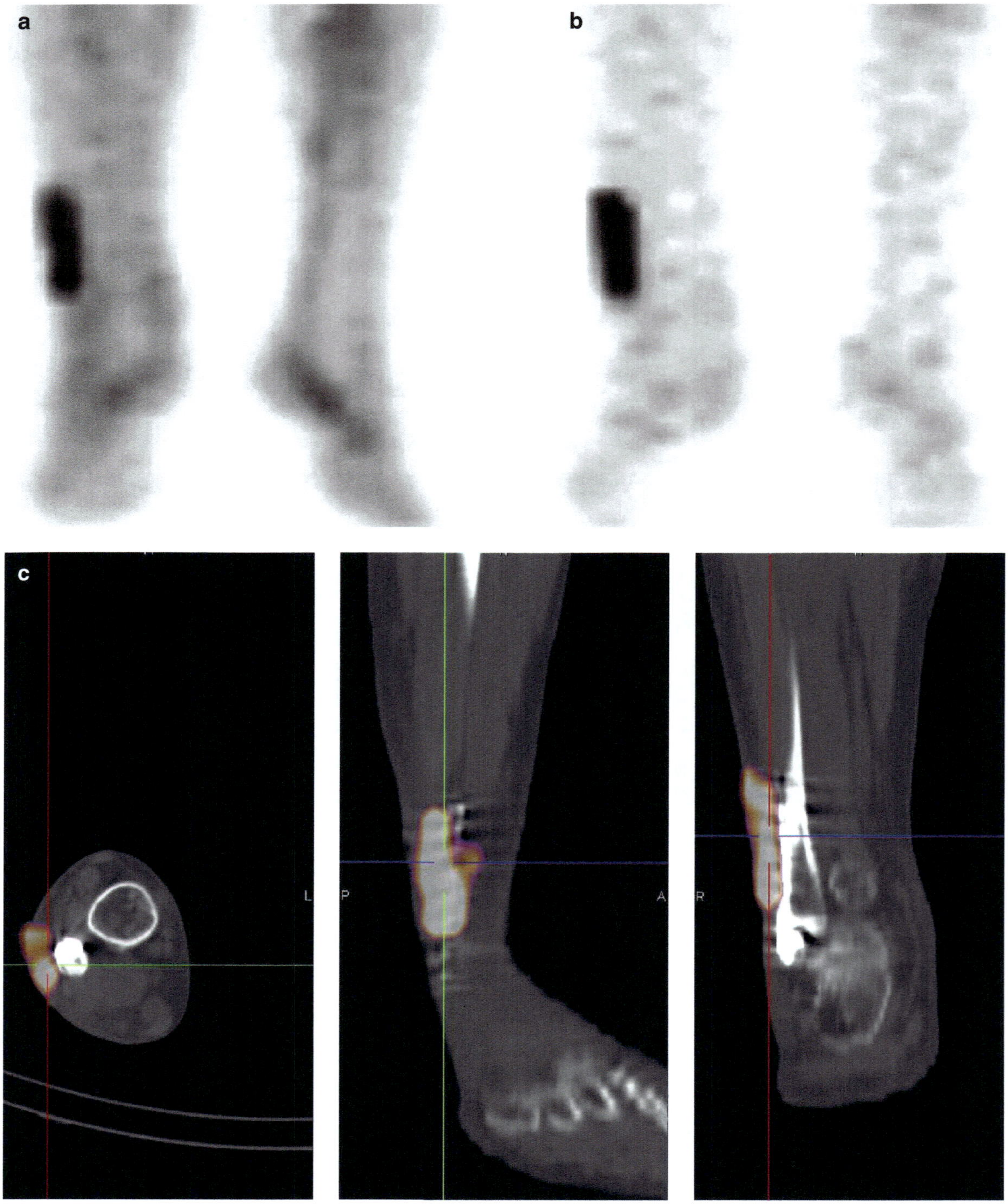

Patient suspected to have an osteomyelitis of the right fibula

^{99m}Tc-HMPAO-WBC scintigraphy findings

(**a**) Early image (3 h) anterior view, (**b**) late image (24 h) anterior view and (**c**) fusion SPECT-CT images in transaxial, sagittal and coronal view show area of high uptake located in the lateral part of the right lower leg, suspected for an infection. SPECT-CT fusion images show the high uptake is clearly located laterally to the bone, and thereby a soft tissue infection was diagnosed.

9.2 Other Tracers for Infection

Elena Lazzeri

In this chapter we describe the use of a new radioactive tracer of infection with SPECT/CT acquisition in patients with infective spinal disease and the use of PET/CT during scintigraphic imaging.

9.2.1 ^{111}In-Biotin SPECT/CT

Biotin, also called vitamin H, is a water-soluble vitamin of the B-complex group of vitamins. Biotin (molecular weight about 224 Da) is a growth factor for the majority of bacteria. In particular, pyruvate carboxylase, a key metabolic pathway for producing energy by ATP cleavage, is biotin-dependent, and bacterial acetyl-coA carboxylase is a biotin-dependent enzyme utilised in the first step of fatty acid synthesis [18, 19]. This vitamin can be labelled and utilised for diagnosis of infection, in particular in those infections where the conventional radioactive tracers are limited. Nowadays the gold standard of nuclear medicine imaging for infection is represented by labelled leukocyte scintigraphy because of its high sensitivity (95%) and specificity in many infectious processes (90%) [20, 21]. In case of vertebral infection, however, labelled leukocyte scans present considerable limits: in the majority of cases we can find a photopenic area in the corresponding infected vertebra, which is not specific for infection [22]; many other pathologies, in fact, such as vertebral crush, Paget's disease or tumors, show a decrease of leukocyte uptake in nuclear medicine imaging [23–32]. More rarely, an increased uptake of labelled leukocytes can be found in the site of vertebral infection that has been correlated to the duration of symptoms: less than 25% of patients who were symptomatic for more than 2 weeks showed presented such findings [22]. Magnetic resonance imaging (MRI) and other radiopharmaceuticals proposed to complement the diagnostic value of MRI, such as bone scintigraphy with ^{99m}Tc-MDP and ^{67}Ga-citrate [33, 34] and ^{18}F-FDG PET [35–41], have shown high sensitivity but variable specificity (ranging from 35.8% to 87.9%), especially in cases in that require differentiating vertebral infection from benign pathologies or septic and aseptic SD in the early post-surgical phase [40–45].

The labelling of biotin with ^{111}In is an easy and fast procedure, and shows high efficiency and stability (>98% until 24 h).

The scintigraphic acquisition protocol is based on planar and SPECT/CT images of the suspected vertebral region 4–6 h after i.v. injection of ^{111}In-biotin (111 MBq).

The main advantage of using ^{111}In-biotin is the absence of uptake of healthy bone marrow of the spine, so it is quite simple to read SPECT/CT images when, in case of spine infection, they show a focal uptake of the tracer in the region of interest (Fig. 1a, b). Another advantage of this scintigraphic procedure is the possibility to study the patients in follow-up during antibiotic treatment without any suspension of the therapy [46, 47].

Rarely false-positive results can be found when a large inflammatory process leads to leakage of the tracer because of the altered capillary permeability. When a false-positive result is present, it can be resolved by comparing early images (4–6 h post injection) with late images (18–20 h post injection).

False-negative results can be found if the infective pathologies of the spine are caused by microorganisms that do not utilise biotin for their own growth or if the microrganisms have a low rate metabolism (e.g. *Mycobacterium tubercolosis*).

The main limit of ^{111}In-biotin scintigraphy is the complete urinary excretion of ^{111}In that results in a relatively high dosimetry for the kidneys.

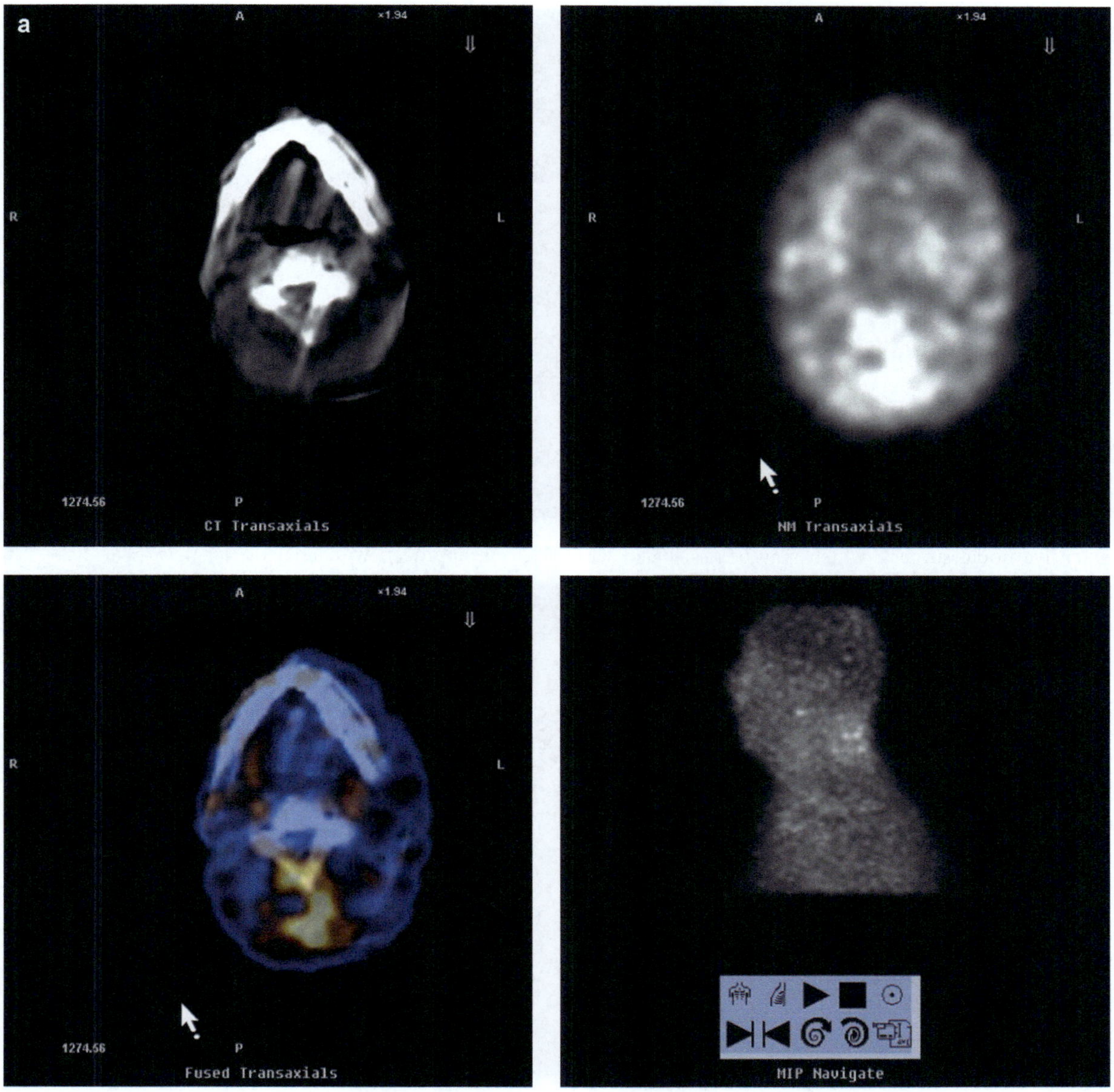

Fig. 1 (**a**) Transaxial reconstructions of CT, scintigraphy and fused images of a paravertebral soft tissue infection of the posterior cervical region in a patient operated on for slipped disc C3-C4. (**b**) Transaxial, sagittal and coronal reconstructions of SPET/CT images of paravertebral soft tissue infection of the posterior cervical region in a patient operated on for slipped disc C3-C4

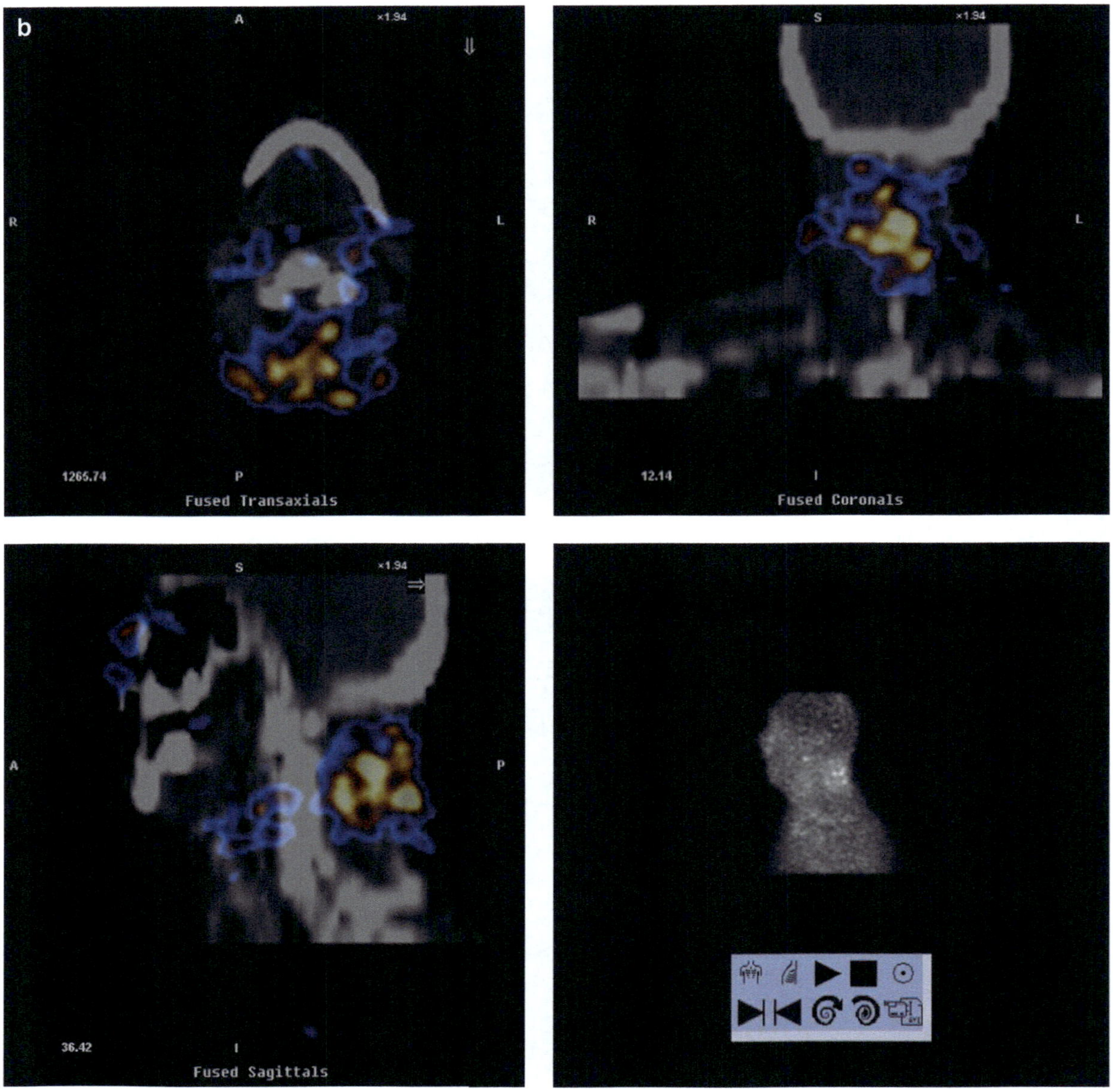

Fig. 1 (continued)

References

18. Yao X, Wei D, Soden Jr C, Summers MF, Beckett D. Structure of the carboxyl terminal fragment of the apo-biotin carboxyl carrier subunit of *Escherichia coli* acetyl-coA carboxylase. Biochemistry. 1997;36:15089–100.
19. Attwood PV. The structure and the mechanism of action of pyruvate carboxylase. Int J Biochem Cell Biol. 1995; 27:231–49.
20. Devillers A, Moisan A, Jean S, Arvieux C, Bourguet P. Technetium-99m hexamethyl-propylene amine oxime leucocyte scintigraphy for the diagnosis of bone and joint infections: a retrospective study in 116 patients. Eur J Nucl Med. 1995;22:302–7.
21. Palestro CJ, Torres MA. Radionuclide imaging in orthopaedic infections. Semin Nucl Med. 1997;27:334–45.
22. Palestro CJ, Kim CK, Swyer AJ, Vallabhajosula S, Goldsmith SJ. Radionuclide diagnosis of vertebral osteomyelitis: indium-111-leukocyte and technetium-99m methylene diphosphonate bone scintigraphy. J Nucl Med. 1991;32: 1861–5.
23. Coleman RE, Welch D. Possible pitfalls with clinical imaging of indium-111 leukocytes. J Nucl Med. 1980;21:122–5.
24. Mok YP, Carney WH, Fernandez-Ulloa M. Skeletal photopenic lesions in In-111 WBC imaging. J Nucl Med. 1984;25:1322–6.
25. Fernandex-Ulloa M, Vasavada PJ, Hanslits ML, Volarich DT, Elgazzar AH. Diagnosis of vertebral osteomyelitis: clinical, radiological and scintigraphic features. Orthopedics. 1985;8:1144–50.
26. Datz FL, Thorne DA. Cause and significance of cold bone defects on indium-111-labelled leukocyte imaging. J Nucl Med. 1987;28:820–3.
27. Whalen JL, Brown ML, McLeod R, Fitzgerald Jr RH. Limitations of indium leukocyte imaging for the diagnosis of spine infections. Spine. 1991;16:193–7.
28. Jacobson AF, Gilles CP, Cerqueira MD. Photopenic defects in marrow containing skeleton on indium-111 leucocyte scintigraphy: prevalence at sites suspected of osteomyelitis and as an incidental finding. Eur J Nucl Med. 1992;19:858–4.
29. Even-Sapir E, Martin RH. Degenerative disc disease. A cause for diagnostic dilemma on In-111 WBC studies in suspected osteomyelitis. Clin Nucl Med. 1994;19:388–92.
30. Roelants V, Tang T, Ide C, Laloux P. Cold vertebra on ^{111}In-white blood cell scintigraphy. Semin Nucl Med. 2002;32:236–7.
31. Gratz S, Dorner J, Oestmann JW, Opitz M, Behr T, Meller J, et al. 67Ga-citrate and ^{99m}Tc-MDP for estimating the severity of vertebral osteomyelitis. Nucl Med Commun. 2000; 21:111–20.
32. Love C, Patel M, Lonner BS, Tomas MB, Palestro CJ. Diagnosing spinal osteomyelitis: a comparison of bone and Ga-67 scintigraphy and magnetic resonance imaging. Clin Nucl Med. 2000;25:963–77.
33. Stumpe KD, Dazzi H, Schaffner A, von Schulthess GK. Infection imaging using whole-body FDG-PET. Eur J Nucl Med. 2000;27:822–32.
34. Kalicke T, Schmitz A, Risse JH, Arens S, Keller E, Hansis M, et al. Fluorine-18 fluorodeoxyglucose PET in infectious bone diseases: results of histologically confirmed cases. Eur J Nucl Med. 2000;27:524–8.
35. Zhuang H, Alavi A. 18-Fluorodeoxyglucose positron emission tomographic imaging in the detection and monitoring of infection and inflammation. Semin Nucl Med. 2002; 32:47–59.
36. Schmitz A, Kalicke T, Willkomm P, Grunwald F, Kandyba J, Schmitz O. Use of fluorine-18 fluoro-2-deoxy-D-glucose positron emission tomography in assessing the process of tuberculous spondylitis. J Spinal Disord. 2000;13:541–44.
37. Gratz S, Dorner J, Fischer U, Behr TM, Behé M, Altenvoerde G, et al. 18F-FDG hybrid PET in patients with suspected spondylitis. Eur J Nucl Med. 2002;29:516–24.
38. De Winter F, Gemmel F, Van De Wiele C, Poffijn B, Uyttendaele D, Dierckx R. 18-Fluorine fluorodeoxyglucose positron emission tomography for the diagnosis of infection in the postoperative spine. Spine. 2003;28:1314–9.
39. Rosen RS, Fayad L, Wahl RL. Increased 18F-FDG uptake in degenerative disease of the spine: characterization with 18F-FDG PET/CT. J Nucl Med. 2006;47:1274–80.
40. Wolansky LJ, Heary RF, Patterson T, Friedenberg JS, Tholany J, Chen JK, et al. Pseudosparing of the endplate: a potential pitfall in using MR imaging to diagnose infectious spondylitis. Am J Roentgenol. 1999;172:777–80.
41. Enzmann DR. Infection and inflammation. In: Enzmann DR, DeLaPaz RL, Rubin JB, editors. Magnetic Resonance of the Spine. St. Louis: Mosby; 1990. p. 260–300.
42. Wagner SC, Schweitzer ME, Morrison WB, Przybylski GJ, Parker L. Can imaging findings help differentiate spinal neuropathic arthropathy from disk space infection? Initial experience. Radiology. 2000;214:693–9.
43. Kylampaa-Back ML, Suominen RA, Salo SA, Soiva M, Korkala OI, Mokka RE. Postoperative discitis: outcome and late magnetic resonance image evaluation of ten patients. Ann Chir Gynaecol. 1999;88:61–4.
44. Van Goethem JW, Parizel PM, van den Hauwe L, Van de Kelft E, Verlooy J, De Schepper AM. The value of MRI in the diagnosis of postoperative spondylodiscitis. Neuroradiology. 2000;42:580–5.
45. Grane P, Josephsson A, Seferlis A, Tullberg T. Septic and aseptic postoperative discitis in the lumbar spine: evaluation by MR imaging. Acta Radiol. 1998;39:108–15.
46. Lazzeri E, Erba P, Perri M, Tascini C, Doria R, Giorgetti J, et al. Scintigraphic imaging of vertebral osteomyelitis with ^{111}In-biotin. Spine. 2008;33(7):198–204.
47. Lazzeri E, Erba P, Perri M, Doria R, Tascini C, Mariani G. Clinical impact of SPECT/CT with In-111 biotin on the management of patients with suspected spine infection. Clin Nucl Med. 2010;35:12–7.

Chapter 10 Red Blood Cell Imaging with SPECT-CT

Cornelis A. Hoefnagel

Contents

S. Fanti et al., *Atlas of SPECT-CT*,
DOI: 10.1007/978-3-642-15726-4_10,

10.1 Introduction

In patients suspected to have an acute bleeding, accurate localization of the bleeding site and assessment of the severity of blood loss are essential for the proper management of the condition.

In gastrointestinal bleeding, a distinction is made between upper and lower gastrointestinal bleeding. The most frequent causes of bleeding in the upper gastrointestinal are: duodenal ulcer, gastric ulcer, gastric erosions, varices and Mallory-Weiss tears. Lower gastrointestinal bleeding is most commonly caused by angiodysplasia, diverticula, polyps or bowel cancer.

Both endoscopy and angiography are mostly used to detect, localize and possibly control the bleeding if it is active at the time these procedures are performed. It has been reported that endoscopy of the upper gastrointestinal tract is accurate in more than 90% of the cases of upper GI bleeding, and that coloscopy can detect or exclude a colonic bleeding site in 70% of the cases. Nevertheless, because of the often intermittent nature of gastrointestinal bleeding, both methods may fail to find the bleeding.

It is in these circumstances that scintigraphy with radiolabeled red blood cells can have a complementary role. The advantages of this technique are the fact that no patient preparation is required, its noninvasiveness and easiness to perform, even in acutely ill patients, and its sensitivity at low bleeding rates. In this respect, the greatest advantage of red blood cell scintigraphy is its ability to detect intermittent bleeding by monitoring the abdomen over a period of time (up to 24 h). Although angiography is successful in localizing the site in 65% of active bleedings with a bleeding rate of >1 mL/min, the handicap is that the bleeding must be active during the 20–30 s of a contrast injection.

Experimentally in dogs, bleeding rates as low as 0.05–0.1 mL/min have been reported to be detected by scintigraphy. Although in patients generally a bleeding rate of 0.4 mL/min is required to produce an intense focus of extravasation in the early scintigrams, detection of foci with a lower bleeding rate is possible, especially if, in addition, SPECT/CT can be performed.

10.2 Indication

The main indication for red blood cell scintigraphy is recurrent intermittent (gastrointestinal) bleeding of unknown origin for which endoscopy and angiography had a negative result. The greatest chance of success is when there is a need for transfusions of more than 500 mL per 24 h. The aim is to find a bleeding site to direct angiography or endoscopy to more specific areas. Rarely, the scintigraphy alone suffices to guide the surgeon.

10.3 Procedure

For scintigraphic imaging of bleeding, the radiopharmaceutical of choice is Technetium-99m-labeled autologous erythrocytes. After pretinning, a blood sample is drawn for ex-vivo labeling with a yield of 90–95%. This is preferred over the in-vivo labeling technique, which may result in varying amounts of free pertechnetate, which, due to uptake in the gastric mucosa, passing into the upper gastrointestinal tract and by excretion via the kidneys, may lead to false-positive results.

Following i.v. administration of 740 MBq ^{99m}Tc-labeled erythrocytes, a dynamic study of 1 frame/s during the first minute is acquired, and subsequently either a dynamic image sequence of 15-s frames for the next 15 or 30 min, or 1-min frames for the next 60 min is recorded, which can be displayed in cine mode. Thereafter, a series of static anterior view images of the abdomen is made, initially frequently, and subsequently at greater intervals for up to 24 h.

X-ray contrast from gastric and bowel imaging may interfere with detection of extravasations and should therefore be avoided.

10.4 Interpretation

The aim of the procedure is to detect and localize extravasation of blood into the bowel, preferably at its earliest appearance. Viewing images in cine mode can be of help in this respect. In subsequent images, extravasation may be seen to be transported both in the distal and proximal direction. Extravasations shown on late images may be more difficult to localize because of the movement of activity within the bowel.

Accumulation of activity that does not move on subsequent images is more likely to be due to vascular abnormalities than to bleeding, although a clot remaining in the bowel can also cause such a finding.

A negative scintigraphic study does not rule out an intermittent bleeding, but does indicate that during the past 24 h the patient had no or hardly any bleeding.

10.5 Role of SPECT/CT

Whenever scintigraphy reveals a clear bleeding site (as shown in Case 1), either immediately or shortly after intravenous administration of ^{99m}Tc-labeled autologous red blood cells, further localization by SPECT/CT is not required and may, depending on the patient's acute condition, actually be contraindicated. It may be safer to transfer the patient immediately to focused angiography and/or surgery to control the bleeding.

However, at slower bleeding rates and extravasations occurring over a period of time (as in Case 2), SPECT/CT is superior to planar scintigraphy to pinpoint the accumulation of ^{99m}Tc-labeled red blood cells to an anatomical structure that can direct radiological or surgical intervention.

In analogy with the experience in sentinel node imaging in which SPECT/CT may detect sentinel nodes not visualized on the planar lymphoscintigram, SPECT/CT may be able to find or confirm extravasation of blood in cases of very low bleeding rates (<0.2 mL/min) for which planar red blood cell scintigraphy is doubtful or even negative.

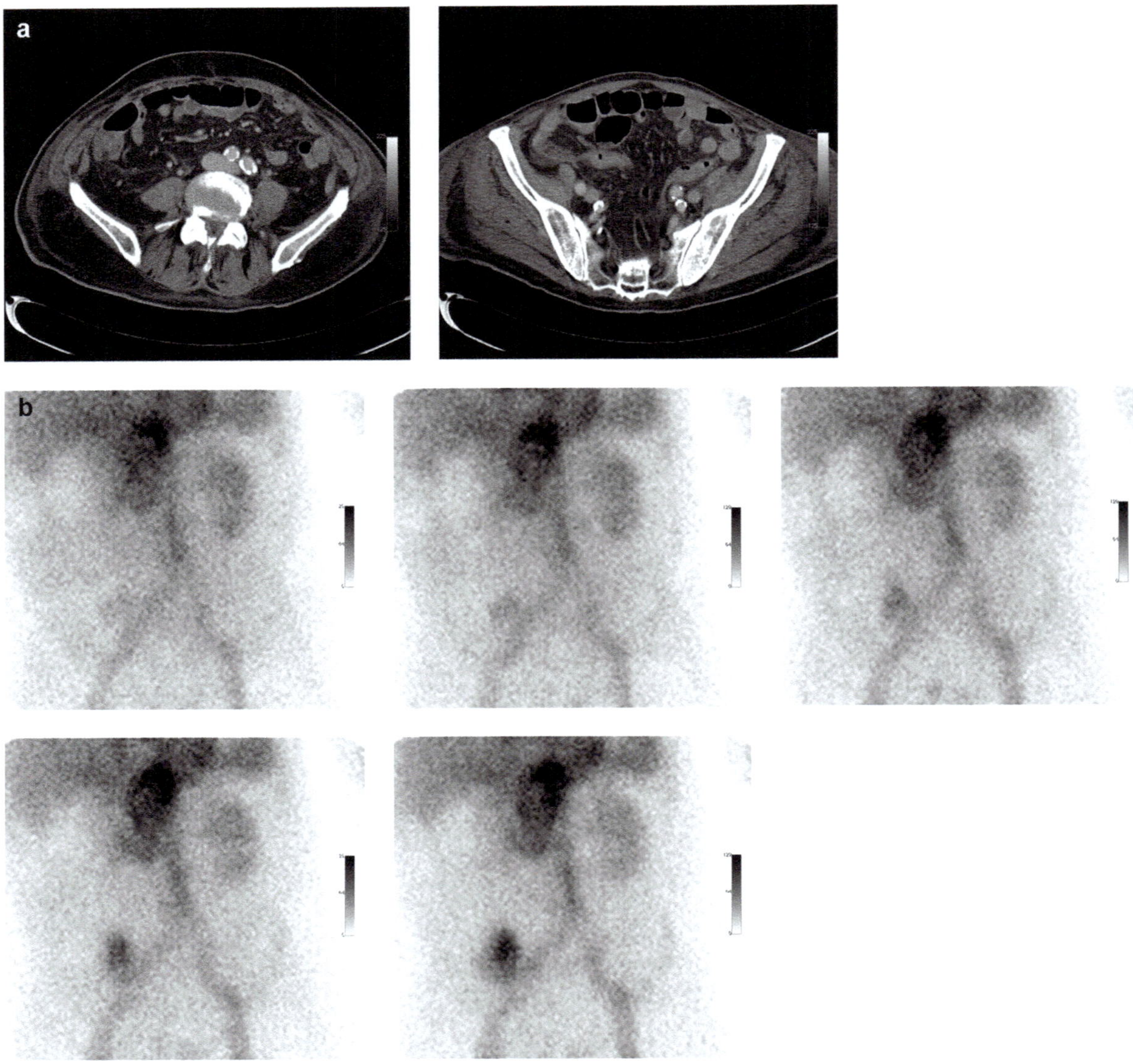
a
b

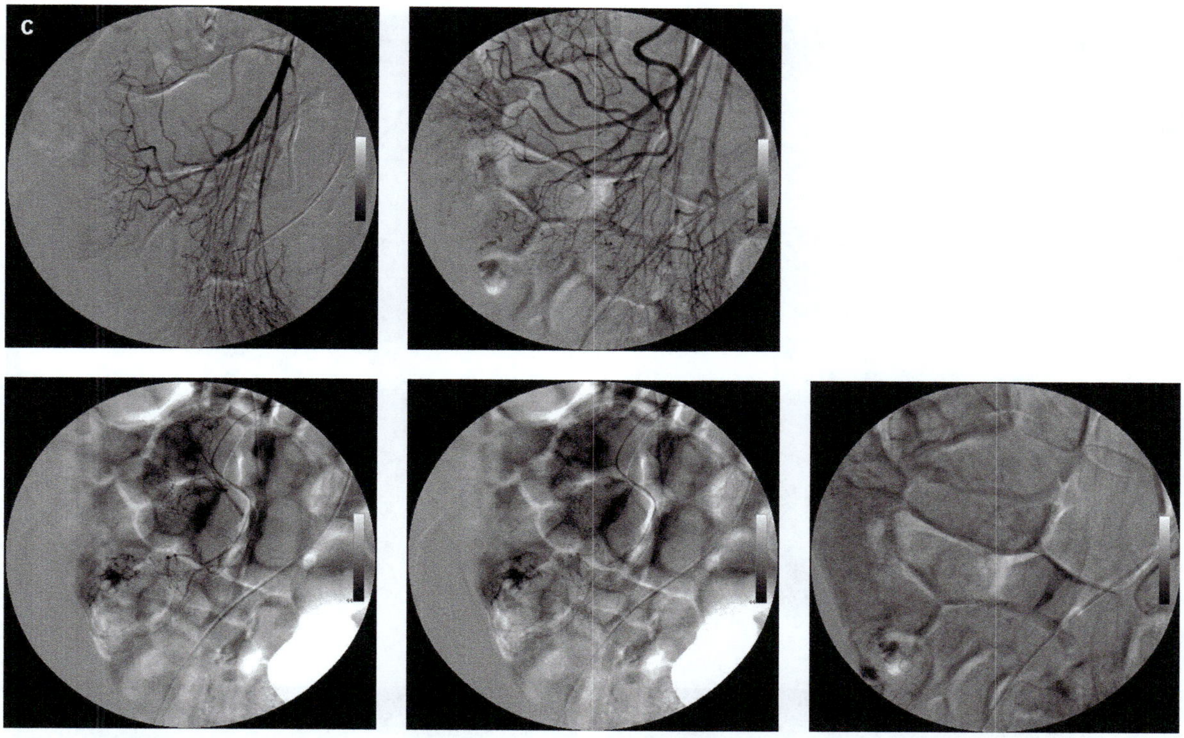

Patient with gastrointestinal blood loss who repeatedly required blood transfusions. CT scan (**a**) reveals no cause for or site of bleeding: possibly intermittent bleeding

Red blood cell scintigrahpy findings

Dynamic scintigraphy with in vivo Tc-99m-labeled erythrocytes (**b**) reveals an extravasation within seconds. Because of the patient's condition and the clear visualization of the bleeding by planar scintigraphy, no SPECT/CT was performed. Guided by the erythrocyte scintigram, the bleeding was further localized and treated by subsequent focused angiography (**c**).

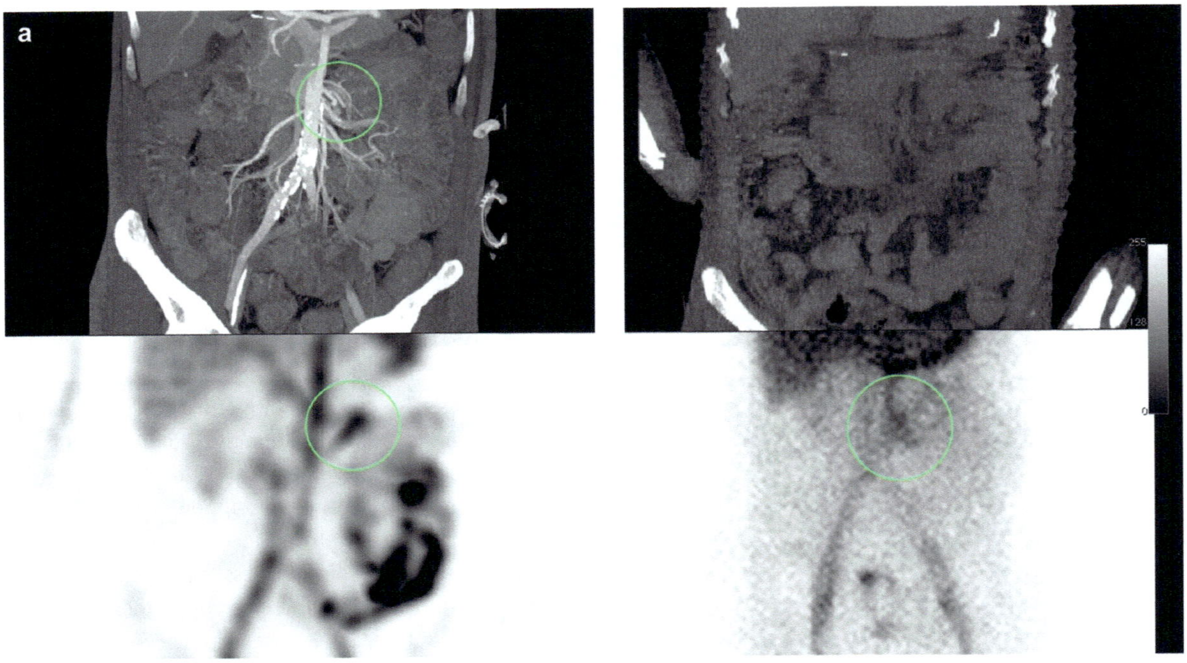
a
255
128
0

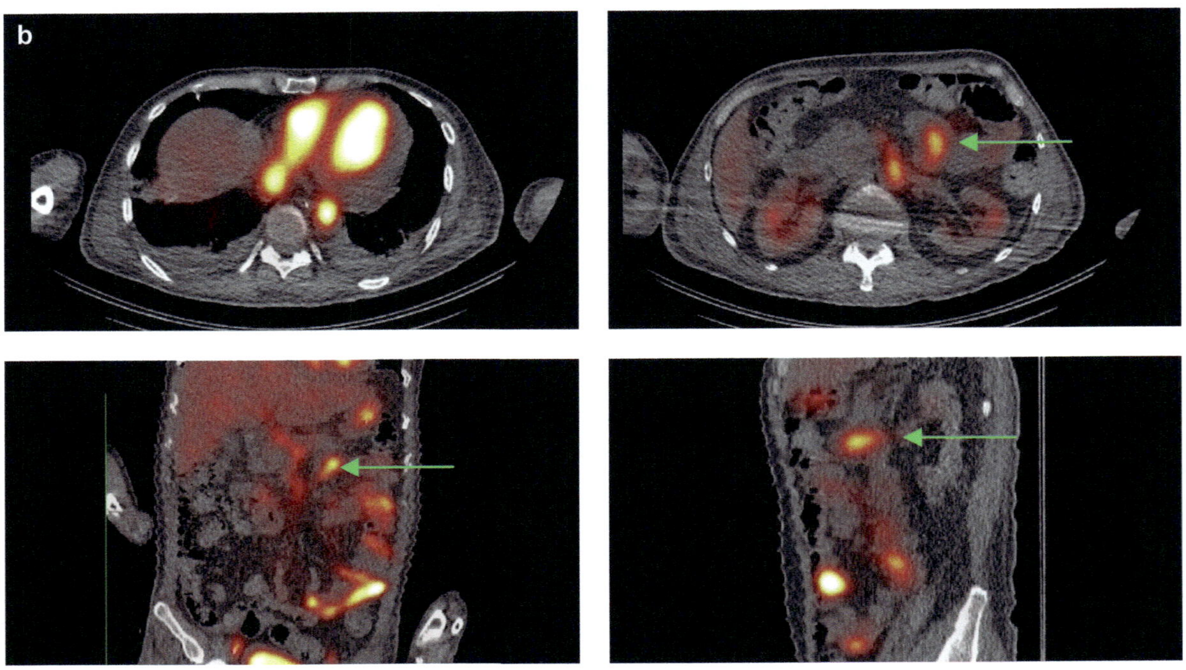
b

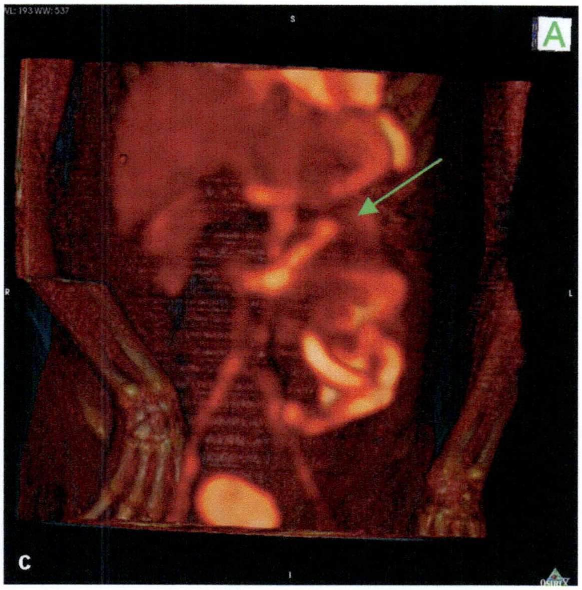

Male patient, 70 years old, with intermittent gastrointestinal blood loss who required blood transfusions. After CT scan with contrast (**a**) had failed to reveal the site of bleeding

Red blood cell scintigraphy findings

Dynamic scintigraphy using in vivo ^{99m}Tc-labeled erythrocytes shows an extravasation in the left median abdomen (*green circle*). Subsequent SPECT/CT (**b**) shows considerable intraintestinal bleeding with transport in the distal direction, but is able to localize the site of the bleeding in the small bowel [*green circle* on coronal SPECT image in (**a**), *arrows* on fusion images in (**b**)]. The 3D volume-rendered image (**c**) gives a good impression of the site and extent of the gastrointestinal bleeding.

Teaching point

SPECT/CT improves the localization and subsequent identification and treatment of gastrointestinal bleeding.

Chapter 11 Ventilation/Perfusion Imaging with SPECT-CT

Henrik Gutte, Jann Mortensen,
and Andreas Kjær

Contents

S. Fanti et al., *Atlas of SPECT-CT*,
DOI: 10.1007/978-3-642-15726-4_11,

Acute pulmonary embolism (PE) is a severe and potentially fatal disease with a mortality rate of approximately 30% if untreated. The incidence is 2 per 1,000 person years in the Western countries. PE is a blockage of the main pulmonary artery or one of its branches by a thrombus, typically a blood clot from the deep veins of the lower extremities. PE reduces the cross-sectional area of the pulmonary blood vessels, resulting in an increase in total pulmonary vascular resistance and pulmonary hypertension.

The clinical presentation of PE is highly variable, and many of its associated symptoms are non-specific, which makes diagnosis difficult. The diagnosis of PE is usually established by a combination of clinical assessment, D-dimer test and imaging with either lung scintigraphy or multidetector computer tomography (MDCT) angiography. Other indications for lung scintigraphy are preoperative regional function before lung cancer surgery, lung volume reduction surgery and cases of pulmonary hypertension.

Pulmonary MDCT angiography has a higher diagnostic accuracy and specificity than conventional planar ventilation/perfusion (V/Q) scintigraphy [1]. Thus, in many institutions MDCT is the first-line imaging test in daily clinical routine in patients suspected of having PE [2–4]. In addition, MDCT has the ability to yield an alternative diagnosis and has a high degree of interobserver agreement [1, 2, 5, 6]. Several studies have demonstrated that MDCT angiography is sensitive with a high specificity [1, 5]. However, the positive predictive value for pulmonary MDCT angiography declines when thrombi are located in smaller pulmonary vessels. Positive predictive values have been reported to be 97% (116 of 120 patients) for PE in a main or lobar artery, 68% (32 of 47 patients) for a segmental vessel and 25% (2 of 8 patients) for a subsegmental branch [2, 3]. However, data are sparse in the subsegmental group. Predictive values vary substantially when clinical probability of PE is taken into account. In patients with high or intermediate clinical probability, the positive predictive value of MDCT is high, but decreases in the case of low clinical probability. The negative predictive value of MDCT is high in patients with low or intermediate clinical probability (96% and 89%, respectively), but is lower in patients with high clinical probability (60%) [2, 3].

A V/Q lung scan involves imaging and evaluation of the distribution of pulmonary blood flow and alveolar ventilation. The ventilation scan can be performed with radioaerosols, Technegas and Krypton (^{81m}Kr), to assess the ability of air to reach all parts of the lungs. ^{81m}Kr is an ultra-short-lived (T½: 13 s) isotope that is eluted from the Rb-Kr generator by oxygen and flows directly to the lungs. By the patient's continuous inhalation of ^{81m}Kr, the scintigram illustrates the distribution of air flow/ventilation.

The perfusion scan shows how blood circulates within the lungs and is most commonly performed in order to check for the presence of decreased perfusion because of an embolism or abnormal blood flow inside the lungs. Perfusion lung scanning is performed after intravenous (i.v.) injection of radiolabeled microparticles (^{99m}Tc-MAA; macroaggregated albumin) that are trapped in the pulmonary precapillaries on a first pass transit. The principle underlying the diagnosis of PE is that whereas pulmonary perfusion is abnormal, the pulmonary alveolar ventilation usually remains intact as a result of its bronchial ventilation supply. On the V/Q scan, it is seen as a mismatch defect.

Among the weaknesses of traditional two-dimensional (2D) planar V/Q scintigraphy when using the Prospective Investigation of Pulmonary Embolism Diagnosis (PIOPED) interpretation criteria are high proportions of equivocal studies [4, 7] as well as only moderate interobserver agreement [1]. Accordingly, in recent years V/Q scintigraphy has had a diminished role in the diagnosis of PE.

At present, many centers use only pulmonary MDCT, but this might not be optimal because of a possible lower sensitivity and higher radiation dose compared with lung scintigraphy. Reasons for extensive use of MDCT may also include its around-the-clock availability, lower cost and high frequency of conclusive results, as well as staff inexperience with V/Q-SPECT. Recently, some proposed algorithms for evaluation of patients suspected of having PE have totally omitted the use of lung scintigraphy in the diagnostic workup. Some guidelines only include lung scintigraphy as an alternative imaging technique when patients cannot have a MDCT performed because of severe renal insufficiency or allergy to intravenous contrast agents, or when a CT-based strategy is inconclusive.

However, the introduction of 3D V/Q-SPECT technology instead of 2D planar V/Q-scintigraphy suggests an improvement in the diagnostic performance of scintigraphy [8–11]. The main advantage of using the SPECT technique compared to planar imaging in relation to V/Q scanning is a higher image "contrast" because superimposing of surrounding normal activity onto lesions is eliminated [12], and the images can then be viewed in sagittal, axial and coronal views.

V/Q-SPECT examinations can be obtained in less than 20 min if ventilation is performed with Technegas (13 min), immediately followed by a perfusion SPECT

(6 min). Alternatively, V/Q-SPECT can be performed as we do simultaneously in 72 steps of 20 s through a 180° projection on a dual-headed gamma camera. Accordingly, the total V/Q-SPECT acquisition time is 13 min. The perfusion study can be performed after, i.e., injection of ~150 MBq of ^{99m}Tc-MAA. The ventilation study can be performed when inhaling ^{81m}Kr; however, other tracers for ventilation, e.g., Technegas, can also be used. At our department, both studies are performed simultaneously with low-energy general-purpose collimators and acquired in a 128 × 128 matrix.

Recently, hybrid gamma camera/MDCT systems have been introduced that allow for simultaneous lung V/Q-SPECT and MDCT angiography, and can be used for diagnosing PE [9, 13]. However, very limited data directly comparing these two 3D modalities are available [10, 14], and a head-to-head comparison of simultaneous V/Q-SPECT and pulmonary MDCT angiography for the detection of PE is warranted.

In our recently performed study, V/Q-SPECT, pulmonary MDCT angiography and low-dose CT were performed in 100 patients suspected of having PE. The first CT acquisition in the study consisted of a low-dose CT scan without contrast enhancement (140 kV, 20 mAs/slice, collimator 16 × 1.5 mm, rotation time 0.5 s and pitch 0.813, 512 × 512 matrix) and was obtained during tidal breathing. The low-dose CT was used for attenuation correction of the V/Q SPECT data and for fusion with the V/Q-SPECT images [11].

V/Q-SPECT alone had a sensitivity of 97% and a specificity of 88%. When adding the information of a low-dose CT scan, the sensitivity was still 97%, but the specificity increased to 100%. A MDCT angiography alone had a sensitivity of 68% and a specificity of 100% [11].

This is in agreement with regard to sensitivity, specificity and accuracy to a previous retrospective study that found values of 97%, 91% and 94%, respectively, for V/Q-SPECT alone and values of 86%, 98% and 93%, respectively, for MDCT [10]. Another study found that the observed percentage of agreement between SPECT V/Q scintigraphy and CTPA data for the diagnosis of PE was 95%. When calculated against the respiratory physicians' reference diagnosis, V/Q-SPECT alone had a sensitivity of 83% and a specificity of 98% [14].

We find that using the PIOPED criteria is inappropriate when classifying PE patients using the SPECT technique, since these criteria were derived from single view ^{133}Xe ventilation and planar perfusion imaging, which is very different from V/Q-SPECT [7]. The best way to report V/Q-SPECT has not been clarified. However, there seems to be consensus about a more simplified reporting scheme in V/Q-SPECT reading [15–18].

The use of the SPECT technique involves a much lower frequency of equivocal tests than is known from traditional planar lung scans, which in previous studies have been reported to result in up to 73% non-conclusive examinations [7]. This is in accordance with previous studies that demonstrated that the use of SPECT in V/Q scintigraphy reduces the frequency of equivocal tests markedly [15, 19, 20].

In one study, the addition of low-dose CT without a contrast agent to the V/Q-SPECT resulted in an even higher confidence of the reading with a reduction of inconclusive studies from 5% with SPECT alone to 0% with SPECT + low-dose CT. In addition, the specificity was improved with fewer false-positive interpretations (from 18% to 0%). This was mainly due to findings on the low-dose CT scan that gave alternative explanations for subtle perfusion defects that otherwise would have been interpreted as PE on SPECT alone. Although a low dose CT scan without a contrast agent is inherently inferior to those acquired by a diagnostic CT scan with a contrast agent, the low-dose CT scan can satisfactorily provide relevant diagnostic information to determine the origin of the V/Q-SPECT lesions. When assessing the V/Q-SPECT datasets alone, mismatched defects on the V/Q-SPECT scans due to interlobar fissures, paraseptal emphysema, pneumonic infiltration, atelectasis and pleural fluid could be well demonstrated on the low-dose CT [11].

The fact that that there is no independent gold standard for establishing the PE diagnosis poses difficulties for the evaluation and comparison of the diagnostic accuracy of different modalities in PE. In order to compare the diagnostic performance of the tested modalities, a combination of composite and head-to-head consensus reading as the criterion standard has been used [11]. The use of this combined method, which includes all tested modalities to classify PE patients, raises methodological and conceptual problems and is controversial. However, this reference is the best currently available. Nevertheless, it is important to keep in mind the possibility that some patients being studied may be incorrectly assigned to a disease category by the examination, which can lead to exaggerated or underestimated accuracies.

With the use of hybrid scanners, V/Q-SPECT in combination with low-dose CT without contrast enhancement has "revitalized" lung scintigraphy and should probably be considered the first-line imaging test in diagnosing PE.

References

1. Blachere H, Latrabe V, Montaudon M, Valli N, Couffinhal T, Raherisson C, et al. Pulmonary embolism revealed on helical CT angiography: comparison with ventilation–perfusion radionuclide lung scanning. Am J Roentgenol. 2000;174(4):1041–7.
2. Stein PD, Fowler SE, Goodman LR, Gottschalk A, Hales CA, Hull RD, et al. Multidetector computed tomography for acute pulmonary embolism. N Engl J Med. 2006;354(22):2317–27.
3. Stein PD, Woodard PK, Weg JG, Wakefield TW, Tapson VF, Sostman HD, et al. Diagnostic pathways in acute pulmonary embolism: recommendations of the PIOPED II investigators. Radiology. 2007;242(1):15–21.
4. Strashun AM. A reduced role of V/Q scintigraphy in the diagnosis of acute pulmonary embolism. J Nucl Med. 2007;48(9):1405–7.
5. Mayo JR, Remy-Jardin M, Muller NL, Remy J, Worsley DF, Hossein-Foucher C, et al. Pulmonary embolism: prospective comparison of spiral CT with ventilation-perfusion scintigraphy. Radiology. 1997;205(2):447–52.
6. Coche E, Verschuren F, Keyeux A, Goffette P, Goncette L, Hainaut P, et al. Diagnosis of acute pulmonary embolism in outpatients: comparison of thin-collimation multi-detector row spiral CT and planar ventilation-perfusion scintigraphy. Radiology. 2003;229(3):757–65.
7. PIOPED Investigators. Value of the ventilation/perfusion scan in acute pulmonary embolism. Results of the prospective investigation of pulmonary embolism diagnosis (PIOPED). The PIOPED investigators. JAMA. 1990;263(20):2753–9.
8. Gutte H, Mortensen J, Jensen C, von der Recke P, Petersen CL, Kristoffersen US, et al. Comparison of V/Q-SPECT and planar V/Q-lung scintigraphy in diagnosing acute pulmonary embolism. Nucl Med Commun. 2010;31(1):82–6.
9. Gutte H, Mortensen J, Jensen C, von der Recke P, Kristoffersen US, Kjær A. Added value of combined simultaneous lung ventilation-perfusion single-photon emission computed tomography/multi-slice-computed tomography angiography in two patients suspected of having acute pulmonary embolism. Clin Respir J. 2008;1(1):52–5.
10. Reinartz P, Wildberger JE, Schaefer W, Nowak B, Mahnken AH, Buell U. Tomographic imaging in the diagnosis of pulmonary embolism: a comparison between V/Q lung scintigraphy in SPECT technique and multislice spiral CT. J Nucl Med. 2004;45(9):1501–8.
11. Gutte H, Mortensen J, Jensen C, Johnbeck CB, von der Recke P, Petersen CL, et al. Detection of pulmonary embolism with combined ventilation-perfusion SPECT and low-dose CT: head-to-head comparison with CT angiography. J Nucl Med. 2009;50:1987–92.
12. Petersson J, Sanchez-Crespo A, Larsson SA, Mure M. Physiological imaging of the lung: single-photon-emission computed tomography (SPECT). J Appl Physiol. 2007;102(1):468–76.
13. Bailey D, Roach P, Bailey E, Hewlett J, Keijzers R. Development of a cost-effective modular SPECT/CT scanner. Eur J Nucl Med Mol Imaging. 2007;34(9):1415–26.
14. Miles S, Rogers KM, Thomas P, Soans B, Attia J, Abel C, et al. A comparison of SPECT lung scintigraphy and CTPA for the diagnosis of pulmonary embolism. Chest. 2009;136(6):1546–3.
15. Bajc M, Olsson CG, Olsson B, Palmer J, Jonson B. Diagnostic evaluation of planar and tomographic ventilation/perfusion lung images in patients with suspected pulmonary emboli. Clin Physiol Funct Imaging. 2004;24(5):249–56.
16. Roach PJ, Bailey DL, Harris BE. Enhancing lung scintigraphy with single-photon emission computed tomography. Semin Nucl Med. 2008;38(6):441–9.
17. Schumichen C. V/Q-scanning/SPECT for the diagnosis of pulmonary embolism. Respiration. 2003;70(4):329–42.
18. Bajc M, Neilly J, Miniati M, Schuemichen C, Meignan M, Jonson B. EANM guidelines for ventilation/perfusion scintigraphy. Eur J Nucl Med Mol Imaging. 2009;36(8):1356–70.
19. Leblanc M, Leveillee F, Turcotte E. Prospective evaluation of the negative predictive value of V/Q SPECT using 99mTc-Technegas. Nucl Med Commun. 2007;28(8):667–72.
20. Bajc M, Olsson B, Palmer J, Jonson B. Ventilation/perfusion SPECT for diagnostics of pulmonary embolism in clinical practice. J Intern Med. 2008;264(4):379–87.

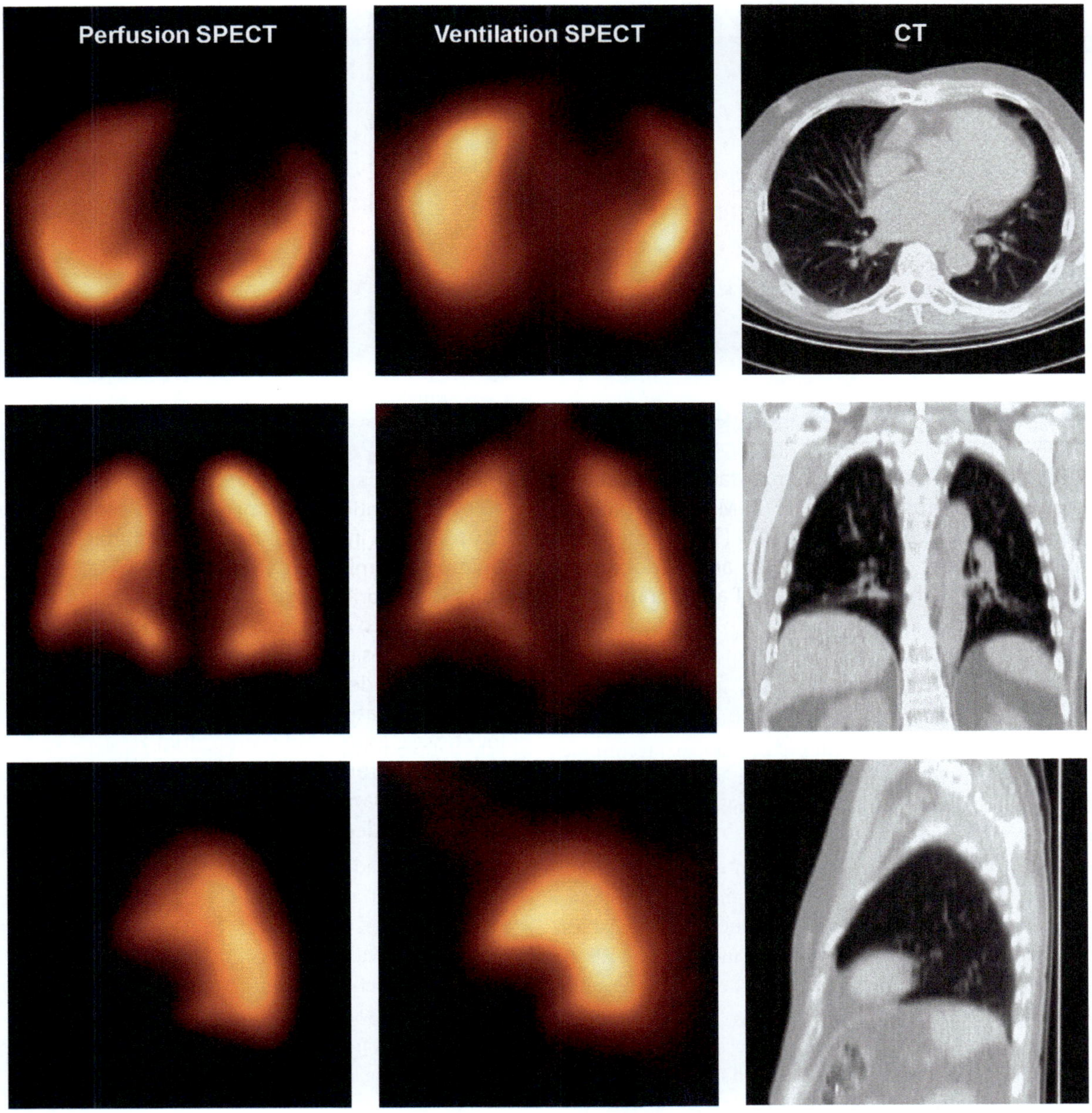

V/Q-SPECT low-dose CT findings

A case of physiologic distribution of V/Q-SPECT using ^{99m}Tc-MAA and ^{81m}Kr in combination with low-dose CT without contrast enhancement.

Teaching point

Normally the CT scan is obtained during a deep inspiration breath hold. However, in order to increase the alignment of the lung borders patients are asked to breathe normally during the low-dose CT scan in order to obtain the best correspondence of the lung borders at the CT and the SPECT modality

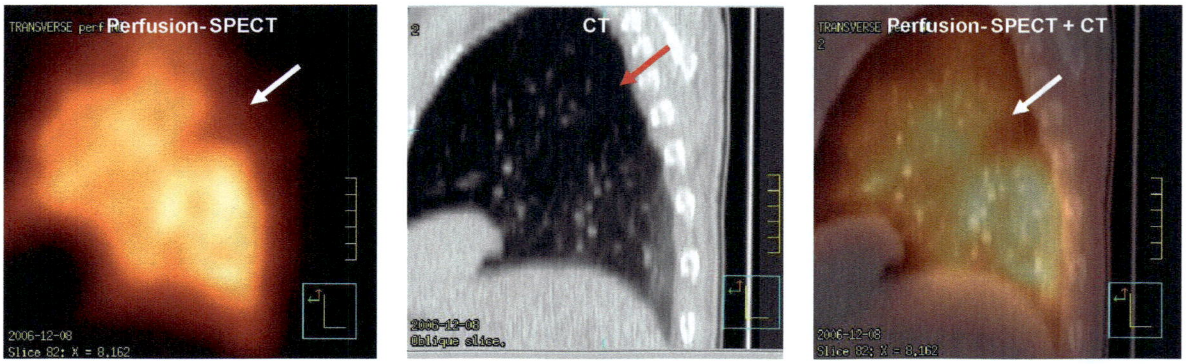

V/Q-SPECT low-dose CT findings

Sagittal view of a small subsegmental defect (*arrows*) seen on the perfusion SPECT (^{99m}Tc-MAA). The patient had a normal ventilation SPECT (^{81m}Kr). The mismatched defect corresponded to an interlobar fissure as seen on the low-dose CT. CT angiography did not reveal PE.

Teaching point

A case of a patient with mismatched defect caused by an interlobar fissure and mimicking pulmonary embolism. The low-dose CT scan can satisfactorily provide relevant diagnostic information to determine the origin of the V/Q-SPECT lesions. Other causes of mismatched defects imitating pulmonary embolism that might be ruled out by the low-dose CT are emphysema, fluid, pneumonia, tumor and atelectasis. Notice the small discrepancy between SPECT and CT of the lung borders

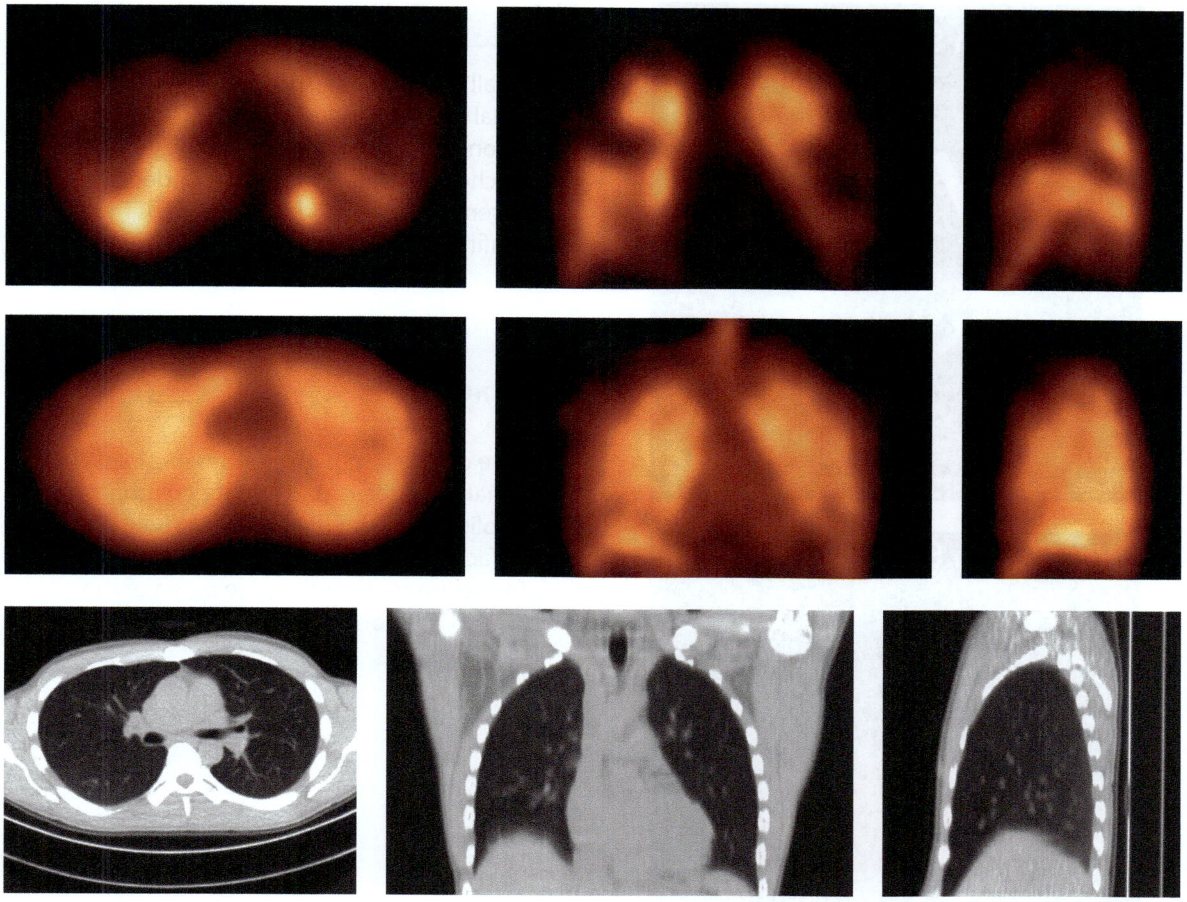

V/Q-SPECT low-dose CT findings

A case with many wedge-shaped mismatched defects as seen on the V/Q-SPECT (^{99m}Tc-MAA and ^{81m}Kr). At the corresponding low-dose CT scan no explainable cause of the defects was found.

Teaching point

Wedge-shaped mismatched defect >0.5 segment is highly suspicious of PE

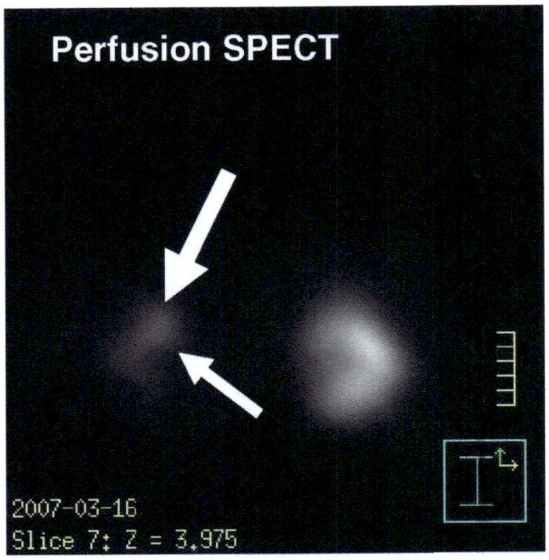

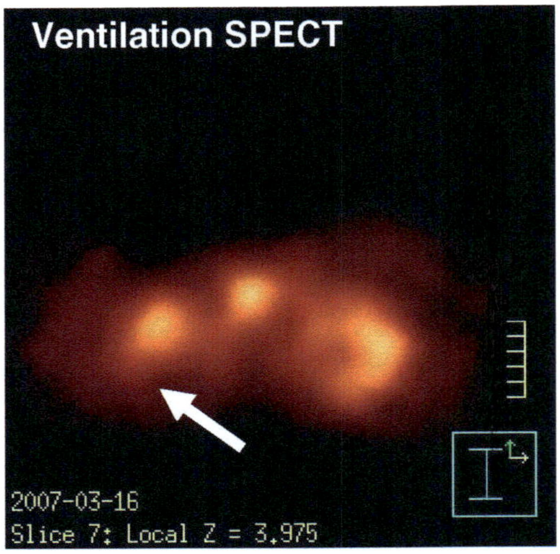

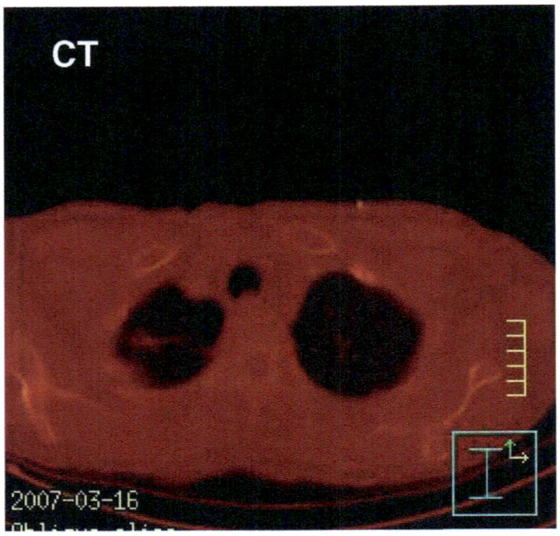

V/Q-SPECT low-dose CT findings

Two small subsegmental defects (*arrow*) seen on the transaxial views of perfusion SPECT (^{99m}Tc-MAA) with corresponding normal ventilation SPECT (^{81m}Kr). The mismatched defect (*arrow*) corresponded to regional emphysema as seen on low-dose CT. CT angiography confirmed that there was no PE.

Teaching point

A case of a patient with emphysema causing mismatched defect and imitate pulmonary embolism. The low-dose CT scan can satisfactorily provide relevant diagnostic information to determine the origin of the V/Q-SPECT lesions.

Chapter 12 Radiation Therapy Planning Using SPECT-CT

Gianfranco Loi, Eugenio Inglese, and Marco Krengli

Contents

S. Fanti et al., *Atlas of SPECT-CT*,
DOI: 10.1007/978-3-642-15726-4_12,

Up to date image-guided radiotherapy extensively involves radiology, nuclear medicine and medical physics for accurate delineation of the volumes of interest (VOIs) and assists physicians to extract the most relevant clinical information. The aim is to precisely identify the gross tumor volume (GTV) and to use the available information to delineate the clinical target volume (CTV) that represents the microscopic invasion of the tumor. The ever-increasing amount of image data acquired (CT, MRI, SPECT and PET) requires the development of a robust image registration process for precise image alignment. This is a prerequisite for obtaining imaging useful for precise target identification that employs multiple modalities with morphological, functional and biological information. The integration of these multiple images may allow identifying target and non-target structures better than using each single imaging modality [1–3].

12.1 Image Fusion (Co-registration) of Functional and Anatomical Data

These can simply be divided into image-based and non-image based co-registration methods.

Image-based registration includes:

- *Extrinsic method*: based on external fiducial markers attached to the body surface, designed to be accurately detectable in all the different imaging modalities. The co-registration of different images is easy and fast, and can usually be automated without the need of complex algorithms. Unfortunately, this method is not suitable for retrospective co-registration tasks and not practical for routine clinical use, especially if patients are studied on different days [4].
- *Intrinsic methods*: the information for the co-registration process is derived from a set of identified landmarks and on the alignment of segmented binary structures (segmentation-based methods), or directly onto measures computed from the image gray values (voxel property-based method). Landmarks can be anatomical (points identified by the operator) or geometric (shapes automatically localized) [5].
- *Segmentation based methods* can be:
  1. Rigid model based, where extracted anatomical structures are co- registered as the only input for the alignment procedure
  2. Deformable model based, where an extracted structure from one image is elastically deformed to fit the same on the other image
  3. Voxel property methods, where intensity-based values in different images are aligned.

The low-resolution nuclear medicine image is the major limitation of these registration techniques.

12.1.1 Non-image-Based Registration Methods (Dual-Modality Devices)

A non-image-based registration is possible if the imaging coordinate systems of the two scanners involved are calibrated to each other. This usually requires the scanners to be brought into the same physical location, with the assumption that the patient will remain motionless between both acquisitions [7].

This method forms the basis for the development of multi-modality devices combining structural and functional measurements.

These new devices, combining PET and SPECT with CT, are able to acquire data in the same session and therefore limit the fusion accuracy problems (positioning and movement of patients) of anatomical modalities outside of the brain, without the need for fiducial markers and complicated mathematical algorithms.

A hybrid imaging device composed of a dual-head variable angle SPECT combined with a CT scanner is now the standard equipment proposed by the industry for cross-sectional fusion imaging and systematic scatter and attenuation correction of gamma ray emission [6, 7].

This hybrid imaging system was used with In-111 pentetreotide scintigraphy to evaluate 73 patients with neuroendocrine tumors. In 40% of the patients with abnormal scintigraphic findings, SPECT/CT improved the accuracy of nuclear medicine studies by providing better localization of SPECT-detected lesions; in particular, in 21 patients, it precisely defined the organ involved and the relationship of lesions to adjacent structures, in 4 patients, it showed unsuspected bone involvement, and in 4 patients, it differentiated physiological from tumor uptake [8, 9].

In-111 pentetreotide can also be used to identify the precise location and the tumor extension of other neoplasms such as meningioma. These images are very suitable for radiotherapy treatment planning, especially when the tumor is located in close proximity to critical structures (Figs. 12.2 and 12.3).

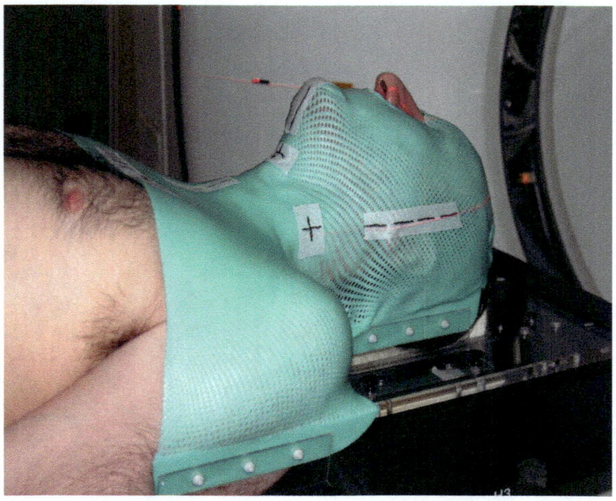

Fig. 12.1 A customized-shape conformed heat deformable mask positioned on the head and neck of a patient affected by oropharyngeal carcinoma, lying on the rigid table of an hybrid machine (SPECT/CT). External anatomical landmarks, exactly coincident with laser beams, are adopted to facilitate the accuracy of repositioning

12.1.2 The Mask Approach

Stereotactic techniques are widely used in neurosurgery, radiosurgery and fractionated radiotherapy. For these treatments, the patient is fixed to a stereotactic frame that defines a coordinate system within the patient. Using tomographic imaging, the positions and shapes of the clinical target volume (CTV) and the organs at risk can be located by special localizers. These tomographic images serve as the basis for the three-dimensional treatment planning process (Fig. 12.1).

In special cases of treatment planning, CT and MRI are co-registered to PET or SPECT for specific reasons: the CT data set reflects the electron density of the tissue and is needed to calculate dose distribution within the patient. When available, MRI provides superior soft tissue contrast and is used to delineate the tumor and the organs at risk. PET and SPECT images can additionally be used to measure the relative metabolic activity for detecting differences in tumor regions or differentiating tumor from necrosis.

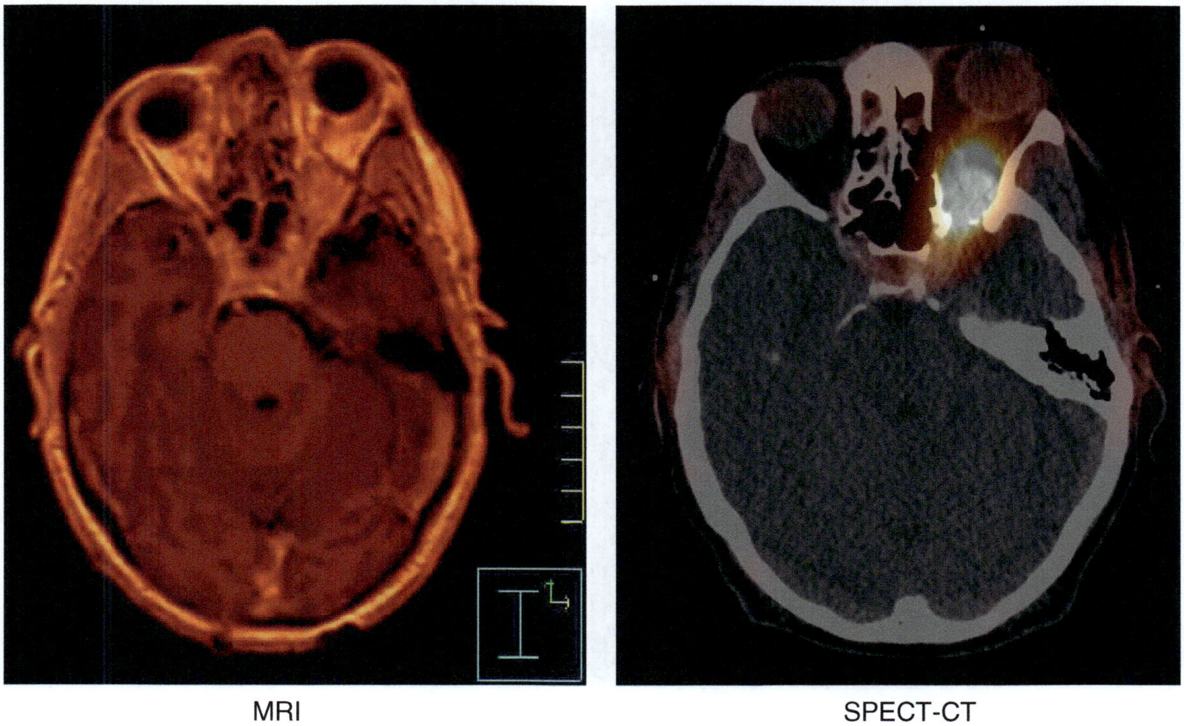

Fig. 12.2 In-111 pentetreotide SPECT-CT images showing tumor relapse in a case of operated meningioma

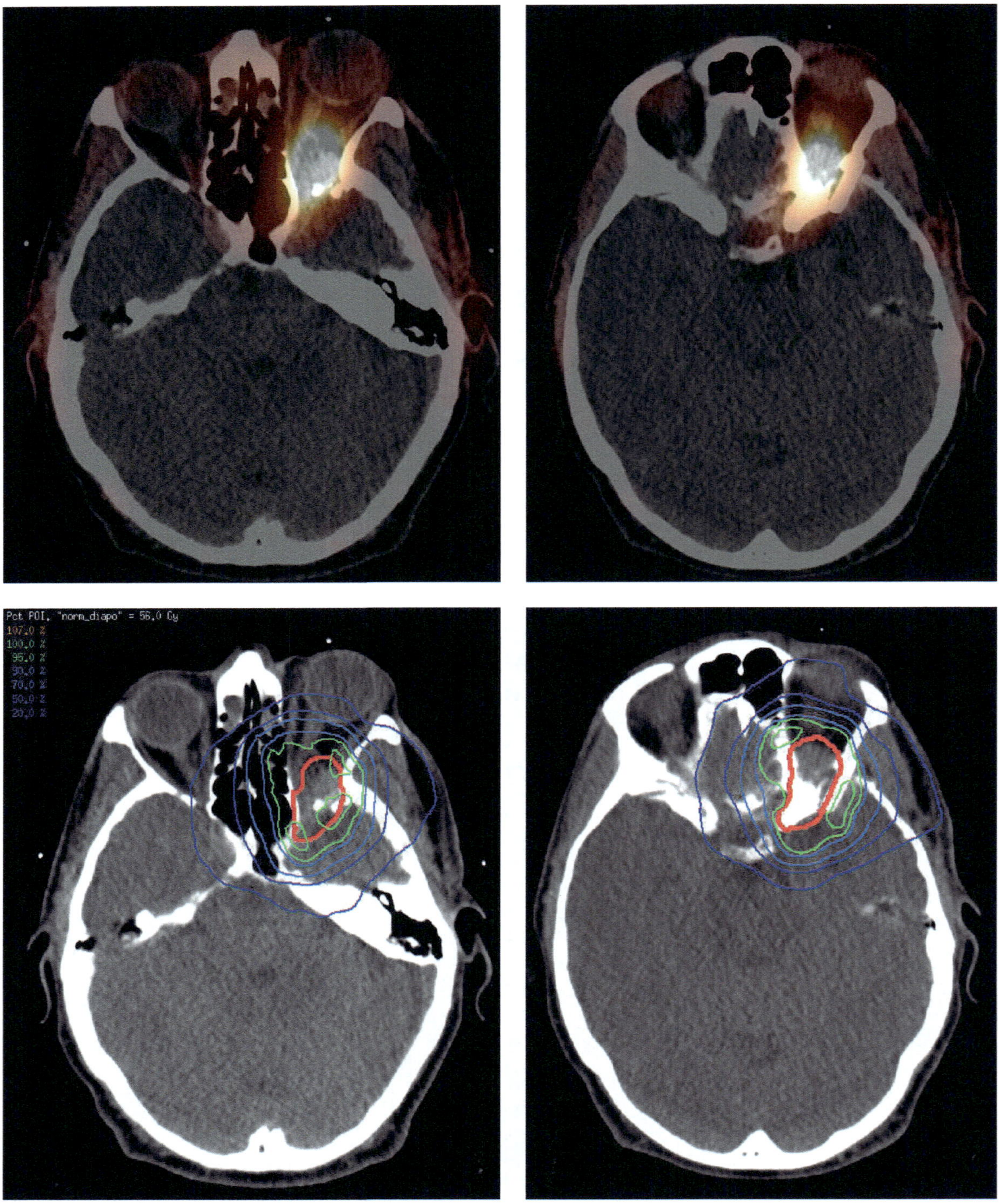

Fig. 12.3 SPECT-CT images and corresponding RT plan images reporting the dose distribution. The GTV is the red ROI delineated on the basis of the tracer uptake

These complementary aspects can be integrated into treatment planning by stereotactic correlation of the images from different modalities. The accuracy of the stereotactic correlation depends on:

1. Distortions of the imaging process itself
2. Mechanical errors of the localization hardware (e.g., the localizers)
3. Errors in the software that calculates the stereotactic coordinates from the positions of the fiducials.

A commissioning test by the customer is part of a QC program prior to the first application to patients.

For PET, the localization accuracy was found by Karger et al. [10] to be device dependent, ranging from 1.1 to 2.4 mm. For SPECT, the mean deviations in space were found to be 1.6 and 2.0 mm. No dependence on device type was observed, and the deviations were well below the physical resolution of SPECT. Therefore, uncertainties due to image distortion can be neglected.

With respect to image distortions, CT is less dependent on target point position, and for MRI the errors may be larger because of larger inhomogeneities of the basic magnet in the off-center region of this device. The physical resolution worsens towards the border of PET and towards the center of SPECT; therefore, different errors can be expected for different modalities. It is therefore of paramount importance to localize errors for each modality and target point position.

12.2 Stereotactic Radiotherapy

When images of different modalities are to be stereotactically correlated for radiotherapy, the combined uncertainty of stereotactic localization, patient fixation as well as possible organ movements has to be considered in the definition of the planning target volume. In fractionated radiotherapy, this uncertainty may be significant. Methods registering anatomical structures have the advantage that the anatomical structures are matched directly, which may compensate for different patient positions within the mask. For radiotherapy purposes, if external markers are placed on the body surface for this purpose, the determined accuracy may not apply for regions within the body where no markers can be fixed.

For stereotactic radiotherapy, it appears more reasonable to use stereotactic imaging with known uncertainty and consider patient and organ movements separately.

12.3 Brain High-Grade Glioma

Despite recent progress in biological knowledge, the prognosis of patients with high-grade glioma remains poor, with a median survival time of about 10–14 months after multimodality treatment, including surgery, radiotherapy and chemotherapy [11–14].

The identification of the target volume for radiotherapy of high-grade glioma is still an unsolved problem, as demonstrated in clinical practice by the high recurrence rate in the marginal region surrounding the volume irradiated to the highest dose [15, 16].

Although a number of recent studies have described the use of PET imaging with ^{18}F and ^{11}C compounds, the role of SPECT is still under investigation, thanks to the variety of molecules and the wide availability of this technique [17–19].

Among the SPECT radiotracers for brain studies, ^{99m}Tc-methoxy-isobutyl-isonitrile (^{99m}Tc-SestaMIBI) has shown a favorable tumor-to-background uptake related to its accumulation in tumor cells [20, 21].

Several studies investigated the use of ^{99m}Tc-MIBI imaging for detecting the biological characteristics of brain tumors, distinguishing between tumor tissue and radiation-induced signal alteration predicting the response to radiotherapy and chemotherapy, and the prognosis as well [22–26].

Major drawbacks of ^{99m}Tc-MIBI, that is, poor morphological resolution and disturbing sites of physiological uptake, can be overcome by dual-modality, integrated systems. In fact, SPECT/CT can distinguish tumor from the skull and other sites of physiological uptake better than SPECT alone (as confirmed by MRI in all cases) and affords a morphological map.

The delineation of gross tumor volume (GTV) by ^{99m}Tc-SestaMIBI SPECT imaging for conformal radiotherapy of high-grade glioma is based on the characteristics of this radiotracer, which is a small lipophilic radioligand that enters cells by diffusion, being preferentially trapped in mitochondria. As a result of the high mitochondrial activity in tumor cells, ^{99m}Tc-SestaMIBI accumulates more in tumor rather than in normal tissue.

In brain tumors, its accumulation is facilitated by disruption of the blood-brain barrier. The role of ^{99m}Tc-SestaMIBI SPECT in the diagnosis and follow-up of brain glioma was investigated during the last decade in several studies [22, 24–28].

These results showed that ^{99m}Tc-SestaMIBI uptake correlates with histological grade and prognosis, and can allow distinguishing tumor recurrence from post-treatment necrosis with a sensitivity of 73–88% and a specificity of 75–100% [27, 29, 30].

Another study correlating ^{99m}Tc-SestaMIBI SPECT and stereotactic biopsy for the detection of tumor recurrence found 90% sensitivity, 91.5% specificity and 90.5% accuracy [31].

We investigated the use of this radiotracer in 21 patients diagnosed with high-grade supratentorial glioma after surgery or stereotactic biopsy. We demonstrated that the fusion of ^{99m}Tc-SestaMIBI SPECT imaging with CT and MRI is useful for target volume delineation in conformal radiotherapy of high-grade glioma, since ^{99m}Tc-SestaMIBI SPECT imaging significantly affected the delineation of the target volume identified by CT and MRI alone [32].

Image registration was obtained by an interactive method based on three-dimensional rigid body transformation using the software of the treatment-planning system Pinnacle® (Philips, Adac Laboratories, Milpitas, CA). CT images were selected as the reference data set, and MRI and ^{99m}Tc-SestaMIBI SPECT images as floating data sets.

Image registration was obtained by translating and rotating the floating images according to CT images. The accuracy of the procedure was verified by several anatomic landmarks. A previous analysis by Jaszczak phantom had shown that the registration error of this interactive procedure was less than 2 mm, according to other literature data [33].

Our study confirmed the high sensitivity of ^{99m}Tc-SestaMIBI SPECT for high-grade gliomas, which is comparable or even higher than that of MRI in detecting remnant tumor tissue. Adding ^{99m}Tc-SestaMIBI SPECT to MRI, it was possible to identify a larger size and to redefine the spatial distribution of GTV, as defined by MRI alone.

Based on these considerations and waiting for a non-Cyclotron-dependent PET brain imaging, SPECT functional images of the brain deserve to be studied more in depth for the treatment planning of gliomas with the purpose of making new imaging modalities available, such as ^{123}I-α-methyl-tyrosine (IMT-SPECT), which could be able to identify the presence, location and possibly the biological features of tumor tissue in order to optimize the delivery of high-dose precision radiotherapy [19].

Our findings on ^{99m}Tc-SestaMIBI SPECT imaging demonstrated that the target volumes for radiotherapy planning of gliomas can be substantially modified (Figs. 12.4 and 12.5). The average target volume on SPECT was actually 33% larger than the average volume on MRI, with greater difference for operated than for inoperable cases. This kind of information can really be of substantial help to focus the high irradiation dose on the tumor area and to spare normal brain tissue in a similar way as the more specific, but more expensive, tracer ^{123}I-α-methyl-tyrosine (IMT-SPECT/CT).

The future of brain glioma imaging for treatment planning of high-precision radiotherapy is most likely related to the integration of multiple biological imaging modalities allowing the highlighting of the various tumor characteristics, following and developing the concept of biological target volume as already proposed by Ling et al. [34]. This concept would include information about metabolism, proliferation, hypoxia, apoptosis and location of tumor stem cells in order to use radiation in such a way as to deliver different dose levels with different fractionation schedules realizing a kind of dose deposition (dose painting) to optimize the control of the various tumor components. In this effort, imaging techniques based on biological tumor characteristics, such as non-conventional MRI sequences, MR spectroscopy, PET and also SPECT images, may find their ideal place.

12.4 Lymph Nodes in Prostate Cancer

The precise identification of the pathway of lymphatic drainage is a very relevant issue when treating prostate cancer with high risk of lymph node involvement by radiotherapy. Typically, internal and external iliac nodes are included in the treatment volume, which is identified more on the basis of anatomical landmarks than on functional information on the real pathway in the single patient. Such information is greatly relevant because nowadays it is possible to optimize the treatment by using intensity-modulated radiation therapy (IMRT), which allows precise shaping of the isodose curves to conform to the delineated target [35]. A quite recent study investigated the anatomic mapping of nodal disease in prostate cancer by using a magnetic resonance lymphangiographic technique [36]. Interestingly, the authors found that nodal metastases tightly mapped relative to the large pelvic vessels leading to a clinical target volume around not only the proximal external and internal iliac, but also the distal common iliac vessels.

The technique of the sentinel node (SN) via ^{99m}Tc-nanocolloid scintigraphy has been studied in prostate cancer in several surgical series with high sensitivity up to 93–96% [37].

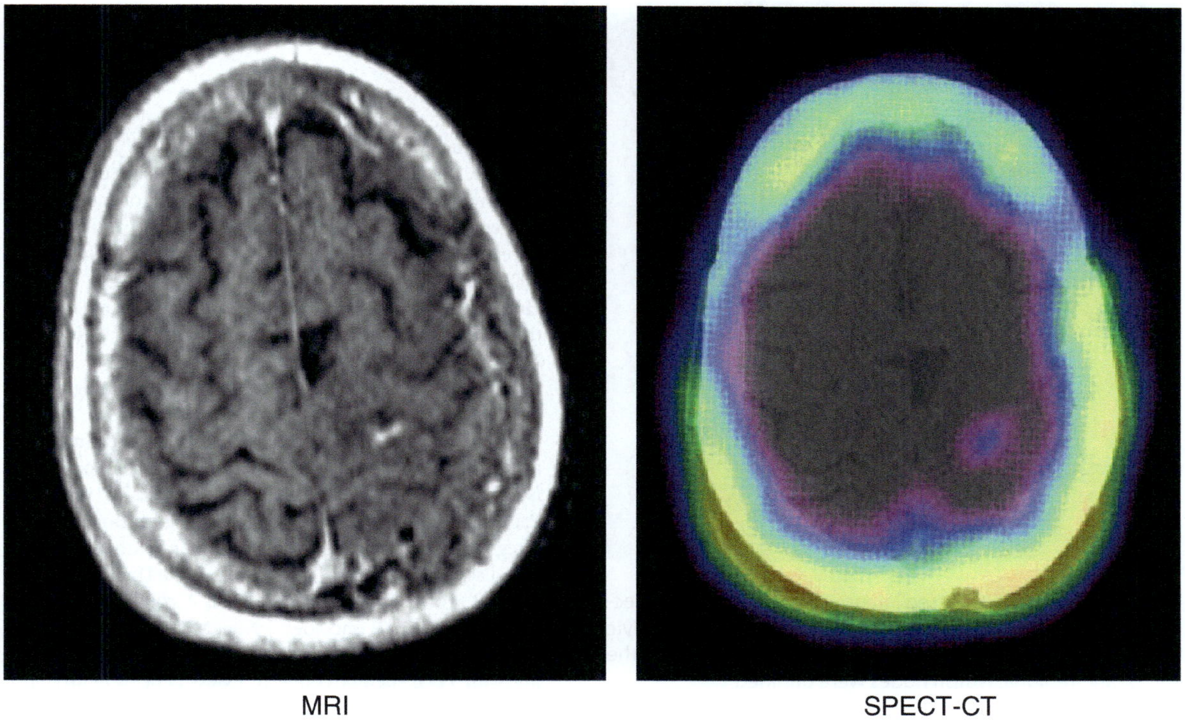

Fig. 12.4 ^{99m}Tc-SestaMIBI SPECT-CT image shows tracer uptake proximal to the surgical cavity, suggesting disease persistence in a case of operated GBM

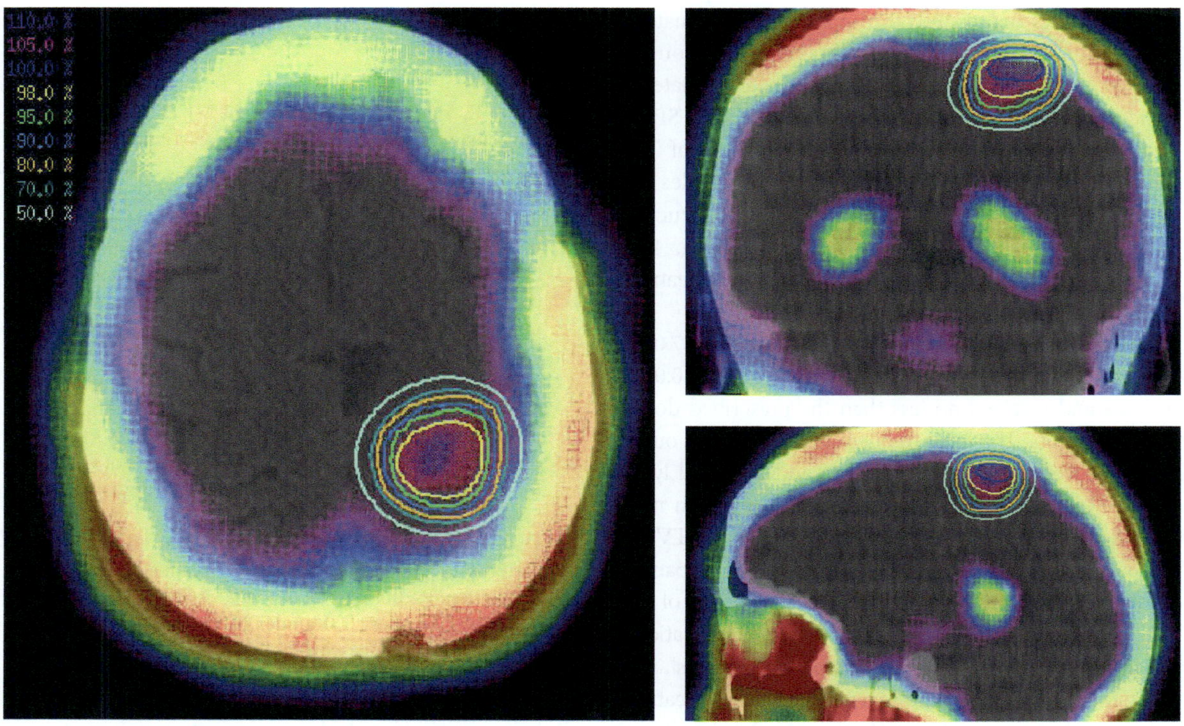

Fig. 12.5 RT plan dose distribution obtained with stereotactic radiotherapy of the target volume identified on the basis of the SPECT-CT images

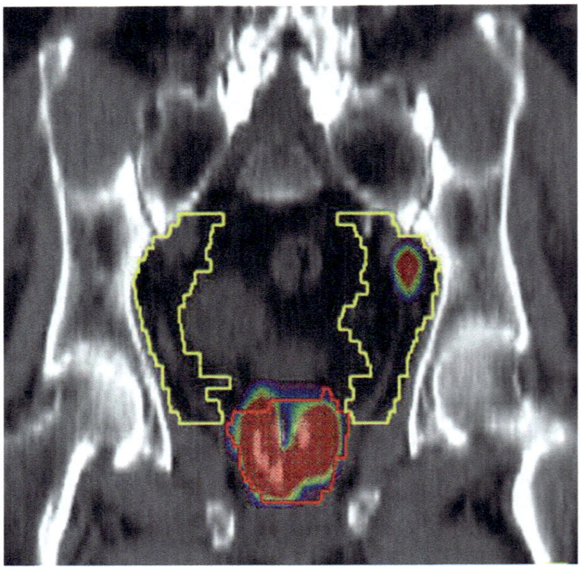

Fig. 12.6 SPECT/CT fused image after intra-prostate injection of 115 MBq of ^{99m}Tc-nanocolloid. The SN and other pelvic lymph nodes were clearly identified and the volumes of the tumor and regional lymph nodes were outlined

We investigated the in vivo drainage pathway of lymphatic spread by using the SN technique and SPECT-CT image fusion to identify the location of the potentially involved nodes and to study the impact that such anatomic information can have on conformal pelvic irradiation [38].

Twenty-three prostate cancer patients, candidates for radical prostatectomy, were studied by CT and SPECT images after intra-prostate injection of 115 MBq of ^{99m}Tc-nanocolloid. The SN and other pelvic lymph nodes were clearly identified, and target and non-target structures were drawn on SPECT-CT fusion images (Fig. 12.6). Subsequently, a three-dimensional conformal treatment plan was performed for each patient.

SPECT lymph nodal uptake was detected in 87.0% of patients. The SN was inside the pelvic CTV in 80.0% of patients and received no less than the prescribed dose in 85% of patients. The most frequent locations of SN outside the CTV were in the common iliac and presacral lymph nodes. Most interestingly, 50% of the other lymph nodes identified by SPECT were found outside the CTV and received less than the prescribed dose in 44% of patients. This study demonstrated that detailed knowledge of lymphatic drainage can contribute to a better identification of the in vivo potential pattern of lymph node metastasis in prostate cancer and can lead to a modification of treatment volume with consequent optimization of pelvic irradiation.

References

Co-registration

1. Weber DA, Ivanovic M. Correlative image registration. Semin Nucl Med. 1994;24:311.
2. Israel O, Keidar Z, Iosilevsky G, et al. The fusion of anatomic and physiologic imaging in the management of patients with cancer. Semin Nucl Med. 2001;24:191.
3. Shreve PD. Adding structure to function. J Nucl Med. 2000;41:1380.
4. Hutton BF, Braun M, Thurfjell L, Lau DYH. Image registration: an essential tool for nuclear medicine. Eur J Nucl Med Mol Imaging. 2002;29:559.
5. Maintz JB, Viergever MA. A survey of medical imaging registration. Med Image Anal. 1998;2:1.
6. Bocher M, Balan A, Krausz Y, et al. Gamma camera mounted anatomical x-ray tomography: technology system characteristics and first images. Eur J Nucl Med. 2000;27:619.
7. Patton JA, Delbeke D, Sandler MP. Image fusion using an integrated-dual-head coincidence camera with x-ray tube-based attenuation maps. J Nucl Med. 2000;41:1364.
8. Beyer T, Townsend D, Brun T, et al. A combined PET/CT scanner for clinical oncology. J Nucl Med. 2000;41:1369.
9. Krausz Y, Keidar Z, Kogan E, et al. SPECT/CT hybrid imaging with 111In-pentetreotide in assessment of neuroendocrine tumours. Clin Endocrinol (Oxf). 2003;59:565–73.
10. Karger CP, Hipp P, Henze M, et al. Stereotactic imaging for radiotherapy: accuracy of CT, MRI, PET and SPECT. Phys Med Biol. 2003;48:211–21.

Brain

11. Stupp R, Mason WP, van den Bent MJ, et al. Radiotherapy plus concomitant and adjuvant temozolomide for glioblastoma. N Engl J Med. 2005;352:987–96.
12. Van Meir EG, Hadjipanayis CG, Norden AD, et al. Exciting new advances in neuro-oncology: the avenue to a cure for malignant glioma. CA Cancer J Clin. 2010;60:166–93.
13. Combs SE, Gutwein S, Schulz-Ertner D, et al. Temozolomide combined with irradiation as postoperative treatment of primary glioblastoma multiforme. Phase I/II study. Strahlenther Onkol. 2005;181:372–7.
14. Schillaci O, Filippi L, Manni C, Santoni R. Single-photon emission computed tomography/computed tomography in brain tumors. Semin Nucl Med. 2007;37:34–47.
15. Aydin H, Sillenberg I, Von Lieven H. Patterns of failure following CT-based 3-D irradiation for malignant glioma. Strahlenther Onkol. 2001;177:424–31.
16. Oppitz U, Maessen D, Zunterer H, et al. 3D-recurrence-patterns of glioblastomas after CT-planned postoperative irradiation. Radiother Oncol. 1999;53:53–7.
17. Chen W, Cloughesy T, Kamdar N, et al. Imaging proliferation in brain tumors with 18 F-FLT PET: comparison with 18 F-FDG. J Nucl Med. 2005;46:945–52.
18. Floeth FW, Pauleit D, Wittsack HJ, et al. Multimodal metabolic imaging of cerebral gliomas: positron emission tomog-

raphy with [18 F]fluoroethyl-L-tyrosine and magnetic resonance spectroscopy. J Neurosurg. 2005;102:318–27.
19. Grosu A, Weber W, Feldmann J, et al. First experience with I-123-alphamethyl-tyrosine SPECT in the 3-D radiation treatment planning of brain gliomas. Int J Radiat Oncol Biol Phys. 2000;47:517–26.
20. Baldari S, Restifo Pecorella S, Cosentino S, et al. Investigation of brain tumors with 99mTc-MIBI SPET. J Nucl Med. 2002;46:330–45.
21. Goethals I, De Winter O, Dierckx R, et al. False-negative 99mTc-MIBI scintigraphy in histopathologically proved recurrent high-grade oligodendroglioma. Clin Nucl Med. 2003;28:299–301.
22. Ak I, Gulbas Z, Altinel F, et al. 99mTc-MIBI uptake and its relation to the proliferative potential of brain tumors. Clin Nucl Med. 2003;28:29–33.
23. Soler C, Beauchesne P, Maatougui K. Technetium-99 sestamibi brain singlephoton emission tomography for detection of recurrent gliomas after radiation therapy. Eur J Nucl Med. 1998;25:1649–57.
24. Yamamoto Y, Nishiyama Y, Toyama Y, et al. 99mTc-MIBI and 201Tl SPET in the detection of recurrent brain tumours after radiation therapy. Nucl Med Commun. 2002;23: 1183–90.
25. Beauchesne P, Pedeux R, Boniol M, et al. 99mTc-sestamibi brain SPECT after chemoradiotherapy is prognostic of survival in patients with high-grade glioma. J Nucl Med. 2004;45:409–13.
26. Prigent-Le Jeune F, Dubois F, Perez S, et al. Technetium-99 m sestamibi brain SPECT in the follow-up of glioma for evaluation of response to chemotherapy: first results. Eur J Nucl Med Mol Imaging. 2004;31:714–9.
27. Lamy-Lhullier C, Dubois F, Blond S, et al. Importance of cerebral tomoscintigraphy using technetium-labeled sestamibi in the differential diagnosis of current tumor vs. radiation necrosis in subtentorial glial tumors in the adult. Neurochirurgie. 1999;45:110–7.
28. Maffioli L, Gasparini M, Chiti A, et al. Clinical role of technetium-99 m sestamibi single-photon emission tomography in evaluating pretreated patients with brain tumours. Eur J Nucl Med. 1996;23:308–11.
29. Nagamachi S, Jinnouchi S, Nabeshima K, et al. The correlation between 99mTc-MIBI uptake and MIB-1 as a nuclear proliferation marker in glioma – a comparative study with 201Tl. Neuroradiology. 2001;43:1023–30.
30. Palumbo B, Lupattelli M, Pelliccioli GP, et al. Association of 99mTc-MIBI brain SPECT and proton magnetic resonance spectroscopy (1 H-MRS) to assess glioma recurrence after radiotherapy. Q J Nucl Med Mol Imaging. 2006;50:88–93.
31. Prigent-Le Jeune FP, Dubois F, Blond S, et al. Sestamibi technetium-99 m brain single-photon emission computed tomography to identify recurrent glioma in adults: 201 studies. J Neurooncol. 2006;77:177–83.
32. Krengli M, Loi G, Sacchetti G, Manfredda I, Gambaro G, Brambilla M, et al. Delineation of target volume for radiotherapy of high-grade glioma by ^{99m}Tc-MIBI SPECT and MRI fusion. Strahlenther Onkol. 2007;183:689–94.
33. Pfluger T, Vollmar C, Wismuller A, et al. Quantitative comparison of automatic and interactive methods for MRI-SPECT image registration of the brain based on 3-dimensional calculation of error. J Nucl Med. 2000;41:1823–9.
34. Ling CC, Humm J, Larson S, et al. Towards multidimensional radiotherapy (MD-CRT): biological imaging and biological conformality. Int J Radiat Oncol Biol Phys. 2000;47:551–60.

Prostate

35. Taylor A, Rockall AG, Reznek RH, et al. Mapping pelvic lymph nodes: guidelines for delineation in intensity-modulated radiotherapy. Int J Radiat Oncol Biol Phys. 2005;63:1604–12.
36. Shih HE, Harisinghani M, Zietman A, et al. Mapping of nodal disease in locally advanced prostate cancer: rethinking the clinical target volume for pelvic nodal irradiation based on vascular rather than bony anatomy. Int J Radiat Oncol Biol Phys. 2005;63:1262–9.
37. Wawroschek F, Vogt H, Wengenmair H, et al. Prostate lymphoscintigraphy and radio-guided surgery for sentinel lymph node identification in prostate cancer. Technique and results of the first 350 cases. Urol Int. 2003;70:303–10.
38. Krengli M, Ballarè A, Cannillo B, Rudoni M, Kocjancic E, Loi G, et al. Potential advantage of studying the lymphatic drainage by sentinel node technique and SPECT-CT image fusion for pelvic irradiation of prostate cancer. Int J Radiat Oncol Biol Phys. 2006;66:1100–4.

Chapter 13 Dosimetry Using SPECT-CT

Chiara Basile, Francesca Botta,
Marta Cremonesi, Concetta De Cicco,
Amalia Di Dia, Lucio Mango,
Massimiliano Pacilio,
and Giovanni Paganelli

Contents

S. Fanti et al., *Atlas of SPECT-CT*,
DOI: 10.1007/978-3-642-15726-4_13, © Springer-Verlag Berlin Heidelberg 2011

13.1 For Targeted Radionuclide Therapy

Marta Cremonesi (✉), Francesca Botta,
Amalia Di Dia, and Giovanni Paganelli

13.1.1 Introduction

The role of dosimetry for radiation therapy is to guide the selection of the optimal treatment design, depending on radiation modality, parameter setting, and clinical needs of the single patient. The best balance between the irradiation of healthy tissues and target tissues allows improving the therapeutic ratio.

Dealing with targeted radionuclide therapy (TRT), external beam radiotherapy (EBRT), or brachytherapy, the common effort is to evaluate the absorbed dose distribution as accurately as possible. This effort requires more or less complex calculations about the interaction of particles with matter, and proper characterization and localization of the tissues involved in the radiation field.

The development of multimodality imaging combining functional and anatomic information allows more accurate identification and spatial localization of uptaking areas. This has been leading to important steps forward in the last years, not only in diagnosis, but also in the dosimetry for treatment planning.

The contribution of PET/CT to the identification of biological target volumes of EBRT is acknowledged. Complementarily to PET/CT, the role of SPECT/CT, offering better attenuation correction, increased specificity, and accurate localization of disease than SPECT alone, is swiftly gaining relevance to tailor treatments [1, 2]. There are in fact many applications – several of which are described in the previous chapters – that can retrieve crucial information for dosimetry from γ-emitting radiotracers. This chapter illustrates the contribution of SPECT/CT to dosimetry for TRT, EBRT, and brachytherapy.

13.1.2 Dosimetry for TRT Using SPECT/CT

The SPECT/CT features can be richly exploited in the field of dosimetry for TRT [3, 4].

TRT consists of the systemic or locoregional administration of a radiolabelled agent that specifically distributes depending on its own pharmacokinetics and metabolism.

Dosimetry studies in TRT require the quantification of the radiopharmaceutical uptake and its variation over time in all tissues of interest, as experimentally derived from patient measurements. This information embodies the input data for dose processing, while the other data needed for dose calculation, namely the parameters describing the physical properties of tissues and radionuclides, are incorporated in computation systems.

A skilled analysis with such a task has to take into account that: (1) a radiotracer is needed that suitably simulates therapy, and not every radiopharmaceutical used for diagnostic purposes is adequate for dosimetry; (2) a sufficient number of serial images should be acquired over a time period and at time intervals that entail all the kinetic phases of the therapeutic agent; (3) the more correct the activity quantification and the spatial association of activity to target/non-target organs are, the more refined the dosimetry estimate.

Hybrid SPECT/CT imaging allows fulfilling the above requisites.

The array of radiopharmaceuticals for consolidated and more recently developed TRT is summarized in Table 1 along with the corresponding radiotracers useful for dosimetry and the possible acquisition modality. Remarkably, the dosimetry can be determined based on SPECT/CT images for all therapeutic applications, but this is not the case for PET/CT. In fact, options to mimic therapy include the use of low activities of the same radiocompound, if also a γ- or β^+-emitter (e.g., ^{131}I, ^{177}Lu, and ^{64}Cu), or of the same therapeutic molecule labeled with a γ- or β^+-emitter isotope of the same radionuclide (e.g., ^{124}I or ^{123}I for ^{131}I), or of a radionuclide with similar chemical behavior (e.g., ^{111}In for ^{90}Y). Moreover, the tracer $T_{1/2,phys}$ has to be compatible with the biological half-life of the therapeutic agent. Thus, besides the less widespread availability β^+-emitters, the too short $T_{1/2,phys}$ of some candidates (e.g., ^{68}Ga) makes SPECT γ imaging and also bremsstrahlung more valuable (e.g., with ^{131}I, ^{111}In, ^{153}Sm, ^{177}Lu, ^{186}Re, ^{188}Re, ^{90}Y, etc).

The impact of image registration of SPECT and CT on dosimetry accuracy is palpable, especially when dealing with a time-sequential SPECT dataset. Dedicated studies have shown that even small mis-registrations might consistently affect absorbed dose estimates, especially for tumors of certain sizes and sites [5]. Thus, the inherent registration of the anatomical and the functional information in SPECT-CT has consistently improved dosimetry, simplifying the mass delineation in each 3D SPECT-CT data set and allowing the generation of registered time-SPECT-CT (4D) datasets based on CT-CT registration [2, 5, 6].

In addition, the quantitative images obtained by CT-based attenuation correction are more accurate than those obtained using conventional SPECT attenuation maps.

Further, the integration of the data collected by multimodality imaging may significantly improve the accuracy of dose distribution calculation in organs at risk and

Table 1 Radiopharmaceuticals for dosimetry in the principle targeted radionuclide therapies

Radiopharmaceuticals for targeted radionuclide therapy	Corresponding radionuclides for dosimetry	3D acquisition for dosimetry	
		SPECT/CT	PET/CT
^{131}I-Chloride; MoAbs; MIBG	^{131}I	Yes	–
	^{123}I	Yes	–
	^{124}I[a]	–	Yes
^{90}Y-MoAbs; peptides	^{111}In	Yes	–
	^{90}Y[b]	Yes	(c)
	^{86}Y[d]	–	Yes
^{90}Y-microspheres	^{99m}Tc[e]	Yes	–
	^{90}Y[b]	Yes	(c)
	^{86}Y[d]	–	Yes
^{177}Lu-peptides	^{177}Lu	Yes	–
^{153}Sm-EDTMP	^{153}Sm		
	^{99m}Tc[f]	Yes	–
^{186}Re-HEDP	^{186}Re	Yes	–
^{188}Re-HEDP; MoAbs; peptides	^{188}Re	Yes	–

[a]124I: high costs, limited availability
[b]90Y-Bremsstrahlung SPECT to confirm the predicted distribution: complex image corrections
[c]90Y-PET imaging: feasibility under evaluation
[d]86Y: short half-life, complex image corrections
[e]99mTc-MAA used to mimic therapy
[f]99mTc-MDP used to mimic therapy

tumor targets: whereas SPECT images alone allow 3D dose calculation only in homogeneous tissues, the availability of combined SPECT and CT images allows 3D dose calculation also in inhomogeneous tissues, provided computational methods are developed based on direct Monte Carlo simulations [7, 8].

The assessment of the absorbed dose delivered during any radionuclide therapy should be mandatory, as is currently the case for EBRT. This is to rationally plan the administered activity and/or to determine the need for additional therapeutic approaches. In addition, such an attitude would help to correlate the absorbed doses to biological effects (toxicity, response) [9], having finally the safety and efficacy of TRT as the future goal.

Among the TRT applications that could benefit dosimetry with SPECT/CT are:

- *Radioiodine treatment of metastatic thyroid cancer*. The contribution of dosimetry and of SPECT/CT has been published in several studies [10, 11], and interesting images are shown in Chap. 3.5.
- *Radioimmunotherapy of lymphoma* and other cancers with ^{90}Y-, ^{131}I-, and ^{188}Re-radiolabelled monoclonal antibodies (e.g., ^{90}Y-ibritumomab tiuxetan, ^{131}I-anti-CD20 rituximab, and ^{131}I-L19SIP), given at standard administered activities or in myeloablative settings. Especially in the latter case, other critical organs other than bone marrow impose special efforts to minimize side effects vs. treatment efficacy [12–15]. Chapter 4 illustrates a few examples.
- *Radiopeptide therapy of neuroendocrine and other tumors* overexpressing somatostatin receptors with ^{90}Y- and ^{177}Lu-peptides. ^{111}In-pentetreotide images allow evaluating patients for recruitment and rough prevision of therapy, but are not adequate for dosimetry. In case of ^{90}Y-peptides, ^{111}In- or ^{86}Y-surrogates are helpful (Table 1), although the latter are more critical because of the complex corrections required and short time available for data collection [16]. Radiopeptide therapy needs to be divided into multiple cycles, this being a peculiar advantage: dosimetry evaluations can be performed before or during the first course of therapy, or even repeated to follow possible dose variations at each cycle (especially in responsive tumors). This has been done with ^{177}Lu-peptides using SPECT/CT [16, 17]. Moreover, the technical advances of hybrid equipments and the improvements in image correction methods have shown the possibility of achieving reasonably accurate activity estimates also from ^{90}Y-bremsstrahlung SPECT/CT [18–20]. Figure 1 illustrates the case of a patient with a pancreatic lesion (red arrow) with a diagnostic SPECT-CT from ^{111}In-pentetreotide and the corresponding bremsstrahlung images acquired during therapy with ^{90}Y-DOTATATE for dosimetric purposes. The different uptakes

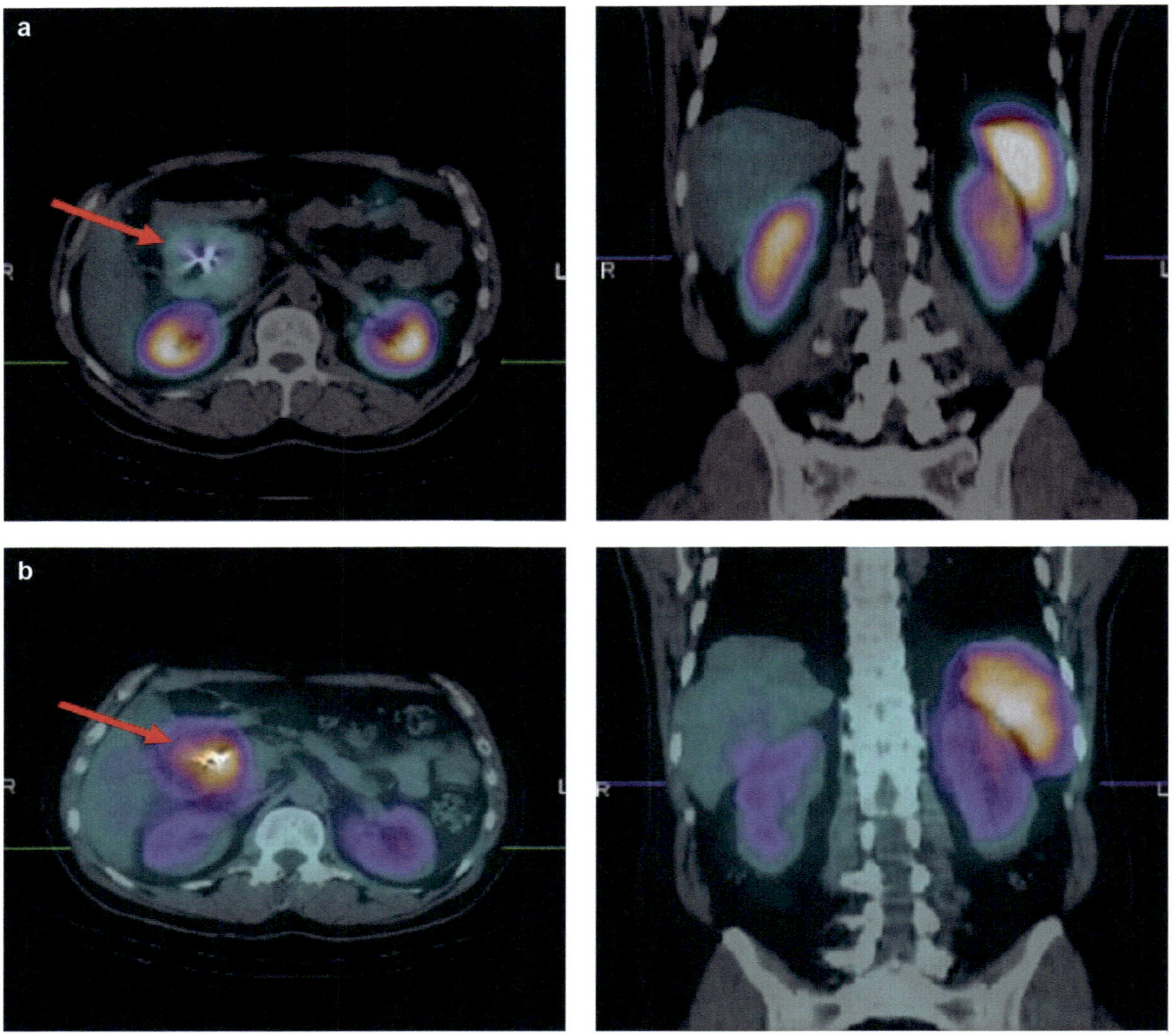

Fig. 1 Dosimetry with SPECT-CT applied to radionuclide therapy. Transaxial and coronal slices of fused SPECT-CT showing uptake in a pancreatic lesion (*red arrow*), the kidneys and the spleen: (**a**) Diagnostic image obtained 24 h after the injection of ^{111}In-pentetreotide; (**b**) bremsstrahlung image obtained during therapy, 24 h after the injection of ^{90}Y-DOTATATE (1.7 GBq) (Reproduced with permission of Ecancermedical science www.ecancermedicalscience.com/tv [19]

(lower in the tumor and higher in the kidneys) of ^{111}In-pentetreotide vs. ^{90}Y-DOTA-TATE because of their different receptor specificities are worth noting.

- *Locoregional and systemic therapy of unresectable and/or recurrent brain tumors*, given as a further boost after EBRT or adjuvant setting. Especially in patients already pre-irradiated, the higher dosimetry accuracy with SPECT/CT can direct the decision-making for a better choice of radionuclide and activity to be administered. Chapter 5 and Fig. 1 of Chap. 13.2 report a few examples of radionuclide therapy for the treatment of meningiomas and high-grade gliomas [21].
- *Therapy with ^{131}I-MIBG addressed to neuroblastoma.* Chapter 3.2 offers clarifying SPECT/CT images. Dosimetry, which can be performed using +^{131}I- or ^{123}I-MIBG as tracers, has special importance in

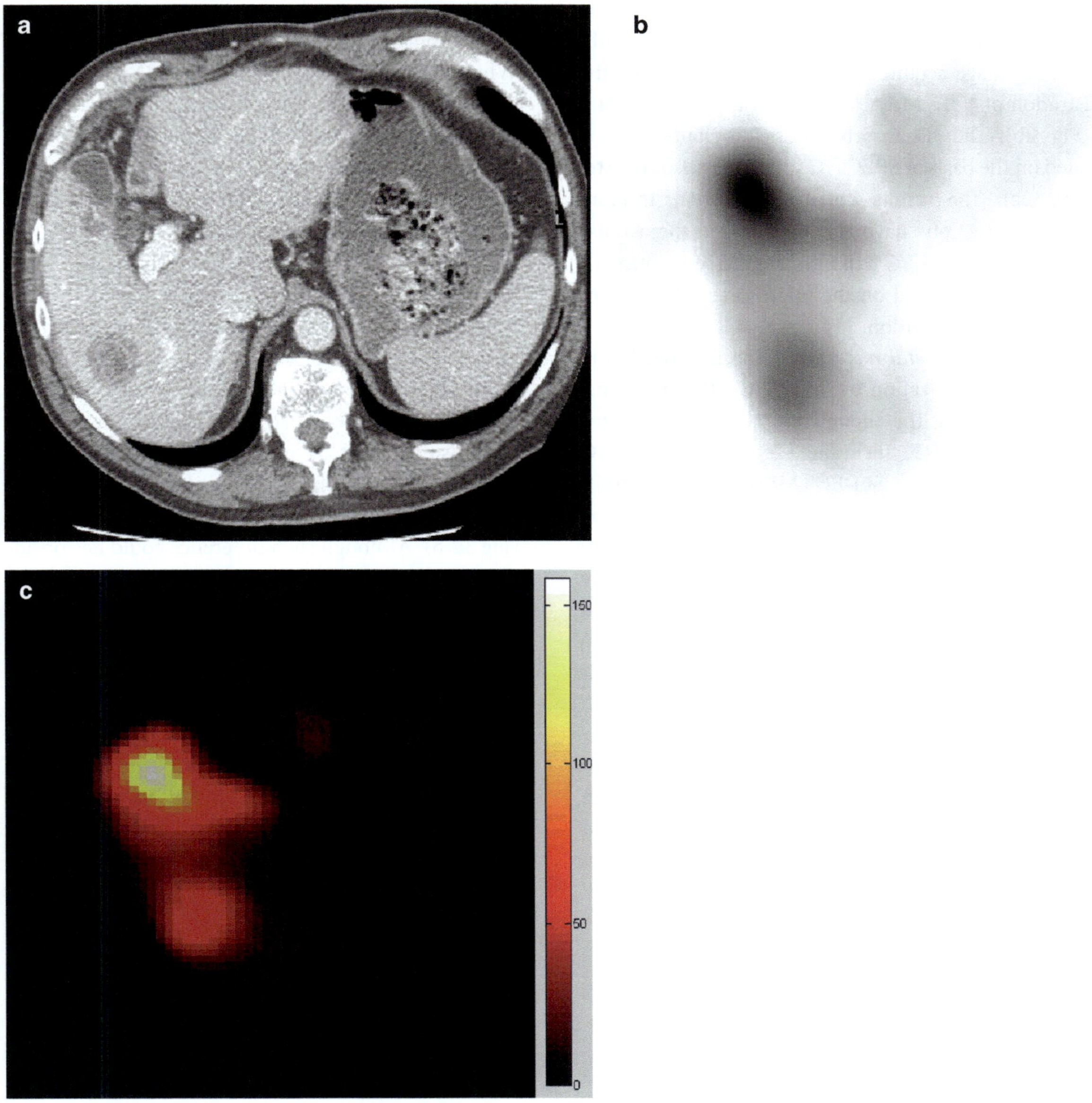

Fig. 2 Dosimetry with SPECT-CT applied to liver radioembolization. (**a**) Transaxial contrast-enhanced CT image of the liver obtained before liver radioembolization showing hepatic metastases; (**b**) SPECT image acquired after the intra-hepatic administration of 99mTc-MAA for pre-therapeutic evaluation; (**c**) absorbed dose distribution (Gy) calculated from SPECT/CT images

children and in patients undergoing high doses and autologous stem cell rescue [22, 23].

- *Radioembolization of primary and metastatic liver cancer by* locoregional administration of ^{90}Y-microspheres. This therapy requires careful planning to maximize the response and minimize hepatic toxicity and complications related to possible shunt. Usually, ^{99m}Tc-macroaggregated albumin (^{99m}Tc-MAA) scans (Table 1) precede ^{90}Y-therapy both to detect any extra-hepatic shunting and to predict absorbed dose distribution to tumor and normal liver [24–27]. SPECT/CT imaging has proven to influence the therapeutic decision, especially in terms of activity for tailored treatments [25, 28]. Figure 2 shows a transaxial contrast-enhanced

CT image of the liver obtained before liver radioembolization showing hepatic metastasis (Fig. 2a) and a SPECT image acquired after the intrahepatic administration of ^{99m}Tc-MAA for pre-therapeutic evaluation (Fig. 2b). The 3D absorbed dose distribution calculated on the basis of SPECT/CT images is also reported (Fig. 2c). The results obtained on bremsstrahlung image corrections have also encouraged the acquisition of ^{90}Y- SPECT/CT to ultimately assess dosimetry estimates [20] based on the microsphere distribution after radioembolization.

- *Treatment of skeletal metastases*. The improved bone lesion characterization by SPECT/CT (Chap. 5) may lead to revising the therapeutic activity of curative or palliative TRT, including, e.g., ^{131}I, ^{131}I-MIBG, ^{90}Y/^{177}Lu-peptides, ^{153}Sm-EDTMP, etc. [29–31]. With the aim to enhance efficacy while keeping red marrow doses acceptable, a refined dose evaluation of bony lesions based on SPECT/CT can make a difference. The possibility to associate the punctual uptake of a therapeutical agent to the anatomical and density information becomes very important. Whether, or in which extent, the tissue density information from CT is relevant for dosimetry is an issue of interest. In principle, sites with variable density or at interfaces might heavily impact on the dose distribution computation, as compared to uniformity. Thus, the integration of the data collected by multimodality imaging may significantly increase the accuracy of dose distribution calculation in organs at risk and tumor targets. Whereas SPECT images alone allow 3D dose calculation only in homogeneous tissues, the availability of combined SPECT and CT images allow 3D dose calculation also in non homogeneous tissues, provided developing computational methods based on direct Monte Carlo simulations [30, 31]. For example, the comparison between the dose distribution maps derived by the same 3D activity distribution in bony lesions, combined with either a uniform water density, or instead the CT-derived spatial tissue density distribution, has evidenced moderate differences between radiation doses. Absorbed doses derived for a patient administered with ^{90}Y-peptides, showed an overestimate around 10% when neglecting the real density in favor of uniform water density approximation (Fig 3a-b). Although such difference could be considered as negligible within the overall uncertainties typical of internal dosimetry, they deserve to be taken into account and better investigated. Further analyses might deepen the impact from various radionuclides and maybe different skeletal composition, lesion dimensions and localization. Conversely, preliminary results in a patient treated with ^{90}Y-peptides have shown underestimate in lesions at the lung-tissue interface when the hypothesis of uniform density was accepted (Fig 3c–e).

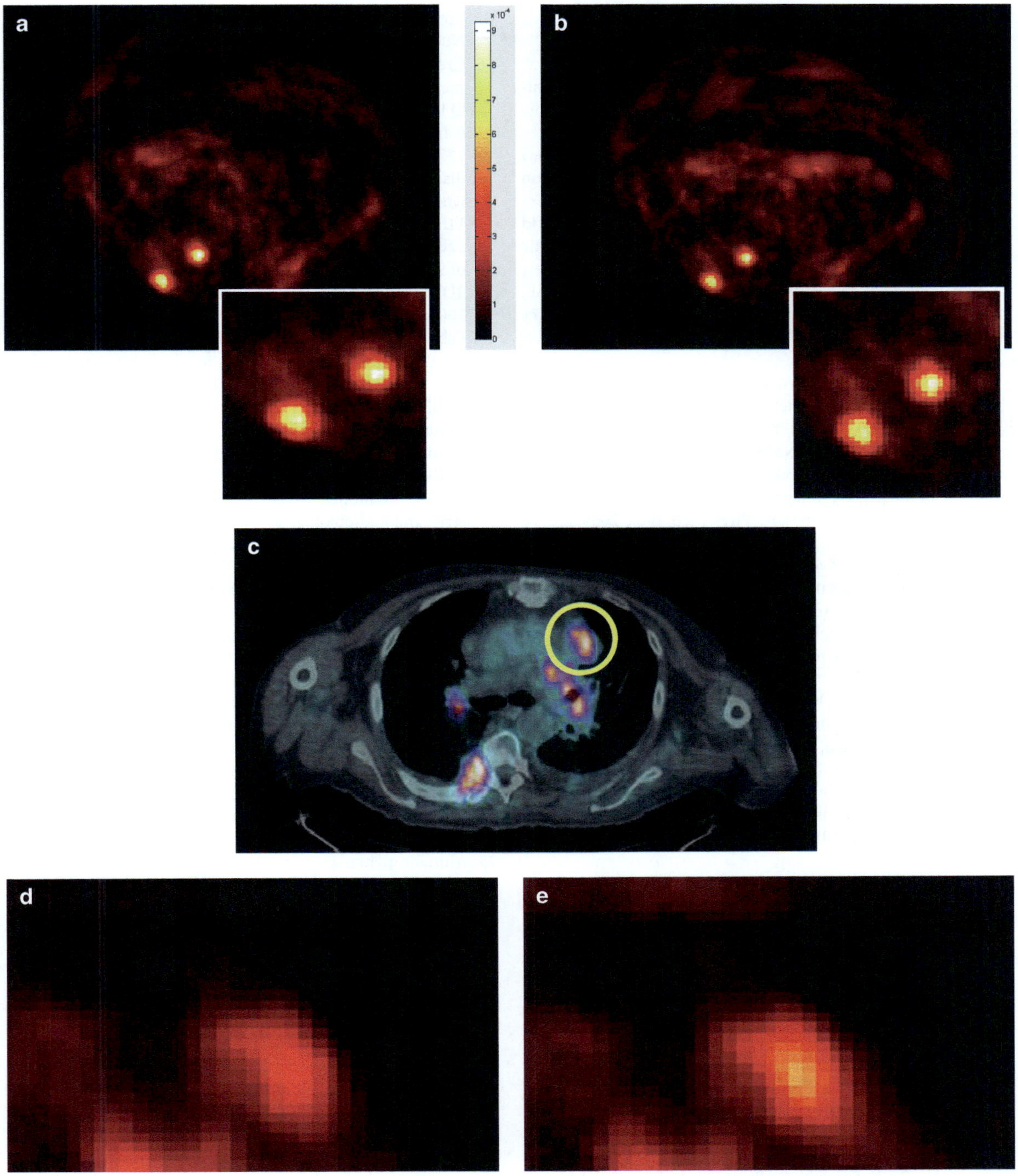

Fig. 3 Impact of SPECT-CT on dosimetry evaluation in heterogeneous tissues in case of radionuclide therapy. Absorbed dose maps showing in particular two bony lesions with positive somatostatin receptors derived from: (**a**) voxel dosimetry method based on SPECT images only (approximation of homogeneous tissue density); (**b**) Monte Carlo simulation based on SPECT/CT images (activity distribution from SPECT, tissue density from CT). Fused SPECT/CT image showing uptake in a positive somatostatin receptor tumor at the lung-tissue interface (**c**). Correspondent absorbed dose maps derived from (**d**) voxel dosimetry method based on SPECT images only (approximation of homogeneous tissue density); (**e**) Monte Carlo simulation based on SPECT/CT images (activity distribution from SPECT, tissue density from CT)

References

1. Mariani G, Bruselli L, Kuwert T, et al. A review on the clinical uses of SPECT/CT. Eur J Nucl Med Mol Imaging. 2010;37:1959–85.
2. Yin LS, Tang L, Hamarneh G, et al. Complexity and accuracy of image registration methods in SPECT-guided radiation therapy. Phys Med Biol. 2010;55:237–46.
3. Delbeke D, Schöder H, Martin WH, Wahl RL. Hybrid Imaging (SPECT/CT and PET/CT): improving therapeutic decisions. Semin Nucl Med. 2009;39:308–40.
4. Flux G, Bardies M, Monsieurs M, Savolainen S, Strands SE, Lassmann M. The impact of PET and SPECT on dosimetry for targeted radionuclide therapy. Z Med Phys. 2006;16: 47–59.
5. Papavasileiou P, Divoli A, Hatziioannou K, Flux GD. The importance of the accuracy of image registration of SPECT images for 3D targeted radionuclide therapy dosimetry. Phys Med Biol. 2007;52:N539–48.
6. Sjögreen-Gleisner K, Rueckert D, Ljungberg M. Registration of serial SPECT/CT images for three-dimensional dosimetry in radionuclide therapy. Phys Med Biol. 2009;54(20): 6181–200.
7. Petoussi-Henss N, Zankl M, Nosske D. Estimation of patient dose from radiopharmaceuticals using voxel models. Cancer Biother Radiopharm. 2005;20:103–9.
8. Bolch WE. MC applied to The Monte Carlo method in nuclear medicine: current uses and future potential. J Nucl Med. 2010;5:337–9.
9. Sgouros G, Frey E, Wahl R, He B, Prideaux A, Hobbs R. Three-dimensional imaging-based radiobiological dosimetry. Semin Nucl Med. 2008;38:321–34.
10. Wang H, Fu HL, Li JN, Zou RJ, Gu ZH, Wu JC. The role of single-photon emission computed tomography/computed tomography for precise localization of metastases in patients with differentiated thyroid cancer. Clin Imaging. 2009;33: 49–54.
11. Song H, Prideaux A, Du Y, et al. Lung dosimetry for radioiodine treatment planning in the case of diffuse lung metastases. J Nucl Med. 2006;47:1985–94.
12. Boucek JA, Turner JH. Validation of prospective whole-body bone marrow dosimetry by SPECT/CT multimodality imaging in 131I-anti-CD20 rituximab radioimmunotherapy of non-Hodgkin's lymphoma. Eur J Nucl Med Mol Imaging. 2005;32:458–69.
13. Sauer S, Erba PA, Petrini M, et al. Expression of the oncofetal ED-B-containing fibronectin isoform in hematologic tumors enables ED-B-targeted 131I-L19SIP radioimmunotherapy in Hodgkin lymphoma patients. Blood. 2009; 113:2265–74.
14. Song H, Du Y, Sgouros G, Prideaux A, Frey E, Wahl RL. Therapeutic potential of 90Y- and 131I-labeled anti-CD20 monoclonal antibody in treating non-Hodgkin's lymphoma with pulmonary involvement: a Monte Carlo-based dosimetric analysis. J Nucl Med. 2007;48:150–7.
15. Pacilio M, Betti M, Cicone F, et al. A theoretical dose-escalation study based on biological effective dose in radioimmunotherapy with 90Y-ibritumomab tiuxetan (Zevalin). Eur J Nucl Med Mol Imaging. 2010;37:862–73.
16. Cremonesi M, Botta F, Di Dia A, et al. Dosimetry for treatment with radiolabelled somatostatin analogues. A review. Q J Nucl Med Mol Imaging. 2010;54:37–51.
17. Garkavij M, Nickel M, Sjögreen-Gleisner K, et al. 177Lu-[DOTA0,Tyr3] octreotate therapy in patients with disseminated neuroendocrine tumors: analysis of dosimetry with impact on future therapeutic strategy. Cancer. 2010; 116(4 Suppl): 1084–92.
18. Fabbri C, Sarti G, Cremonesi M, et al. Quantitative analysis [of 90Y Bremsstrahlung SPECT-CT images for application to 3D patient-specific dosimetry. Cancer Biother Radiopharm. 2009;24(1):145–54.
19. Fabbri C, Sarti G, Agostini M, Di Dia A, Paganelli G. SPECT/CT 90Y-Bremsstrahlung images for dosimetry during therapy. Ecancermedicalscience. 2008; 2:n.106 www.ecancermedicalscience.com/tv.
20. Minarik D, Sjögreen Gleisner K, Ljungberg M. Evaluation of quantitative (90)Y SPECT based on experimental phantom studies. Phys Med Biol. 2008;53:5689–703.
21. Botta F, Cremonesi M, Di Dia A, et al. Monte Carlo dosimetric and radiobiological evaluations for 131I-, 90Y- and 177Lu- locoregional treatments of high grade gliomas. Eur J Nucl Med Mol Imaging. 2009;36(S2):OP514.
22. Monsieurs M, Brans B, Bacher K, Van De Putte S, Dierckx RA, Thierens H. Patient dosimetry for neuroendocrine tumours based on 123I-MIBG pretherapy scans and 131I-MIBG post therapy scans. Eur J Nucl Med. 2002; 29:1581–87.
23. Matthay KK, Quach A, Franc BL, et al. 131I-Metaiodobenzylguanidine (131I-MIBG) double infusion with autologous stem cell rescue for neuroblastoma: a New Approaches to Neuroblastoma Therapy (NANT) phase I study. J Clin Oncol. 2009;27:1020–25.
24. Sangro B, Gil-Alzugaray B, Rodriguez J, et al. Liver disease induced by radioembolization of liver tumors: description and possible risk factors. Cancer. 2008;1 12:1538–46.
25. Ahmadzadehfar H, Sabet A, Biermann K, et al. The significance of 99mTc-MAA SPECT/CT liver perfusion imaging in treatment planning for 90Y-microsphere selective internal radiation treatment. J Nucl Med. 2010;51:1206–12.
26. Cremonesi M, Ferrari M, Bartolomei M, et al. Radioembolisation with (90)Y-microspheres: dosimetric and radiobiological investigation for multi-cycle treatment. Eur J Nucl Med Mol Imaging. 2008;35:2088–96.
27. Gulec SA, Sztejnberg ML, Siegel JA, Jevremovic T, Stabin M. Hepatic structural dosimetry in 90Y microsphere treatment: a Monte Carlo modeling approach based on lobular microanatomy. J Nucl Med. 2010;51:301–10.
28. Di Dia A, Botta F, Cremonesi M, et al. Dosimetric evaluation in 90Y-microspheres treatment of liver metastasis: comparison of planar, standard 3D-dosimetry and voxel dosimetry methods. Eur J Nucl Med Mol Imaging. 2010; Accepted as oral presentation of the EANM congress 2010.
29. Horger M, Bares R. The role of single-photon emission computed tomography/computed tomography in benign and malignant bone disease. Semin Nucl Med. 2006; 36: 286–94.

30. Bianchi L, Baroli A, Marzoli L, Verusio C, Chiesa C, Pozzi L. Prospective dosimetry with 99mTc-MDP in metabolic radiotherapy of bone metastases with 153Sm-EDTMP. Eur J Nucl Med Mol Imaging. 2009;36:122–9.
31. Loeb DM, Hobbs RF, Okoli A, et al. Tandem dosing of samarium-153 ethylenediamine tetramethylene phosphoric acid with stem cell support for patients with high-risk osteosarcoma. Cancer. 2010;116(23):5470–8.

13.2 For External Beam Radiation Therapy and Brachytherapy

Massimiliano Pacilio (✉), Chiara Basile, Concetta De Cicco, and Lucio Mango

The role of SPECT/CT in treatment planning procedures for EBRT and brachytherapy has grown considerably in the last few years (see also Chap. 12). The contribution of SPECT/CT is greatly appreciated for some well-defined radiation therapy applications with external sources; a brief overview is reported here, with mention of some specific problems concerning tumor and organ delineation on SPECT/CT images.

- *High-grade brain gliomas and other cerebral mass treatments.* Even though contrast-enhanced CT and T1-weighted MRI allow accurate delineation of brain tumor margins, anatomical imaging can fail in differentiating residual tumor infiltration versus surrounding edema, as well as recurrent tumor versus radiation necrosis and gliosis, after surgery and/or radiotherapy treatments [32]. In some cases PET with [^{18}F]FDG may not be adequate, but several PET tracers are now available, such as ^{11}C-choline, ^{18}F-FDOPA, ^{11}C-methionine, ^{18}F-fluoroethyl-L-tyrosine and ^{18}F-fluorocholine [33–36]. Nevertheless, when the availability of PET/CT is limited, as reported in Chap. 12, SPECT/CT can be employed for these clinical indications using various radiopharmaceuticals, such as ^{201}Tl-chloride, ^{99m}Tc-tetrofosmin, ^{99m}Tc-sestamibi and L-3-^{123}I-α-methyltyrosine. Several studies have demonstrated the usefulness of SPECT/CT for accurate preoperative detection and localization, and for radiotherapy planning and treatment monitoring [37]. SPECT/CT allows good accuracy in the anatomical localization of viable tumor lesions versus adjacent sites with physiological tracer uptake, such as the ventricles, choroid plexus and venous sinuses [38–39], with a proven clinical impact on management in 43% of patients [38]. Figure 1 illustrates an example of a SPECT/CT acquisition of a glioblastoma multiforme grade IV astrocytoma.
- *Prostate cancer treatment.* Among patients undergoing radiotherapy, pre-treatment ProstaScint® SPECT/CT of extra-periprostatic metastatic prostate cancer independently and significantly predicted an increased risk of biochemical failure in those presenting a clinical diagnosis of localized adenocarcinoma of the prostate [40]. Furthermore, ProstaScint® SPECT/CT was reported to accurately identify biological target volumes for treatment planning in brachytherapy seed implants: in a dose-escalation study in patients with T1c-T3b N× M0 prostate adenocarcinoma, pretreatment SPECT/CT permitted achieving dose intensification to occult tumor targets, without increasing rectal toxicity [41]. Also, a significant impact of ProstaScint® SPECT/CT imaging has been demonstrated to modify the delineation of the prostate fossa clinical target volume (CTV) in patients scheduled for external beam radiation therapy after prostatectomy [42].
- *Functioning organ sparing in lung cancer treatment.* SPECT/CT-guided intensity-modulated radiation therapy (IMRT) for lung cancer is currently under investigation to establish a methodology for selecting the beam arrangement able to reduce the dose to the SPECT-defined functioning lung [43–45]. In a recent study, the influence of the number of beams used in the IMRT plan on V5, V15, V20 and V30 for the lungs (the percent functional lung volume receiving a dose greater or equal to 5, 15, 20 and 30 Gy, respectively) has been quantified. A sensible reduction of V5 and V15 (recently associated with radiation pneumonia) has been reported when using fewer beams in IMRT planning [43]. Preplanning SPECT scanning may contribute to assessing the ventilated lung volume included in PTV, and thus to estimating the dose delivered to the functional lung, and possibly to optimizing the treatment depending on the patient's case history [44]. Figure 2 reports an example of the differences in the treatment planning strategy considering functioning lung sparing [44]. The CT images from a hybrid SPECT/CT system are useful for localization and attenuation correction, but treatment planning must be performed on the images obtained from a CT system commissioned for RT treatments. Proper co-registration methods of the functional images on

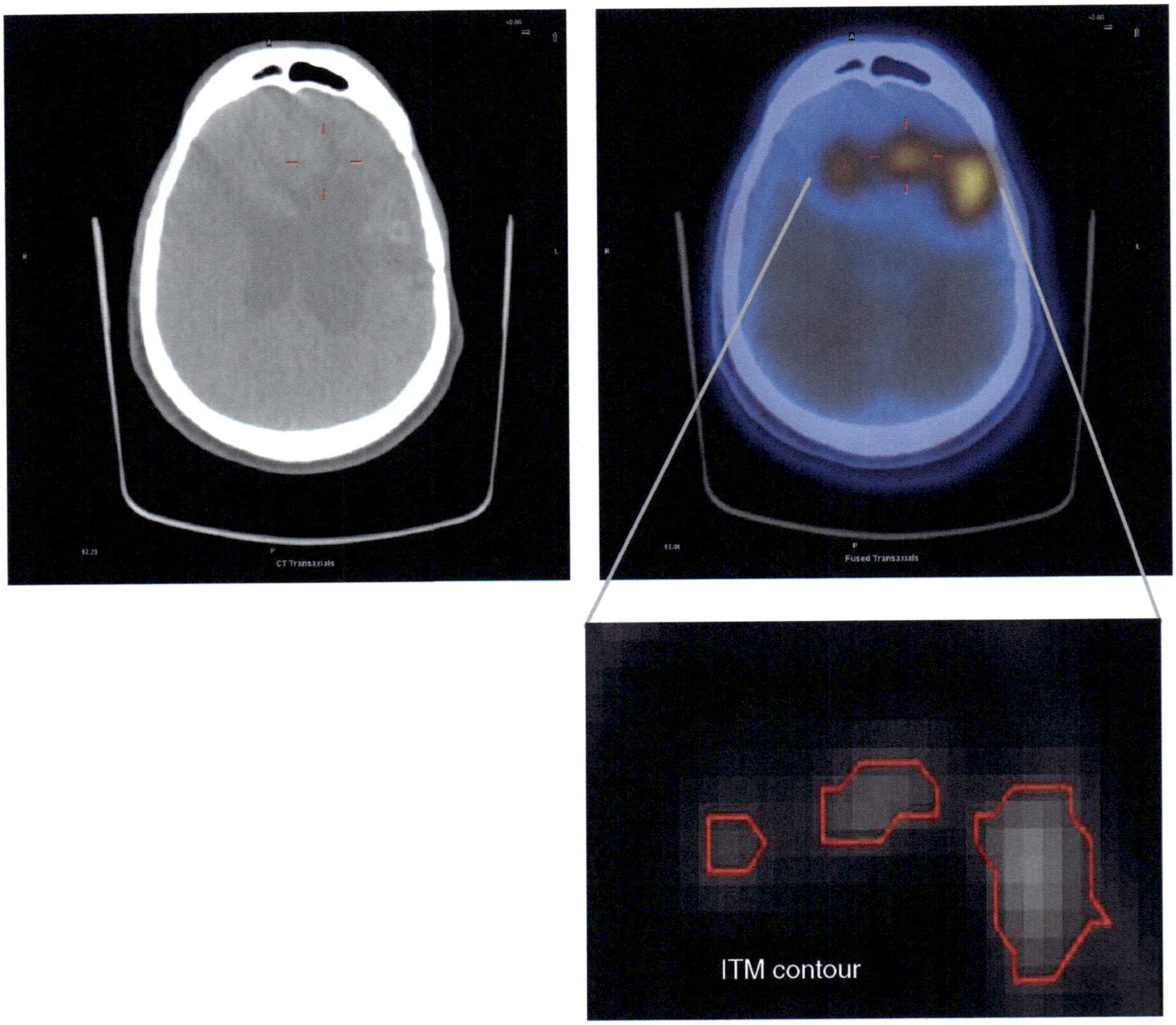

Fig. 1 SPECT/CT for biological target volume contouring (automatic segmentation) in radiotherapy of brain lesions: glioblastoma multiforme grade IV astrocytoma (images obtained with a GE Infinia Hawkeye 4 SPECT/CT system)

the CT images used for RT planning are currently under study. CT images from a hybrid SPECT/CT scanner have to be registered to the planning CT, and then the same transformation has to be applied to the SPECT images. However, new problems are emerging: it has been reported that the application of non-rigid registration methods (which generally provide a higher degree of accuracy than rigid methods) may result in unacceptable changes to the SPECT intensity distribution that would preclude its use in RT planning [46].

- *Follow-up for cardiac complications from thoracic EBRT treatments.* In some cases, SPECT/CT can be also employed for follow-up studies of radiation-induced toxicity effects, helping to better define dose constraints for treatment planning. For instance, the incidence and prevalence of radiation-induced cardiac complications could be better established, including: acute and chronic pericardia, coronary artery disease (CAD), conduction abnormalities, valvular insufficiency and cardiomyopathy. Most of the follow-up data are referred to the older RT techniques. In the last

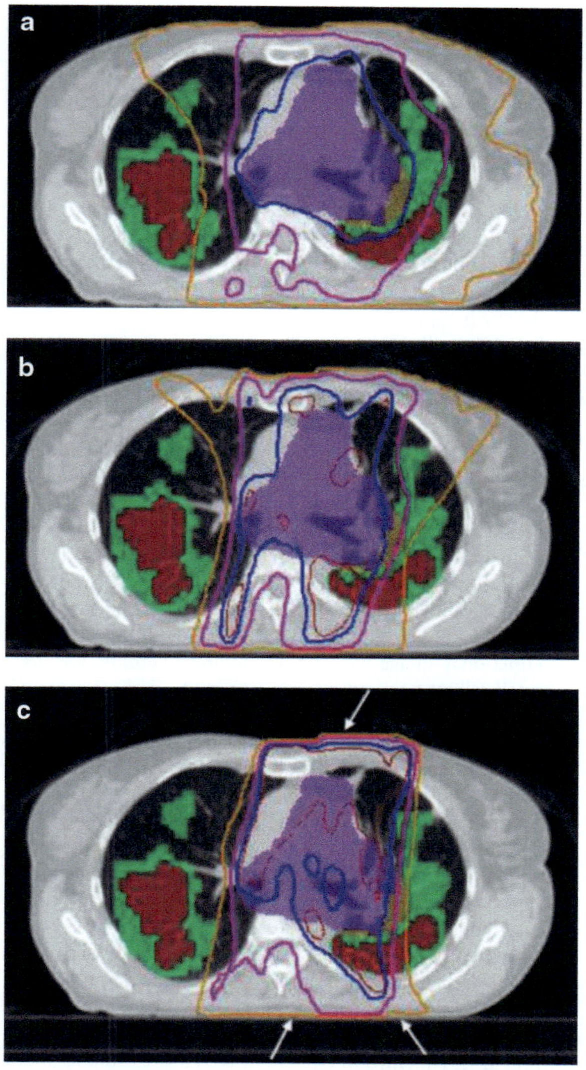

Fig. 2 SPECT/CT for lung perfusion for tissue sparing in radiotherapy. Isodose distributions on an axial CT image of the nine-field IMRT plan with no ventilated lung avoidance (**a**), nine-field IMRT plan with ventilated lung avoidance (**b**) and a three-field IMRT plan with ventilated lung avoidance (**c**): the 66.5 Gy isodose line (95% of prescription dose, *blue line*) conforms to the PTV (*purple*) on this slice for all three plans; ventilation volumes segmented with SPECT/CT by 50% (*green*) and 70% isocount curve (*brown*) are also represented (Reproduced with permission of Munawar et al. [44])

decades, several improvements have been made to EBRT techniques from the 3-dimensional conformal RT (3DCRT) to IMRT and proton therapy, also including respiratory gating. For thoracic irradiations (such as left-side breast cancer, esophageal cancer, lymphoma, etc.), the incidence and prevalence of radiation-induced cardiac complications with each of these RT techniques have not yet been investigated adequately [47–49]. SPECT/CT-gated myocardial perfusion imaging (see Chap. 6) has great relevance for investigations on the prevalence, pattern and location of myocardial perfusion abnormalities.

- *Delineation of biological target volume (BTV) and/or functioning organs on SPECT/CT.* The capability to identify tumors based on functional characteristics, including metabolism, proliferation, hypoxia, and the concentration of specific antigens and metabolites, is highly important for radiation therapy. To this aim, accurate segmentation may help to better customize the radiotherapy treatments, improving radiation targeting. Moreover, better tissue differentiation allows providing more correct dosimetry data, which is associated with eventual response and/or side effects. Tumor volume estimations and segmentations are also important for treatment monitoring. Furthermore, as mentioned above, in some cases delineation of functioning parts of critical organs is of great importance for SPECT/CT-guided radiation therapy. Delineation on CT or MRI images is usually based on visual contour assessments. Conversely, the utilization of PET or SPECT for accurate quantitative measurements of uptake distribution can be more critical because of the high noise and low spatial resolution of these images. Even though a good signal-to-noise ratio is present, when the observed volume is less than twofold the spatial resolution of the scanner, the uptake measurements can be very inaccurate because of partial volume effects. This might compromise the use of SPECT systems in some cases, since the spatial resolution is known to be relatively poor. In any case, new processing algorithms and methods may help to recover information. Studies on PET images have led to the development of different segmentation methods. Their use also for SPECT needs to be carefully evaluated since the source of errors and limitations is more emphasized for SPECT images compared to PET.

Visual segmentation using different window level settings and look-up tables is the most common and widely used technique for PET images, but the method has low reproducibility and is highly operator-dependent [50–51]. Segmentation adopting a fixed threshold (i.e., the use of a given percentage of the maximal activity) is also widespread; however, a fixed threshold value in the range of 40–50% (as in most applications reported in the literature) might lead to significant errors in the volume estimation, depending on the lesion size and the lesion-to-background contrast [52–54]. In the last few years, additional image segmentation approaches have been proposed. These include adaptive thresholding, region growing, classifiers, clustering, edge detection, Markov random field models, artificial neural networks, deformable models, atlas-guided, and many other approaches [51, 55–61]. Despite the remarkable progress that automated image segmentation has made, performance validation in the clinical setting remains the most challenging issue [51, 62]. Adaptive thresholding is considered the most accurate, and it has also been validated thoroughly using histological data for PET segmentation [51, 57, 63]. For SPECT/CT, a new adaptive thresholding method based also on recovery coefficients has been proposed and is currently under study for clinical validation [64–65]. Figure 1 illustrates an example of high-grade glioma contours obtained with an iterative thresholding method (ITM, bottom right of figure).

References

32. Brandes AA, Tosoni A, Spagnolli F, et al. Disease progression or pseudoprogression after concomitant radiochemotherapy treatment: pitfalls in neuro-oncology. Neuro Oncol. 2008;10:361–7.
33. Spaeth N, Wyss MT, Weber B, et al. Uptake of 18F-fluorocholine, 18F-luoroethyl-L-tyrosine, and 18F-FDG in acute cerebral radiation injury in the rat: implications for separation of radiation necrosis from tumor recurrence. J Nucl Med. 2004;45:1931–8.
34. Astner S, Grosu A, Weber W, Wester H, Schwaiger M, Molls M. O-(2-[18F] fluorethyl)-L-tyrosine compared to L-(methyl-11C) methionine in positron emission tomography for tumor volume delineation of gliomas and metastases. Int J Radiat Oncol Biol Phys. 2005;63:S65.
35. Chen W, Silverman DHS, Delaloye S, et al. 18F-FDOPA PET imaging of brain tumors: comparison study with 18F-FDG PET and evaluation of diagnostic accuracy. J Nucl Med. 2006;47:904–11.
36. Huang Z, Zuo C, Guan Y, et al. Misdiagnoses of 11C-choline combined with 18F-FDG PET imaging in brain tumours. Nucl Med Commun. 2008;29:354–8.
37. Mariani G, Bruselli L, Kuwert T, et al. A review on the clinical uses of SPECT/CT. Eur J Nucl Med Mol Imaging. 2010;37:1959–85.
38. Filippi L, Schillaci O, Santoni R, Manni C, Danieli R, Simonetti G. Usefulness of SPECT/CT with a hybrid camera for the functional anatomical mapping of primary braintumors by[Tc99m] tetrofosmin. Cancer Biother Radiopharm. 2006;21:41–8.
39. Schillaci O, Filippi L, Manni C, Santoni R. Single-photon emission computed tomography/computed tomography in brain tumors. Semin Nucl Med. 2007;37:34–47.
40. Ellis RJ, Zhou EH, Fu P, et al. Single photon emission computerized tomography with capromab pendetide plus computerized tomography image set co-registration independently predicts biochemical failure. J Urol. 2008;179:1768–73.
41. Ellis RJ, Zhou H, Kaminsky DA, et al. Rectal morbidity after permanent prostate brachytherapy with dose escalation to biologic target volumes identified by SPECT/CT fusion. Brachytherapy. 2007;6:149–56.
42. Jani AB, Spelbring D, Hamilton R, et al. Impact of radioimmunoscintigraphy on definition of clinical target volume for radiotherapy after prostatectomy. J Nucl Med. 2004; 45:238–46.
43. McGuire SM, Marks LB, Yin FF, Das SK. A methodology for selecting the beam arrangement to reduce the intensity-modulated radiation therapy (IMRT) dose to the SPECT-defined functioning lung. Phys Med Biol. 2010;55:403–16.
44. Munawar I, Yaremko BP, Craig J, et al. Intensity modulated radiotherapy of non-small-cell lung cancer incorporating SPECT ventilation imaging. Med Phys. 2010;37:1863–72.
45. Bates EL, Bragg CM, Wild JM, Hatton MQ, Ireland RH. Functional image-based radiotherapy planning for non-small cell lung cancer: a simulation study. Radiother Oncol. 2009;93:32–6.
46. Yin LS, Tang L, Hamarneh G, et al. Complexity and accuracy of image registration methods in SPECT-guided radiation therapy. Phys Med Biol. 2010;55:237–46.
47. Gallucci G, Capobianco AM, Coccaro M, Venetucci A, Suriano V, Fusco V. Myocardial perfusion defects after radiation therapy and anthracycline chemotherapy for left breast cancer: a possible marker of microvascular damage. Three cases and review of the literature. Tumori. 2008;94:129–33.
48. Gayed IW, Liu HH, Yusuf SW, et al. The prevalence of myocardial ischemia after concurrent chemoradiation therapy as detected by gated myocardial perfusion imaging in patients with esophageal cancer. J Nucl Med. 2006;47(11):1756–62.
49. Boivin JF, Hutchinson GB, Lubin JH, et al. Coronary artery disease mortality in patients treated for Hodgkin's disease. Cancer. 1992;69:1241–7.
50. Yaremko B, Riauka T, Robinson D, et al. Thresholding in PET images of static and moving targets. Phys Med Biol. 2005;50:5969–82.
51. Vees H, Senthamizhchelvan S, Miralbell R, et al. Assessment of various strategies for 18F-FET PET-guided delineation of target volumes in high-grade glioma patients. Eur J Nucl Med Mol Imaging. 2009;36:182–93.
52. Yaremko B, Riauka T, Robinson D, et al. Threshold modification for tumour imaging in non-small-cell lung cancer using positron emission tomography. Nucl Med Commun. 2005;26:433–40.
53. International Atomic Energy Agency. The role of PET/CT in radiation treatment planning for cancer patient treatment. 2008 IAEA-TECDOC-1603, pp. 33.
54. Geets X, Lee J A, Bol A, et al. A gradient-based method for segmenting FDG-PET images: methodology and validation. Eur J Nucl Med Mol Imaging. 2007;34:1427–38.

55. Daisne JF, Sibomana M, Bol A, Doumont T, Lonneux M, Gregoire V. Tri-dimensional automatic segmentation of PET volumes based on measured source-to-background ratios: influence of reconstruction algorithms. Radiother Oncol. 2003;69:247–50.
56. Nestle U, Kremp S, Schaefer-Schuler A, et al. Comparison of different methods for delineation of 18F-FDG PET-positive tissue for target volume definition in radiotherapy of patients with non-small cell lung cancer. J Nucl Med. 2005; 46:1342–8.
57. Jentzen W, Freudenberget L, Eising EG. Segmentation of PET volumes by iterative image thresholding. J Nucl Med. 2007;48:108–14.
58. Schinagl DA, Vogel WV, Hoffmann AL, van Dalen JA, Oyen WJ, Kaanders JH. Comparison of five segmentation tools for 18Ffluoro-deoxy-glucose-positron emission tomography-based target volume definition in head and neck cancer. Int J Radiat Oncol Biol Phys. 2007;69:1282–9.
59. Hatt M, Lamare F, Boussion N, et al. Fuzzy hidden Markov chains segmentation for volume determination and quantitation in PET. Phys Med Biol. 2007;52:3467–91.
60. Montgomery D, Amira A, Zaidi H. Fully automated segmentation of oncological PET volumes using a combined multiscale and statistical model. Med Phys. 2007;34:722–36.
61. Brambilla M, Matheoud R, Secco C, Loi G, Krengli M, Inglese E. Threshold segmentation for PET target volume delineation in radiation treatment planning: the role of target-to-background ratio and target size. Med Phys. 2008;35:1207–13.
62. Jannin P, Fitzpatrick JM, Hawkes DJ, Pennec X, Shahidi R, Vannier MW. Validation of medical image processing in image guided therapy. IEEE Trans Med Imaging. 2002;21:1445–9.
63. Daisne JF, Dupers T, Weygand B, et al. Tumor volume in pharyngolaryngeal squamous cell carcinoma: comparison at CT, MR imaging, and FDG PET and validation with surgical specimen. Radiology. 2004;233:93–100.
64. Basile C. Delineazione del volume neoplastico funzionalmente attivo per scope radioterapici: analisi e sviluppo di algoritmi per la segmentazione di immagini PET o SPECT. Biomedical Engineering Degree Thesis, University of Rome, Tor Vergata, pp. 122.
65. Pacilio M, Basile C, Shcherbinin S, et al. An innovative iterative thresholding algorithm for tumour segmentation and volumetric quantification on SPECT images: monte carlo-based methodology and validation. Submitted to Med Phys. 2010.

Index

S. Fanti et al., *Atlas of SPECT-CT*,
DOI: 10.1007/978-3-642-15726-4, © Springer-Verlag Berlin Heidelberg 2011

S

T

V

Y

GPSR Compliance

The European Union's (EU) General Product Safety Regulation (GPSR) is a set of rules that requires consumer products to be safe and our obligations to ensure this.

If you have any concerns about our products, you can contact us on ProductSafety@springernature.com

In case Publisher is established outside the EU, the EU authorized representative is:

Springer Nature Customer Service Center GmbH
Europaplatz 3
69115 Heidelberg, Germany

Batch number: 10684389

Printed by Printforce, the Netherlands